THE VULVA

&

VAGINA MANUAL

GRAEME DENNERSTEIN

JAMES SCURRY

JOHN BRENAN

DAVID ALLEN

MARIA - GRAZIA MARIN

With a foreword by
PETER LYNCH MD

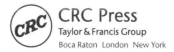

CRC Press
Taylor & Francis Group
Boca Raton London New York

CRC Press is an imprint of the
Taylor & Francis Group, an **informa** business

THE VULVA

&

VAGINA MANUAL

CRC Press
Taylor & Francis Group
6000 Broken Sound Parkway NW, Suite 300
Boca Raton, FL 33487-2742

First issued in paperback 2019

© 2005 by Taylor & Francis Group, LLC
CRC Press is an imprint of Taylor & Francis Group, an Informa business

No claim to original U.S. Government works

ISBN-13: 978-0-646-44531-1 (hbk)
ISBN-13: 978-0-367-39198-0 (pbk)

**Visit the Taylor & Francis Web site at
http://www.taylorandfrancis.com**

**and the CRC Press Web site at
http://www.crcpress.com**

About the Authors

Graeme Dennerstein RFD, MBBS, FRCOG, FRANZCOG, is a Melbourne-based, currently practicing obstetrician and gynecologist whose special interest in this field started with research into the cytology of the vulva as part of his postgraduate studies in obstetrics and gynecology. He was the Head of the Dermogynaecology Clinic at the Mercy Hospital for Women in East Melbourne. He is a member of the International Society for the Study of Vulvovaginal Disease

James Scurry MD, FRCPA, qualified as an anatomical pathologist in 1986 and currently works in that field. He developed a research interest in vulvovaginal disorders while reporting for 10 years for the Dermogynaecology Clinic, Mercy Hospital for Women, Melbourne. He has been a member of the International Society for the Study of Vulvovaginal Diseases since 1991. He published his thesis on the relationship of lichen sclerosus to squamous cell carcinoma in 2000.

John Brenan MBBS [Hons], FRACP, FACD, is a dermatologist and consultant dermatologist to St. Vincent's Hospital, Melbourne. He was Chief Censor and subsequently President of the Australasian College of Dermatologists. He is a life member of the American Academy of Dermatology, a member of the European Academy of Dermatology and Venereology and was Honorary President of the World Congress of Dermatology in 1997. He was the consultant dermatologist to the Mercy Hospital for Women and the original dermatologist for the Dermogynaecology Clinic at that hospital.

David Allen MBChB, MMed, PhD, FCOG(SA), FRANZCOG, CGO, is a certified gynecological oncologist currently practicing at the Mercy Hospital for Women and the Peter MacCallum Cancer Centre, East Melbourne. He is an Associate Professor in the Department of Surgery at the University of Melbourne. He is a member of the International Society for the Study of Vulvovaginal Disease

Maria - Grazia Marin MAPS, is a psychologist in private practice in Melbourne and past committee member and Education Officer of the Victorian Psychosexual Society. She is also a member of the International Society for the Study of Vulvovaginal Diseases and is currently serving on its Patient Education and Sexual Difficulties committees. She was the psychologist to the Dermogynaecology clinic at the Mercy Hospital for Women from 1989 to 2001.

Foreword

Is this the best textbook available on vulvovaginal disorders? Probably it is. This judgment is based on the achievement of excellence in the four areas of erudition, extension, editing and graphics.

Erudition has occurred through an astute choice of authors. Other textbooks in this area have primarily been written by either gynecologists or dermatologists and understandably neither specialist can cover the other's specialty with complete competence. The co-authors for this book not only include specialists in gynecology and dermatology but also those certified in oncology, pathology and psychology. With this wide range of backgrounds, the text delivers authoritative dissertation in all of the areas covered.

The inclusion of specialists from multiple areas also allows for extension: nearly 300 disorders have been included. Most previous books on vulvar disease have been limited to benign disorders and in situ malignancy. Here, essentially all benign and malignant disease has been covered. With a sole exception, other books in this area have dealt almost exclusively with vulvar disease and have ignored vaginal disorders; this book covers both. For those of us working in vulvology, the importance of this dual coverage was acknowledged a few years ago when the members of the International Society for the Study of Vulvar Disease (ISSVD) changed its name to the International Society for the Study of Vulvovaginal disease to better reflect the continuity of structure and function possessed by these two organs. Likewise, histopathology, with one major exception, has generally been given short shrift. It surely seems crucial to me that clinicians and pathologists not only work together as a team but also that each understands enough of the other specialty to achieve the best in clinicopathological correlation. In this text, histological discussion and depiction are included for almost every entity. And, in perhaps one of this book's most attractive features, a psychologist has added highly important and useful insight into the all-too-often ignored intertwining roles of organic disease and psychosexual dysfunction.

Despite having five co-authors, this book, through aggressive editing has avoided two major pitfalls found in most multi-authored texts: conflicting information and unnecessary duplication. The Vulva and Vagina Manual demonstrates both uniformity and conciseness. It reads seamlessly as if a single author had written the whole of it.

For most clinicians, the illustrative aspects of a textbook are of utmost importance. The graphics found in this book are numerous and excellent. There are 301 photographs, equally divided between the clinical and histopathological aspects of the diseases covered. All are reproduced in excellent color and detail. And, while other books have illustrated the most common diseases well, this book includes otherwise unavailable photos of seldom-encountered disorders.

I believe that this book achieves a most outstanding goal: Clinicians, regardless of specialty, who utilize this book, will undoubtedly be able to provide better care for the women they serve.

Peter J. Lynch, MD. Frederick G. Novy, Jr. Professor of Dermatology and Training Program Director of the Department of Dermatology, University of California, Davis.

Acknowledgements

In 1989, Professor Norman Beischer AO, then the Chairman of the Melbourne University Department of Obstetrics and Gynaecology at the Mercy Hospital for Women, decided that the hospital needed a vulva clinic. As a result, the Dermogynaecology Clinic was formed, bringing together the five authors of this book. We are most grateful to Professor Beischer for his foresight.

Many others have contributed to the collection of much of the material used in this manual. In particular, we must thank the gynecologists, dermatologists and pathologists who have been associated with the Dermogynaecology Clinic. Others who have contributed include Dr. Robert King PhD, who assisted with the psychology research, the dedicated nursing and clerical staff of the clinic and the librarians of Sunshine Hospital. We trust that this manual helps justify their efforts.

Contents

Introduction 12

Chapter 1. Gynecologist's perspective 13
    Clinical assessment of lower female genital tract complaints 14
    Office pathology 17

Chapter 2. Dermatologist's perspective 21
    Epidermis, dermis 22
    Basement membrane zone 23
    Clinical features 23
    Treatment of vulvar dermatoses 26

Chapter 3. Oncologist's perspective 29
    Benign and premalignant conditions 30
    Malignant conditions 31

Chapter 4. Psychologist's perspective 33
    Multifactorial nature of chronic vulvar disease 34
    Human behavior and chronic vulvar disease 36
    Management of patients with chronic vulvar disease 39
    Instructions for self care 44

Chapter 5. Pathologist's perspective 47
    Clinical aspects relevant to the pathologist 48
    Pathologist's report 50
    Communication 53
    Classification 55

Chapter 6. The basics 59
    Embryology 59
    Anatomy 61
    Histology 65
    Ecology 75

Table of Modes of Clinical Presentation 79

Chapter 7. Normal variations 91
    Vulva 91
    Vagina 93

Chapter 8. Developmental abnormalities 97
    Malformations that do not lead to sexual ambiguity 97
    Malformations with ambiguous external sexual organs 104

Chapter 9. Infections 109
    Parasites 109
    Fungi 117
    Bacteria 125
    Viruses 136

Chapter 10. Non-infectious dermatoses 149
    Spongiotic 149
    Psoriasiform 153
    Lichenoid 160
    Vesicobullous 174
    Granulomatous 181
    Vasculopathic 184
    Others 188

Chapter 11. Endocrine and metabolic disorders and disorders of pigmentation 195

Chapter 12. Trauma 205

Chapter 13. Neoplasms 215
    Vulva - epithelial 215
    Vulva - melanocytic 235
    Vulva - mesenchymal 239
    Vulva - hemopoietic and lymphoid 246
    Vulva - secondary tumors 248
    Vagina 249
    Urethra 256

Chapter 14. Non-neoplastic cysts and swellings 263

Chapter 15. Functional disorders 283
    Disorders of sensation 283
    Sexual disorders 286

Index 291

Classification of vulvovaginal disease (Last page)

Introduction

The purpose of this manual is to provide clarity where confusion has reigned. We have all experienced this confusion first hand and bad results of inappropriate treatment. Examples are when psoriasis or lichen planus manifest firstly on the vulva and are referred to the gynecologist or when recurrent candidiasis is referred to the dermatologist, particularly when it is complicating the management of other genital disorders. The oncologist is familiar with the sometimes lethal consequence of under treatment of genital malignancy or preneoplasia but also the unnecessary production of a sexual 'cripple' by its over treatment. Pathologists too have had their share of confusion. An example occurred in the 1980's when the intracellular edema of spongiosis was misinterpreted as the koilocytosis of papillomavirus infection resulting in women being subjected to ablative treatments with severe untoward sequelae. If these problems do not impact immediately on the woman's psychological and sexual well-being, it is only a matter of time before they will. The counseling psychologist has much to offer in the management of many of these cases. These are reasons why a multidisciplinary approach will be necessary for the optimal management of many of the more difficult vulvovaginal complaints.

The backbone of this manual is the classification of disorders affecting the vulva and vagina (inside back cover). We have agonized over it for several years, as others have done before us. It is a very difficult task to produce such a classification in an area where different disciplines have their own nomenclature and where conflict occurs between the clinical and etiological approaches to these disorders. Our aims have been to produce a classification based on etiology as much as possible and to have no disorder appearing more than once. Nomenclature has been restricted to the Systematized Nomenclature of Medicine of the American College of Pathologists.

In addition to the classification, is a listing of disorders according to their modes of presentation. Controversial terms such as 'vestibulitis syndrome' and 'vulvodynia' fit more comfortably within this section.

The first part of the manual (Perspectives), summarizes the experience of the 5 authors within areas in this field which have needed special consideration. We have worked as a team but obviously with different emphases.

The second part of the manual lists the disorders themselves according to the classification. Their description is intended to contain sufficient information to diagnose and treat them accurately, by the most expedient means.

We trust the reader will find this manual practical and useful and would welcome suggestions for future editions. Suggestions used would be suitably acknowledged.

Chapter 1

THE GYNECOLOGIST'S PERSPECTIVE

The management of many vulvar and vaginal complaints can present difficulties for gynecologists because of the complexity of vulvovaginal conditions and gynecologists' relative lack of training and experience in dermatology, pathology and psychosexual disorders. Nevertheless, the gynecologist will most commonly be the specialist to which the more difficult vulvovaginal cases are referred. Furthermore, vulvovaginal complaints are present incidentally in many obstetric and gynecologic patients who rightly expect a high standard of care from their specialist for these disorders. This chapter provides an approach to all but the simplest of problems in this area. The requirements are an appropriate history, clinical examination and usually collection of specimens for microbiology and/or biopsy. Optimal management may be facilitated if, during the consultation, the clinician is able to perform the special investigations also outlined in this chapter.

Clinical Assessment of Lower Female Genital Tract Complaints

When vulvar and vaginal complaints present management difficulties, the solution is most likely to arise from revision of the diagnosis rather than the treatment. Of all the diagnostic techniques to be discussed, clinical assessment remains the primary method. In fact, in some areas, for example 'vestibulitis syndrome', experience has taught us that clinical methods provide the most information.

The Presenting Complaint

It is important to get the patient to begin at the beginning - to think back to how the complaint began and when. Usually the onset can be related to puberty, first intercourse, pregnancy, menopause, some major event such as surgery or an episode of particular emotional stress. Obviously, the last may be the key to the diagnosis of a stress-related disorder.

For example, recurrent candidiasis generally starts a few years after puberty or in pregnancy or following a course of antibiotics. Atrophic vaginitis follows ovarian failure by a year or so and the epithelial disorders are of gradual onset unrelated to any of the above.

When these complaints extend over many months or years, a sameness may develop but it is essential to determine exactly what is disturbing the patient at the time of the consultation. This may differ from the complaint at onset. It is particularly important to determine if the complaint is related to sexual activity. Thus, the vulvar dermatoses may not cause dyspareunia but psychosexual problems will invariably interfere with intercourse. When trying to assess the likelihood of dyspareunia having an organic or functional cause, it is useful to know whether intercourse has ever been enjoyable and whether or not the complaint is now intermittent or with every act of intercourse.

Pruritus is by far the commonest symptom of vulvar disease but is quite nonspecific. It can result from a multitude of causes and merges with other common descriptions such as discomfort, burning, stinging, soreness, vulvodynia and burning vulva syndrome. Treatment should never be initiated on this symptom alone, even if the patient has been shown to have, say, candidiasis in the past.

Inflammation in the vestibular region may result in discomfort from contact with urine. This results in the symptom of vulvar dysuria and is one of the reasons why women should never be treated for urinary infection, when dysuria is the only complaint, without at least performing a micro-urine.

'Splitting' usually equates with fissuring. Inflamed epithelium develops intraepidermal edema (spongiosis) rendering it prone to tearing like wet tissue paper. These fissures can be exquisitely painful because they expose the nerve endings in the dermis. They occur most frequently in the interlabial sulci, fourchette and perineum. Candidiasis is by far the commonest cause but it can be a nonspecific clinical feature of any inflammatory disorder of the vulva.

Discharge is the commonest symptom of vaginal and cervical disease. Unlike the highly pain sensitive vulva, even extreme inflammatory disorders of the vagina and cervix may only manifest by discharge because of the relative absence of pain fibres at this level. A large minority of patients complaining of discharge will be free of pathogens. The diagnoses in these cases include cervical ectropion (eversion, the old term 'erosion'), atrophic vaginitis, erosive disorders, foreign body, cancer and a very important group, namely those whose discharge is physiological in origin. Discharge caused by pathogens will be discussed elsewhere.

The important features of a discharge are duration, quantity and associated inflammatory symptoms such as itch or soreness. Blood staining is of obvious importance, otherwise color can be misleading due to alteration with drying. Odor is highly subjective and therefore may be unhelpful. It is the leading symptom of bacterial vaginosis and few things upset a woman more than when her odor is commented upon by the sexual partner.

Related History

A general obstetric and gynecologic history is essential for good management. It should include parity, gravidity, mode of delivery, contraception, fertility requirements and a detailed menstrual history. For instance, it is no use suggesting depot medroxyprogesterone acetate (see page 121) in the management of recurrent candidiasis if the woman wishes to conceive. The woman with premature menopause may present with atrophic vaginitis. Lactating women seldom suffer from candidiasis but may be sore from atrophic vaginitis and/or vulvar and perineal trauma. Anxiety and/or depression associated with fear of pregnancy or infertility frequently result in sexual problems, which in turn can present as vulvar complaints.

Intercurrent disease may be relevant and, very importantly, whether or not there are skin or mucosal disorders elsewhere. Thus, atopic dermatitis can affect the vulva and is associated with hay fever and asthma. Likewise the clue to vulvar psoriasis may be the more characteristic extragenital lesions. Lichen planus, the commonest vulvovaginal erosive disorder, also affects the mouth in some patients.

Topical Treatment History

Contact dermatitis of the vulva is one of the commonest diagnoses made in these patients so it is essential to know what prescribed and over-the-counter medications the patient has been applying. Getting the information can be difficult but has potential use in subsequent management. Unfortunately, anti-candidals can now be obtained without a prescription in many countries. These potentially irritating substances are also the commonest cause of a falsely negative swab in recurrent candidiasis. Many chemicals in preparations well promoted for female genital use have the potential to result in an inflammatory response by this sensitive epithelium.

A history of any vulvar or vaginal surgery should be recorded and whether or not biopsy has been performed elsewhere. Diathermy, cryotherapy and laser can also have long term sequelae in this area.

Systemic Therapy

Contraception has already been mentioned, but in the older woman the presentation may be directly related to the use of hormone replacement therapy. That is, atrophic vaginitis may result from underdosage or poor absorption of estrogen. Conversely, candidiasis may result from too high a dose. Treatments for sexually transmitted infections may fail for a variety of reasons including poor compliance, failure to treat a partner or the use of the wrong drug. The relationship between antibiotics and candidiasis is unarguable. Finally, orally active candidacides are being used increasingly but with varying success.

Examination

The vulva is best examined with the patient in the dorsal position and the light at the foot of the examination couch. A gynecological chair or the lithotomy position have advantages but are not necessary in most instances. If the examiner is standing on the patient's right, the gloved left hand can be used to separate the labia leaving the right hand free for taking specimens, palpation and detailed examination without obscuring the view. If the patient is menstruating or there is much discharge, it may be necessary to clean the area with wet cotton balls, otherwise erythema, fissures and small ulcers may be missed.

A useful addition to the examination is to hand the patient a swab stick and to instruct her to use the end of it to indicate exactly the site of maximum discomfort. This may be the best way of selecting the site to take a biopsy and is also useful diagnostically. The patient with 'vestibulitis syndrome' will place the swab stick in the region of the minor vestibular glands and the woman with vulvar dysesthesia will merely indicate a wide, ill-defined area, often with a display of emotion.

This author's preference for vaginal examination is to use a Sims' speculum in Sims' position because only a minimum of vagina is obscured. However, the important point is not to overlook the rest of the gynecological examination. Because of the lack of vaginal pain sensation, vaginal causes of vulvar symptoms are often seen, candidiasis being by far the commonest. Bimanual examination, in addition to detecting any pelvic pathology, will permit an appreciation of vaginismus.

Magnification may be useful. The colposcope is only essential in a relatively small number of cases, for example, delineating intraepithelial neoplasia. Incidentally, not only is the application of acetic acid unnecessary in most cases but can cause the sufferer of chronic vulvar disease intense pain. A 4 x loupe can be a most useful tool in this area, particularly when looking for seedling warts.

Important points to remember

- Laboratory investigations will be required for the optimal management of all but the simplest disorders of the vulva and vagina.
- Skilful and thorough history taking and clinical examination remain essential for success.

OFFICE PATHOLOGY

The microscope is a particularly useful tool in the clinical setting when differentiating vulvovaginal complaints. Formal microbiology, cytology and histology will still be required in most cases but the woman is likely to greatly benefit from the rapid narrowing of the differential diagnosis provided by a clinician using this tool. A simple technique of smear preparation is to separate the labia with one hand and insert a cytology brush (intended for endocervical sampling) into the vagina and smear the material on a glass slide. It may be fixed and stained as described below or simply examined after adding a drop of saline, preferably using a phase contrast microscope. However, good results can be obtained without phase contrast, merely by closing the microscope condenser diaphragm. To fix, stain and apply a cover slip is not difficult and has the added advantage of providing a permanent record.

Wright's Stained Smears

Wright's stain is a member of the Romanowsky group of stains which includes Giemsa and Leishman - stains used by the hematologist for blood films. Wright's stain is quick (less than 5 minutes) and easy to use. Host cell and microorganism morphology is readily apparent and preserved indefinitely.

Examination of such smears has produced the following diagnostic categories in our patients complaining of symptoms referrable to the vagina and vulva.

The Preparation of a Wright's Stained Smear

1. Wipe the vaginal wall and/or introitus with a cytology brush or wooden spatula and smear the material on a glass slide.
2. Fix with the usual Pap smear fixative.
3. Apply 10-15 drops of Wright's stain to the slide on a level surface and leave for one minute.
4. Add an approximately double volume (20-30 drops) of water and leave for three minutes.
5. Rinse with tap water for 10 seconds and dry (a hair dryer is ideal).
6. Examine with immersion oil or make the slide permanent by immersing it in xylene and covering it with mounting medium and a cover slip.

Normal

Physiological vaginal contents consist mostly of mature vaginal squames (Fig. 1.2). Polymorphs are few or absent and usually contained within strands of recognizable cervical mucus. Cervical mucus normally contains polymorphs after ovulation. Bacteria are mostly bacilli (rods).

Smears with normal findings may be obtained from patients complaining of discharge, pruritus or dyspareunia. They may also be obtained from patients with known vulvar dermatoses when it is important to know whether or not vaginitis is contributing to the symptomatology. In 493 consecutive smears made from our clinic patients, apparently normal secretion was the most common finding (76%). However, culture of swabs from these patients grew Candida albicans in 59 (16%), Gardnerella in 9 (2%) and Candida glabrata in 2. These smears should be considered complimentary to routine microbiology.

Atrophy

Without estrogen, the vaginal epithelium does not mature (differentiate) so that cells from the deepest layer (parabasal cells) are found on smears (Fig. 1.1). Parabasal cells are easily recognized because they are relatively small, rounded and contain an open nucleus occupying about one half of the cell. In ovulating women, only cells from differentiated epithelium are obtained. These are called intermediate, if some nuclear detail is visible, or superficial if the nucleus has become pyknotic. Cells from mature epithelium are much larger than parabasal cells and the cytoplasmic border tends to be angulated. The ratio of parabasal to intermediate to superficial is known as the maturation or karyopyknotic index and is a fairly reliable indicator of estrogen levels.

Of our smears examined, 10 % indicated atrophy with or without inflammatory cells. Many of these women had used estrogens and it was useful to know that administration had been insufficient. Furthermore, atrophy is associated with a very low incidence of candidal infection although trichomonads are in no way inhibited by estrogen deficiency.

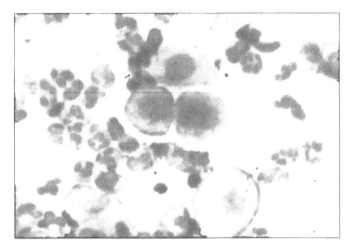

Figure 1.1. Wright's stained vaginal smear from a lactating woman, complaining of dyspareunia, showing pronounced atrophic and inflammatory changes: parabasal cells and polymorphonuclear leucocytes.

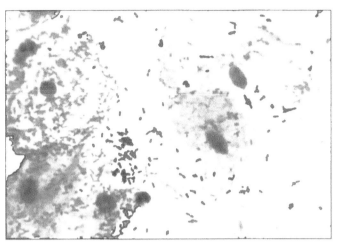

Figure 1.2. A smear has been made by the same technique from the same patient two weeks after the nightly insertion of a vaginal applicator of estrogen cream. Note the change to the normal with the disappearance of the polymorphs and parabasal cells and their replacement with superficial squamous cells and lactobacilli.

Infection

Candida albicans is characterized by basophilic filaments with a non-staining capsule and often budding (Fig. 9.17).

Trichomonads appears as well demarcated, small cells, oval, round or tapered at both ends, which stain as deeply as, or slightly deeper than, the surrounding epithelial cells (Fig. 9.9). They contain a small, purple-staining, oval or sometimes pointed nucleus to one side of the cell. The flagellae will probably not be visible other than under oil immersion. In diameter, they are smaller than the smallest epithelial cells but a little larger than a polymorph. However, trichomonads are best identified in a wet mount because of their characteristic movement.

Epithelial Erosion

It is possible to make a fairly confident diagnosis of an erosive disorder (e.g. desquamative inflammatory vaginitis or lichen planus) on these smears. The characteristics are, in addition to inflammatory changes (numerous polymorphs), the mixture of superficial cells (indicating premenopausal oestrogen levels) with parabasal cells from the depths of the epithelium. Regenerative atypia will be apparent in severe cases.

Bacterial or Anaerobic Vaginosis (*Gardnerella Vaginalis* Infection)

This condition can be confidently diagnosed on these smears so that culture confirmation may be unnecessary. There is a profusion of coccoid flora, imparting a dirty appearance to the smear and a relative absence of polymorphs. The absence of vaginitis is a feature of bacterial vaginosis. The bacteria adhere to many of the epithelial cells so that their borders may appear ragged, the so called 'clue cell' (Fig. 9.34).

Inflammation, no pathogens

This generally refers to smears showing polymorphs in excess of differentiated epithelial cells but with no identifiable pathogen. Causes include trauma, epithelial erosion (Fig. 10.46) or cervicitis. When the discharge is from a cervical eversion (ectropion), the polymorphs are mostly arranged in rows or clumps within the identifiable strands of mucus. Areas of epithelial cells unassociated with polymorphs are also present if cervical eversion is the only disorder.

References

Benign diseases of the vulva and vagina. Gardner HL and Kaufman RH. First edition: The C.V. Mosby Company 1969 and subsequent editions including the 5th edition by Kaufman RH, Faro S and Brown D: Elsevier Mosby 2005.

Chapter 2

THE DERMATOLOGIST'S PERSPECTIVE

Over the years, dermatologists have tended to look upon vulva and vagina as the exclusive domain of gynecologists who were equally uninformed about dermatology. It is only in recent times that dermatologists and gynecologists have formed an increasing partnership leading to the rationalization of diagnosis, classification, investigation and treatment in this area. The following, are the fundamentals of dermatology applicable to vulva and vagina that need to be understood by health practitioners treating these disorders.

The skin, which is the interface with the environment, consists of the cellular epidermis overlying the supportive dermis of stromal tissue containing blood vessels, nerves and appendages.

Epidermis

The epidermis consists of three populations of cells:

Keratinocytes
Basal cells divide to form squamous cells. These move towards the surface and undergo an ordered process of differentiation to synthesize groups of proteins including keratins, keratohyaline granules and cornified cell envelopes. This process results in the stratum corneum which acts as a semi-permeable membrane retaining tissue fluid and acting as a barrier against infection and irritants. Cohesion between cells is provided by adhesion molecules in the cell wall plates known as desmosomes.

Melanocytes
These dendritic cells, derived from the neural crest, transfer melanin to the keratinocytes in packets known as melanosomes. This protects DNA from ultra violet light damage. In black skin, melanosomes are larger and the melanocytes more active. Abnormalities may result in increased pigmentation or in depigmentation, for example, that seen in lichen sclerosus or vitiligo.

Langerhans' Cells
These are dendritic cells and constitute 5% of epidermal cells. They derive from the monocyte macrophage series and are immunocompetent cells acting as the afferent limb of the immune system.

Dermis

The dermis consists of two layers. The first of these is the upper papillary dermis made up of fine bundles of connective tissue, the function of which is to nourish the overlying epidermis. It has a rich supply of capillaries, lymphatics and nerve endings. Beneath the upper papillary dermis is the reticular dermis made up of thick bundles of collagen, elastic tissue and ground substance (a proteoglycan) produced by fibroblasts. This is the supportive structural layer of the skin and contains the pilosebaceous follicles and eccrine sweat glands.

Basement Membrane Zone (BMZ)

The BMZ is a complex layer, defined by electron microscopy and molecular biology. It provides cohesion between the epidermis and dermis and allows transfer of tissue fluid upward into the epidermis. The BMZ is often the site of deposition of immunoreactants and resultant damage to basal cells will result in thinning of the epidermis clinically, seen as **atrophy** (eg. lichen sclerosus, lupus erythematosus).

Clinical Features

The diagnosis of inflammatory diseases of the vulva depends initially on the history. This should include questions on how the condition began, how it has been treated and the symptoms produced. It is essential to know whether skin or mucosa elsewhere is involved or whether there is a past or family history of relevant skin conditions or associated medical conditions. Careful attention must be paid to psychological and social factors as these can play a major role in the patient's concerns.

Clinical dermatology is the interpretation of the macroscopic pathology of the skin. Both the epidermis and the dermis can only react in a limited number of ways. Diseases that alter keratinocyte function will often lead to a thickened, abnormal stratum corneum, which is seen as surface scale. For example inflammation with edema (spongiosis) of the epidermis, as in tinea or dermatitis, will be reflected by **surface scale**. Acute edema (spongiosis) in acute dermatitis will be one of the causes of **blisters**. Genetic disorders of keratinization, such as the various types of ichthyosis, will lead to scaly skin. If the keratin barrier is breached, tissue fluid will escape and micro-organisms can penetrate. Coagulation of tissue fluid on the surface leads to **crust**.

Loss of cohesion between keratinocytes (acantholysis) will also lead to blisters. As the roof of these blisters is made of only part of the epidermis, they break easily to cause **erosions** or **ulcers**. Erosive disease is a non-specific result of several disease processes. When there are erosions in the vagina the term often used is desquamative vaginitis. To determine the cause of these macroscopic changes it is often essential to biopsy the area.

As the dermis is a meshwork of collagen, it allows aggregation of large numbers of cells. Such collections seen in chronic granulomas give rise to localised **plaques**. Conditions which result in excessive production of collagen are manifested by thickening or **sclerosis**. Dilatation of vessels in inflammatory processes gives rise to **erythema** while leakage of blood from capillaries, seen often in conditions such as vasculitis or lichen sclerosus, gives rise to **purpura** or **ecchymoses** (hemorrhage in the skin). A compromised circulation with necrosis of the epidermis is one of the causes of ulcers. Transient dermal edema constitutes a **wheal** (as in urticaria).

The main symptoms of vulvar skin disease are itch or pruritus and burning, stinging or rawness often referred to as 'vulvodynia'.

Pruritus will induce scratching and/or rubbing. Continued scratching produces linear excoriations or erosions. Rubbing manifests as skin thickening, pigmentation and exaggerated skin markings, known clinically as **lichenification** ("magnifying glass skin").

Lichenification may be superimposed on an underlying skin disease or occur as a primary event with a psychogenic basis. This disorder is known as lichen simplex. These changes in the vulva may be subtle or show marked thickening with a gross white appearance. Whiteness reflects the formation of a thickened epithelium and stratum corneum macerated with fluid. Any condition which gives rise to thickening of the stratum corneum will, on a mucosal surface, be reflected as white patches or plaques.

The clinical assessment of the patient, which must include adequate visualization, is based on the observation and interpretation of the various physical signs previously elaborated. These signs, together with their diagnostic significance, tend to fall into the following groups.

Erythemato-squamous (red and scaly) **lesions** may have a non-infectious or infectious etiology. Dermatitis, the commonest example of the former, frequently displays lichenification from rubbing. Findings may be minimal but, in acute contact reaction, there may be small blisters or vesicles. In psoriasis, sharply demarcated areas of erythema are seen but flexural psoriasis loses its characteristic scale and tends to form fissures, particularly in the natal cleft. Tinea is characterised by asymmetric circinate areas with an active scaly edge and clearing centre. This appearance may be masked by the use of topical corticosteroids producing the so-called "tinea incognito". Well demarcated shiny red areas with fine scale and small surrounding satellite lesions are found in candidiasis. A spectrum from fern-like white areas with fine scale to extensive erosions is seen in lichen planus. Cutaneous T cell lymphoma often starts around the buttocks, inner thighs and perineum with erythema, fine scale, atrophy and telangiectasia and may be mistaken for dermatitis or psoriasis. Sharply marginated reddish brown areas, which fluoresce under Wood's Light, are features of erythrasma, an uncommon genital infection.

Hypo-pigmentation (white lesion) suggests, among others, lichen sclerosus and lichen planus. In the former, ivory white areas are found with fine wrinkling and occasionally scale and skin fragility, leading to purpura. Unfortunate confusion with sexual abuse may occur when this appearance is found in children. In lichen planus, white areas with a lacy fern-like appearance, often associated with atrophy and erosions, are found, involving the inner surface of the labia minora and vestibule. Vitiligo demonstrates white areas which are often symmetrical with a well marked border but the skin is otherwise normal.

Atrophy (thinning) is also seen in lichen sclerosus and lichen planus. With the former, 'cigarette paper' thinning with hypopigmentation and purpura occur. Resorption of the labia minora and clitoral hood, and occasional introital narrowing, are characteristic as the disease progresses. Similar changes can be seen in lichen planus with erosions. Lupus erythematosus is rare on the vulva. Atrophy with hypopigmentation may lead to late scarring and loss of the labia minora. Overuse of potent corticosteroids may cause atrophy with telangiectasia, which is reversible when the topical corticosteroid is ceased. Irradiated skin becomes atrophic and hypopigmented with damaged telangiectatic vessels. It is subject to erosion and secondary infection.

Blisters break easily on mucosal surfaces to form erosions, which may be transient. Grouped blisters on an erythematous base are found in herpes simplex. Recurrences occur in the same area and often the buttock is involved. Blisters break to form erosions. With associated human immunodeficiency virus infection, the lesions are severe and chronic. With herpes zoster, groups of blisters on an erythematous base also occur, with a unilateral nerve root distribution usually preceded by pain. Occasionally, acute (usually contact) dermatitis forms blisters, but the lax tissue of the labia absorb edema and only small vesicles form.

The immuno-bullous diseases, pemphigus, pemphigoid, erythema mutiforme and toxic epidermal necrolysis involve the vulva as part of a generalised eruption. All these blisters break easily to form erosions. Cicatricial pemphigoid involves the vulva with erosions and surrounding white thickened skin. There may be loss of labia minora and scarring of clitoral hood. Vaginal involvement is a cause of desquamative vaginitis. Mouth and conjunctiva are also involved.

The genetic acantholytic disorder, Darier's disease, is part of a generalised process and gives rise to brownish crusts and vesicles which allow secondary infection. Hailey-Hailey disease involves axillae and groin and gives rise to crusted lesions induced by friction and infection, which may be mistaken for eczema or candidiasis.

Impetigo, an infection with *Streptococcus* or *Staphylococcus*, gives rise to a flaccid blister on an erythematous base. The blister breaks easily to form crusts. It is rare on the vulva but may be superimposed on an underlying skin condition or seen as part of impetigo elsewhere.

Erosions and ulcers may have the following important causes (in addition to blistering conditions where the blisters have ruptured): Lichen planus is an erosive disorder associated with desquamative inflammatory vaginitis and oral lichen planus. Crohn's disease causes 'knife cut' linear ulcers in the interlabial folds. It may be associated with abscesses and fistulae. Behcet's disease is characterised by deep painful ulcers with necrotic slough. The same process also affects the mouth. Major apthous ulcers are painful with a yellow base and red areola.

Other important causes of female genital ulceration include the sexually transmitted infections, syphilis (with its painless chancre), chancroid (soft chancre), donovanosis and lymphogranuloma venereum. In endemic areas, amebiasis and diptheria can present with ulceration. Finally, glucagonoma and Langerhan's cell histiocytosis are rare causes of ulceration.

Treatment of Vulvar Dermatoses

Resting inflamed skin is an important facet of any treatment regimen. In some cases this may be best achieved by a period of complete rest in hospital.

Wet soaks help with immediate relief for inflamed skin by causing swelling of tissue and closure of painful fissures and cracks. Saline soaks are applied for 15 minutes, 2 to 4 times daily. The effect is transient and must be followed by lubrication with creams, usually a corticosteroid cream. However, creams contain preservatives which may irritate at times.

Local corticosteroids are used for their anti-inflammatory effect, usually twice daily. The bioavailability of the glucocorticoid depends on the vehicle (usually cream bases are more acceptable on the vulva), the potency of glucocorticoid (see Table 1) and the concentration of the glucocorticoid.

Peri-orificial dermatitis, skin atrophy and striae are complications of long term usage of topical steroids and are directly proportional to the potency of the steroid used. Peri-orifical dermatitis is a rosacea-like rash with erythema, scale, papules and pustules. It is caused by the potent and super-potent steroids, the use of which must be stopped when the above changes occur. It is treated with emollients and oral tetracycline. The skin atrophy reverses with cessation of the steroid but the striae are permanent.

It is reasonable to use potent or intermediate steroids for short periods (4 to 6 weeks) to control conditions such as psoriasis, lichen sclerosus and lichen simplex. When adequate control is achieved, hydrocortisone can be substituted. Awareness of the complications and moderate use of steroids should prevent the above problems. Corticosteroids may also cause folliculitis and worsening of dermatophyte and *Candida albicans* infections. Any superimposed infection must be treated with the appropriate local or parenteral agent.

Intralesional corticosteroids (such as triamcinolone acetonide 10mg per ml diluted with lignocaine) are useful for single lesions, recalcitrant lesions or ulcers of complex aphthosis.

Control of the itch-scratch cycle is very important, particularly at night. Patients may need to be sedated with, for example, methdilazine 4 to 8 mg or doxepin 10 to 25 mg.

Table 1. Commonly used topical corticosteroids

Class I Super-Potent	Class II, III Potent Steroids	Class IV, V Mid-strength Steroids	Class VI, VII Mild Steroids
Clobetasol propionate 0.05%	Betamethasone dipropionate 0.05%	Betamethasone valerate 0.02%	Hydrocortisone acetate 1%
Augmented betamethasone dipropionate 0.05% (Available in an optimised propylene glycol vehicle)	Mometasone furoate 0.1%	Triamcinolone acetonide 0.02%	
	Triamcinolone acetonide 0.1%	Alclometasone dipropionate 0.05%	
	Betamethasone valerate 0.1% or 0.05%		
	Methylprednisolone aceponate 0.1%		

Important points to remember

- Always search for more than one cause – vulvar disease is often multifactorial.
- Candida albicans infection may complicate any condition and may be aggravated by corticosteroids.
- Look at the whole skin and in the mouth for evidence of dermatoses elsewhere.
- Dermatoses often flare because of infection or aggravation produced by local medication.
- If therapy is not proving effective, reconsider the diagnosis. DO NOT JUST CHANGE THERAPY.
- A BIOPSY is often essential to make the diagnosis

References

Fischer G. Vulval disease in prepubertal girls. Aust J Derm 2001; 42:225-236.

Halbert A, Chan J. Anogenital and buttock ulceration in infancy. Aust J Derm 2002; 43:1-8.

Chapter 3

THE ONCOLOGIST'S PERSPECTIVE

The subspecialist gynecologic oncologist is specifically trained in the management of premalignant and malignant gynecologic conditions. A comprehensive knowledge of and experience with advanced surgical techniques, as well as chemotherapy and radiotherapy, place the gynecologic oncologist in a good position to manage all types of neoplastic lesions of the vulva and vagina.

Cancers of the vulva and vagina are uncommon, with a lifetime risk of about 1:500 women (compared with breast cancer 1:10, endometrial cancer 1:80, cervix cancer 1:200). The surgical work in this area includes benign and pre-malignant disorders. Managing women with malignancies within a multidisciplinary team of medical, paramedical and nursing staff and social workers results in the best outcomes.

The relationship between the gynecologic oncologist and the pathologist is of paramount importance when it comes to diagnostic and management decisions. Sharing clinical information and intra-operative findings can be invaluable. The pathologist must have a special interest in gynecology and understand what needs to be included in the histology report to enable the necessary management decisions. A mutual understanding of the tissue preparation, cut-up and what constitutes adequate sampling and staining is also important. Reviewing any histology or cytology slides with the pathologist is often necessary prior to management decisions. A reliable frozen section service is also essential. Good communication between the oncologist and the pathologist cannot be over-emphasised if the optimal diagnosis and management of the patient is to be obtained.

Benign conditions

Benign masses are sometimes referred to the gynecologic oncologist because of his/her expertise with colposcopy and surgery in this area. Most benign masses are removed with excision biopsy or wide local excision.

Lichen sclerosus (LS) is a dermatosis that, although often associated with vulvar carcinoma, has a low risk of progression to carcinoma. It is usually excised with the cancer, but can be a particular problem when it recurs or persists. Thickened LS may need further excision under these circumstances to exclude recurrent cancer. Excisions near the clitoris and urethra can present special problems.

Condylomata acuminata of the vagina and vulva are also often referred for management. Surgical treatment (CO_2 laser, excision, diathermy, cryotherapy) is often successful when chemical applications have failed. Again, the clitoris and urethra can be difficult treatment areas.

Premalignant conditions

Vulvar intraepithelial neoplasia (VIN) and vaginal intraepithelial neoplasia (VAIN) are accepted precursors to cancers of the vulva and vagina, respectively. The malignant potential of VIN has been shown to be far greater than initially thought. Only a small percentage (<5%) of treated VIN will progress to cancer, but untreated VIN progresses to cancer in greater than 80% of cases. The premalignant changes on the vulva or vagina can take many forms and guises and biopsy plays an important role. Compared to the cervix, colposcopic features of premalignant changes on the vulva or vagina are not well defined. Aceto-white epithelium, after the application of 5% acetic acid, and iodine-negative areas may nevertheless help to direct the biopsy site. For vaginal lesions a punch biopsy forceps can be used and usually no local anesthesia is required. For vulvar biopsy a scalpel or a 4mm or 6mm dermal biopsy punch can be used. Local anesthetic is necessary. This is injected slowly and subcutaneously below the lesion. Monsell solution or silver nitrate is applied after the biopsy or a suture (5/0 absorbable) may be inserted.

When performing a colposcopy for an abnormal cervical smear, the whole lower genital tract must be examined. This is especially important if no significant lesion is found on the cervix, as the source of the abnormal cells may be from a vaginal lesion.

Experience with different treatment methods for premalignant lesions allows the correct choice for each situation, for example, CO_2 laser or surgical excision. VAIN is well suited for treatment with CO_2 laser. VIN is best excised in hair-bearing areas because dysplastic epithelium can be found deeply placed in skin appendages. CO_2 laser can be used in non-hair bearing areas, especially in the clitoral and peri-clitoral areas where a good therapeutic and cosmetic result can be obtained. A non-surgical approach with immuno-modifiers may be worth a try in some circumstances before resorting to surgery (for example, widespread areas, clitoris). Long-term follow-up is essential as recurrence rates for the squamous dysplasias, and especially Paget's disease, can be high.

Malignant conditions

Women with vulvovaginal malignancies are often elderly and require sensitive care. The management of these cancers almost always affects the patient's perception of self-image and femininity, and may limit further sexual function. The psycho-sexual implications associated with the treatment demands full explanation and a sympathetic approach from the attending gynecologist and the management team. A supportive attitude is always necessary.

The early detection of vulva and vagina malignancies is limited by late presentation, the lack of screening tests and poor physician and patient education. Many of these malignancies are diagnosed after significant delays, and this impacts upon outcome.

A knowledge of radical surgery, split skin grafts, myo-cutaneous flaps and radiotherapy are all essential ingredients for the decision making process. The management of recurrent vulva malignancies, especially after previous radiotherapy, always required a considered approach as treatment options can be limited and complicated.

Although malignancies of the vulva and vagina are uncommon, there are many conditions discussed in Chapter 13 that are exceedingly rare. Sarcomas of the vulva and vagina are one such rare group. They are classified under the mesenchymal diseases and listed here for convenience (tables 1 and 2).

The sarcomas of the vulva constitute 1-2% of the vulva cancers. These malignancies develop in the deep soft tissues of the vulva and paravagina. Most present in the labia majora and macroscopically there are no specific distinguishing features between the different types. All are treated with radical local excision. Post-operative radiotherapy may help to reduce local recurrences.

Of the vaginal sarcomas, leiomyosarcoma is most common in adults and sarcoma botryoides (embryonal rhabdomyosarcoma) is seen mostly in children under the age of 5 years. Surgical resection is recommended as the primary treatment in adults, but chemotherapy now plays a predominant role in children with sarcoma botryoides.

Table 1. Sarcomas of the vulva.

Leiomyosarcoma	Rhabdoid tumor
Rhabdomyosarcoma	Epithelioid sarcoma
Fibrosarcoma	Kaposi's sarcoma
Angiosarcoma	Malignant peripheral nerve sheath tumor
Liposarcoma	Malignant granular cell tumor
Dermatofibrosarcoma protuberans	Alveolar soft part sarcoma
Synovial sarcoma	

Table 2. Sarcomas of the vagina.

Rhabdomyosarcoma	Mullerian adenosarcoma
Angiosarcoma	Kaposi sarcoma
Leiomyosarcoma	Malignant peripheral nerve sheath tumor
Endometrial stromal sarcoma	

Important points to remember

- Biopsy any abnormal vulvar lesions early on in their management.
- Discuss the pathology with a pathologist who has a specific interest in vulvovaginal disease.

Chapter 4

THE PSYCHOLOGIST'S PERSPECTIVE

Managing patients with gynecological difficulties requires a great deal of sensitivity as well as an understanding of female sexuality, psychosocial and cultural issues. For most human beings the reproductive system is closely bound to self esteem, one's concept of the self and where one fits into society. The genitals have many social, religious, emotional and moral connotations and, along with sexual behavior, still carry many taboos. Therefore, working in this field requires an extra effort, a sound knowledge base, patience and inquiry skills.

This chapter aims to clarify some of the nonmedical factors influencing the complicated jigsaw puzzle that chronic vulvar symptoms can be. To assist in patient management there is a description of special categories of patients and a section on communication between the doctor or nurse practitioner and patients.

The Multifactorial Nature of Chronic Vulvar Disease

It is now widely accepted that human behavior and emotions play a part in the onset, course and outcome of many diseases. This observation also applies to diseases of the lower female genital tract but this is often overlooked. A full medical history cannot be undertaken without the inclusion of behavioral and stress factors. The absence of a patient's full history may then lead to misdiagnosis and prolonged, inefficient management, including surgery.

There are many causes for the onset and maintenance of chronic vulvar disease. Figure 5.1 is one way of pictorially representing those many complex factors. The arrows describe how each factor can interact with and affect others. For example, a patient may develop an infection (*Organic*) which may produce an itch and might not respond to topical medication. These two factors may lead to rubbing or scratching due to the patient's lack of tolerance to discomfort or a heightened perception of bodily sensations. The result of this behavior could lead to frictional trauma, excoriations (*Organic*), and chronic symptoms.

The lack of effective initial treatment may lead to continuous treatment with creams and lotions (*Medical Treatment*), excessive hygiene and inappropriate self care (*Hygiene, Self Treatment*). The latter can include damaging naturopathic or herbal preparations not appropriate for sensitive vulvar epithelium (*Organic*). This turn of events may lead to chronic contact dermatitis (*Organic*) and much distress (*Emotional Distress*). If the patient is in a sexual relationship, dyspareunia (*Sexual Difficulties*) may occur and may become self-perpetuating, leading to impaired sexual response and ongoing symptoms.

Another avenue for the onset and maintenance of symptoms can be the pathway that begins with *Emotional Distress*, which may impact on a patient's sexual life. For example, a patient may experience some life change or other sudden stress. If she is in a sexual relationship she may find herself losing interest in sex. If she continues to have sex, but in an unaroused state, she may develop frictional trauma due to penetration of an unlubricated, unrelaxed and ill-prepared vagina. This situation may lead to dyspareunia and possibly vaginismus (*Sexual Difficulties*). If a sexual and/or stress history is not undertaken, the patient may be misdiagnosed and a course of topical medication initiated (*Medical Treatment*). As this will not resolve symptoms caused by unaroused sex, the patient usually finds herself returning to the doctor and receiving further prescriptions, possibly leading to contact dermatitis (*Organic*) or 'vestibulitis syndrome'.

Sometimes a stressful experience can initiate symptoms. Here, a patient may experience a situation that has particularly negative meanings for her such as a death of a loved one, divorce or financial ruin. Symptoms may begin spontaneously, very close in time to the stressful event. Some patients have insight into the relationship between symptoms and the stressor but even so, many women will seek a medical solution. As topical medication is not likely to resolve the symptoms, often more treatment is sought, eventuating in contact dermatitis (*Organic*), further distress (*Emotional Distress*) and possibly dysesthesia ('vulvodynia').

The direct link between psychological distress and physical symptoms is unclear. In psychodynamic terms, such incidents may occur when the patient physically expresses psychic pain which she is unable to express in more appropriate verbal or emotional ways. This may occur in a part of the body which is psychically significant to her or has some predisposing vulnerability.

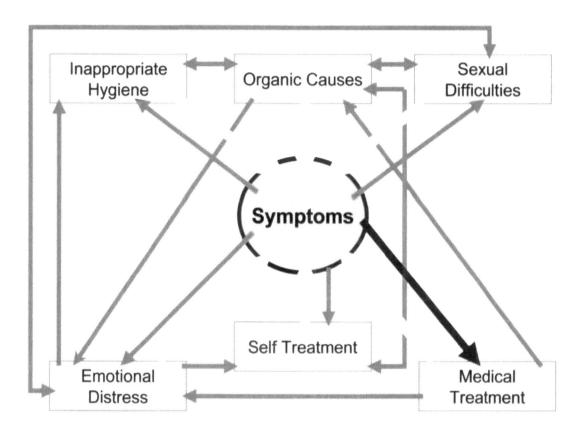

Figure 5.1. Factors affecting vulvar disease. The interaction between a number of factors can initiate and/or maintain symptoms in chronic vulvar disease.

Therefore, we can see how the chronicity of vulvar symptoms can occur and how an appreciation of behavior and stresses is important for good medical management.

Important Points to Remember

- Many vulvovaginal problems have more than one cause.
- Vulvar diseases may become chronic for many reasons.
- It is important to be aware of the variety of causes of symptoms and take a broad history from patients, which should include a medical history (including self treatment), behavioral history (see the following section) and a stress history.

Human Behavior and Chronic Vulvar Disease

This section will focus on patient behavior. Damaging patient behavior is defined as anything a patient does that may adversely affect, induce, maintain, or be a reaction to symptoms. Three foci of damaging behavior are self care, sexual behavior and scratching.

Damaging Self Care

In this context, damaging self care includes excessive hygiene as well as self-treatment. Excessive hygiene is regarded as 'damaging' when it includes practices known from clinical experience to be associated with contact dermatitis. These practices include cleaning with potentially irritating agents and/or the use of excessive friction. Also included in the concept of excessive hygiene is inappropriate frequency of washing.

Among substances known to be used directly on the vulva by patients as part of their hygiene ritual are: diaper cleaning solution, shampoo, disinfectants, antiseptics, nylon wire body sponges and soap substitutes. The use of terry towelling washcloths and the patient's own fingers, pushed high into the vagina in a digging or scraping motion, have also been reported. Many patients wash themselves a number of times a day and often rub the vulva vigorously. The use of harsh products and techniques reported by women is often their response to irritation or a crawling sensation on the surface of the epithelium. Many women also report a belief that their condition is caused by poor hygiene, which is seldom the case.

Damaging self treatment includes self medication with the use of previously prescribed or over-the-counter preparations. Other preparations used include 'natural', homeopathic and herbal preparations (usually not subjected to vigorous scientific testing), prolonged, inappropriate use of topical antifungal agents and other substances that are a potential source of chemical irritation. Their effect will be worse in the presence of inflammatory changes, which undermine the integrity of the epithelium.

Further examples of preparations often used by patients are: concentrated naturopathic substances, moisturizers, 'feminine' (deodorant) products which 'burn' irritated skin in some cases, bleaches, creams prescribed for other women, home remedies, sexual lubricants, petroleum jelly, vitamin creams and baby oil.

There are many reasons why patients treat their bodies in such a risky manner. However, this is a behavioral response which is difficult to research and quantify. When asked, most women cannot explain the reasons for their behavior and have never questioned themselves about the logic of such behavior. The power of the popular press is a contributing factor. Newspapers and women's magazines carry convincing advertisements for various products in an attractive and tempting manner. Often magazines print articles advocating the use of inappropriate products. Popular women's magazines do not always publish the authors of such articles as the emphasis in these magazines is the marketing of products, not unbiased, scientific information. This fact is not understood by most readers. It is therefore suspected that women's health is being manipulated and influenced by unrefereed writers with little knowledge and training in health matters.

From in depth conversations with patients with chronic vulvar disease, it has become apparent that one aspect of poor health behavior is the adage we are all taught from childhood, 'if you have a sore, put something on it'. However, this does not apply to the skin of the vulva and vagina. Other factors may be the embarrassment and shame surrounding the genitals and the reluctance many patients have to see a doctor as soon as symptoms begin. Patients may prefer to try their own remedies firstly. Lately, there have been a number of television advertisements promoting the use of short term antifungal creams, which can be purchased over the counter. These advertisements prey on the above anxieties and may exacerbate contact dermatitis and undiagnosed complaints.

Damaging Sexual Behavior

Damaging sexual behavior includes behavior that causes chemical or physical trauma to vulvar epithelium. Patients may allow painful penetration, have unaroused (unlubricated) intercourse or use potentially irritating chemicals, such as topical anesthetics and lubricants.

In the absence of genital disease, sexual penetration at a heightened state of sexual arousal should be painless and pleasurable. This is due to transudation of natural lubricating fluid, relaxation of the muscles surrounding the vagina, engorgement and separation of the labia and enlargement of the vaginal space. The latter refers to the 'ballooning' of the vagina and the lifting of the base of the cervix, allowing the vagina to accommodate the erect penis.

If any of the above changes are not allowed to develop before penetration, superficial as well deep pelvic pain may occur. Such pain may be caused by frictional trauma during entry and thrusting and deeper pressure of the penis against pelvic structures. The latter may also produce the sensation of a full bladder.

When a woman experiences dyspareunia, some kind of disturbance has occurred. To continue to allow painful intercourse will usually exacerbate problems, physically and emotionally. Common responses to dyspareunia are the increase in expectation of pain, fear and then vaginismus (see chapter 15).

It may seem incomprehensible that a woman experiencing painful sexual penetration would continue to allow penetration. However, this behavior is quite common and occurs for a number of reasons. Initially when asked why, some women cannot explain and some do not see this behavior as contributing to symptoms, although painful, highly distressing and depressing. With further discussion, it was discovered that many women are fearful of perceived consequences of stopping penetrative intercourse. Often, women unconsciously fear reinforcement of their feelings of inadequacy and expect rejection and/or abandonment if they do not have penetrative sex. They may also fear the sense of failure as a person.

Some patients have expressed feelings of guilt if they do not "give" their partners sex. Others are too timid and inhibited to assert themselves or had simply never thought of saying "no". A patient's partner and her doctors may encourage a woman to "keep trying" to continue with penetrative sex, often with the aid of a local anesthetic. However, this is not helpful to the woman or her condition and creates a situation where the woman learns that sex will not provide pleasure for her. Lubricants and anesthetics do not eliminate or treat the problems and may only serve to mask the real problem. Apart from these potential sequelae, urging women to continue with painful sex is unproductive and the couple and the doctor may unconsciously collude in ways that prolong symptoms, create negative attitudes to sex and lead to psychosexual problems.

Many people suffering depression and/or anxiety show distorted thinking, aptly described by cognitive-behavioral theories of psychology. These people do not appear to be able to think rationally about some aspects of their lives. They do not appear to have the ability to discriminate between various sources of information coming from the environment and often have quite unrealistic expectations. Sometimes 'magical', irrational thinking is apparent. This more often occurs when the situation is confusing. The person may then provide himself/herself with a rationale that fits in with his/her lifelong belief system. Women with chronic vulvar disease are often anxious and tense people who may have this style of thinking. For example, some women who have experienced dyspareunia for many months (and sometimes always) keep hoping that the next time they have sex it will not hurt. Realistically, improvement is not likely to happen but this does not seem to occur to these women.

Pruritus and the Itch-Scratch Cycle
Scratching of the vulva, perineum and anal areas is very difficult to stop, although few patients admit to this even when asked. Anecdotally, very tense women experiencing life stresses report instigating an itch-scratch cycle if they perceive sensations on the vulva which they cannot tolerate. Scratching may be an attempt to relieve the sensation but can also be an attempt to relieve tension. If left unattended, this cycle can be difficult to break and may require the administration of some form of sedation.

Pruritus is often reported as being worse at night, in bed, when the woman has no distractions, when body temperature rises and when she is tired and has a lowered tolerance to body sensations. Scratching during sleep is also common and difficult to avoid. Some women admit to scratching until they bleed but still cannot stop themselves from doing so. There seems to be little self control in these cases.

Important points to remember

- Self-treatment, hygiene, sexual behavior and scratching can all impact on vulvar health.
- Often patients use substances on the vulvar and vagina which can produce contact dermatitis.
- Fear of penetration, medical examination and/or pain can lead to vaginismus especially if the patient has experienced dyspareunia.
- Dyspareunia may be caused by unaroused sex, genital pathology, vaginismus or the topical use of irritating substances.
- Scratching is important as it may cause damage to vulvar and anal epithelium. It is difficult to assess and control.

Management of Patients with Chronic Vulvar Disease

Apart from medical management, good patient care should involve support, counseling and preventive education aimed at improving patients' genital health behaviors. The following section describes an approach to patient management that may assist to this end.

Often patients hold irrational and superstitious beliefs about what is appropriate for vulvar health. As a group, these patients appear to be tense. They may display perfectionist tendencies, obsessionality, have difficulty coping with life - and sexual difficulties are common.

Some patients have an over optimistic view that certain behaviors are not damaging. Some health behaviors fail to improve the disorder, especially when health promotion becomes ideological rather than scientific. An example of this is when patients use naturopathic substances just because they are called 'natural' and so take on a special significance not based on science.

Other relevant general health behavior issues are: avoidant coping strategies, complex self-care regimens, non-adherence to doctors' instructions (which can be affected by factors including lack of understanding of the treatment regimen), presence of life stress and feelings of anger in the face of a sense of losing control over one's life.

Strategies in Effective Patient Management

Detailed history taking may uncover relevant information regarding onset and maintenance of symptoms that perhaps patients do not initially believe is relevant or would not think of providing to a doctor.

Preventive instructions on self care help avoid exacerbation of patients' symptoms. To achieve this it is important to find out past treatments and what has been the patient's experience of, and behavioral response to, her disorder. This information is needed to target specific poor health behaviors and make the consultation relevant for her. If this is not achieved the patient may not comply.

Education of patients includes factual information on sexual physiology, the use of topical medication and hygiene. This information is basic material that every woman should have access to, but especially if she has vulvar symptoms. It also assists patients to understand the logic and importance of the prevention instructions. To prevent non-compliance, a rationale for the instructions needs to be provided and all information should be simple and concrete.

Counseling aims to assist patients to vent feelings, gain insight and can sometimes provide an opportunity to find solutions to problems that are impacting on genital health in some way. This includes sexual counseling because of the frequency of sexual difficulties in patients with gynecological disorders.

Important considerations for effective patient management
The rest of this section outlines ways of enhancing doctor patient communication and treatment compliance, often essential to help prevent vulvar diseases from becoming chronic and complicated.

Behavior which interferes with treatment compliance may not change if the purpose of that behavior is not addressed in some way. Often the unconscious purpose is avoidance of anxiety. For example, a woman who lacks self confidence, believes having sex means she is a fully functioning, desirable human being, or believes she will lose her partner if she does not regularly provide him with sex, may not stop having painful sex. If a woman only feels acceptable, wholesome and clean if she vigorously washes her genitals, she may not stop doing this just because a doctor says so. The function or purpose of a person's behavior has a very strong influence and needs to be gently probed.

Although a majority of patients reveal similar patterns of behavior and psychological vulnerabilities, each patient is an individual with a unique history. Consultations therefore need to adjust to the individual. It is important not to draw conclusions about a patient or what she does without first 'checking it out', that is, asking clarifying questions. Expectations or 'mind sets' in the health professional can lead us down the wrong path.

Including the patient's partner in the consultation may be beneficial for a number of reasons. For example, the partner's questions can be addressed, sexual facts can be given to both and the partner can aid in compliance. Relationship issues, which may be impacting on the symptoms, may come to light.

Some knowledge of counseling and interviewing techniques is essential for communicating with patients. For example, establishing a non-threatening environment and the use of open, general questions may produce far more information than closed, specific questions. However, there are occasions when closed questions are needed for specific information. A closed question is one requiring only a 'yes' or 'no' answer. Open questions are those that use the words: 'how', 'why', 'what' or 'when'.

Many patients are difficult to communicate with. Resistance and emotional distress are common. Such patients cannot hear much of what is being said nor can they fully communicate information. Emotions such as anger or distress are very distracting. It is better to address these early in the consultation and allow the patient to vent those feelings. Only then can she focus on the task at hand.

The dynamic and cognitive models of psychological therapy help us understand the power that anxiety and depression have over our reactions to life events. These emotions can lead to life long maladaptive responses to any difficult situation. Anxiety governs the way people deal with difficulties and often makes people do things that worsen their situation.

Anxious people may also have difficulty accepting information or points of view that do not coincide with their own or do not seem relevant to their experiences. From a treatment perspective, this means that changing an anxious person's beliefs and behaviors (for example, a mistaken belief that extensive washing of the vulva is best) is very difficult and could mean the difference between acute and chronic conditions.

Visual aids in the form of diagrams of the vulva and the pelvic floor muscles allow the doctor to demonstrate certain instructions such as irrigating the vulva with saline for hygiene, the physiological responses to sexual arousal and the application of topical medication. Diagrams also help patients become familiar with their bodies.

As a large amount of information may need to be provided, a pamphlet, highlighting the major points, should be supplied to patients to aid their memory (an example is supplied at the end of this chapter). People can only remember small chunks of information.

Patients with Particular Difficulties

Patients who do not speak your language require a professional interpreter if their language skills are insufficient to discuss medical issues and personal problems. Often a woman who does not speak the country's language can be overlooked or ignored, especially if she is timid. Professional interpreters should be specially trained to be a non-interfering go-between. Office or general hospital staff may not have this ability. With the use of family members or friends to interpret, much is lost in the translation and often the interpreter vetoes the information. Patients' children often do not have sufficient knowledge of their parent's language to be of help and perhaps should not be hearing information about their mother's sex life or other intimate details.

The menopausal woman experiences disconcerting changes to her body and often to her emotions. Sex may become very uncomfortable due to hormonal changes and may also become psychologically distasteful to her. Menopausal women need to have these changes explained, warned what to expect and be given information about changing her sexual routine to adjust to her changing body. An example of this may be suggesting longer foreplay and better couple communication about what is exciting for her.

The angry patient is very difficult to communicate with. Anger prevents good hearing on both sides and can be very effective in blocking a doctor's attempts to be open, especially if the information is not what the patient is expecting. Often anger stems from a need to control the environment to make it predictable and 'safe'. This may be due to perceived emotional 'threat' or the emotional 'chaos' the person feels. The person is often a perfectionist, goal orientated and cannot cope with unresolved situations. However, vulvar conditions are often not resolved easily and so the patient becomes angry with the medical profession for not "doing its job". This anger then stems from anxiety. The patient may have an anxious personality style or even an anxiety disorder.

The anger needs to be addressed as soon as possible by the doctor asking such questions as: "Has something upset you? ... Could you tell me about it?" The doctor must be prepared to accept the anger that may be unleashed, even though it can be intimidating. It may help to remember that the anger may not be caused by the doctor, nor necessarily directed at the doctor, but may result from the patient's distress. The way this patient makes the doctor feel might be the way she functions with others in her life. These patients may be non compliant and may not trust the doctor. They may firmly believe that their own opinions about their treatment are more correct.

The hearing impaired patient may be used to medical consultations. Many deaf patients have learned lip reading or may have a sign language interpreter. With a hearing impaired patient sit squarely in front of her, speak clearly and simply and ask her if she understands. When pointing to diagrams, give the patient time to look at the diagram and then back at you before continuing your communication. Direct the questions to the patient at all times regardless of who else is in the room. As with all other patients, explain to her what you are about to do and why.

The homosexual patient does not need to be treated any differently to the heterosexual patient. With all patients, talk openly about sex even if they are not sexually active. Many patients keep their sexuality to themselves out of shame, timidity or fear. This may not be helpful to their management.

If the patient is a member of a celibate religious order, it is still appropriate to ask her if she would like sexual information. The investigation of symptoms in the patient belonging to some religious orders may not include a sexual history but often they do experience stress in their cloistered life. This may be a factor in symptomatology.

Some patients from Middle Eastern countries may be reluctant to be examined without a chaperone if the doctor is a male. For religious reasons, Muslim women have the habit of washing the genitals after each use of the toilet. This habit usually only includes the use of water. However, some women, especially after vulvar symptoms have developed, may be excessive in their hygiene routine. Some women may use depilatory creams to remove pubic hair. This may also have some relevance to their symptomatology.

The depressed patient is often not forthcoming with information. She may not respond to some questions at all and may be passive in her attempts to resolve her problems. If a depressed patient begins to weep she must be given time to gain some control before the consultation continues. It is important to assess whether a depressed patient may be suicidal. Again, the depression should be addressed early in the consultation. If such patients require psychotherapy or medication they should be referred to the appropriate professional quickly.

Important points to remember

- Complete history-taking is essential so as to address all aspects of symptomatology.
- The education of patients is important for a number of reasons including increasing compliance, replacing irrational beliefs, prevention of symptom exacerbation and reducing anxiety.
- Counseling is often required by gynecological patients especially when sexually active or when stressed. Partners should be included. Effective patient management requires an understanding of female sexuality, psychosocial problems and cultural issues.
- Many patients resist treatment for one reason or another and there are many patients with special needs.

Instructions for Patients

A pamphlet has been provided at the end of this section, which can be given to patients as their aide-de-memoir.

Hygiene is usually less threatening so could be discussed first. Most patients are very interested in this topic. The next section is sexual functioning. Often patients are self conscious discussing sex and will sometimes go into denial or withdraw. As the lower female genital tract is primarily a sexual organ, this topic is important in patient management and patients need to take part in this section. The last section is on topical medication as this is very important for the patient to understand. Many patients do not apply medication correctly. Although no specific instructions about stress are supplied here, this is an area that needs assessment.

Instructions for self care

GENITAL HYGIENE
- Treat genital skin gently.
- While you have symptoms, clean only with normal saline solution (2 teaspoons of salt in 1 litre of water) applied with wads of cotton wool.
- When you are better, plain water is sufficient for hygiene purposes.
- Gently pat dry the outside areas only.
- Do not over wash the genitals. Never use soaps, perfumes, perfumed talcs, deodorants, 'feminine' products.
- Do not use douches (internal washing).
- Do not use moisturisers.
- Try not to scratch the skin if it feels itchy.

PREVENTION OF SEXUAL PROBLEMS
- See a doctor if you feel pain during intercourse or have any sexual difficulties.
- It is important to explain your condition to your partner. Ask our help if this is a problem.
- Ensure proper arousal before penetration (which means you are producing your own natural lubrication and the pelvic floor muscles are relaxed). Teach your partner how to help you become aroused (he cannot read your mind).
- Seek out information if you need help.
- Deal with any stresses or marital problems as they will interfere with sexual activity and reduce the quality of your life.
- When you have recovered from your condition and wish to attempt intercourse again, it is suggested you adopt a position during intercourse which will allow you to control the rate and depth of penetration to prevent discomfort.
- Do not use artificial lubricants (such as 'KY' or petroleum jelly).
- Avoid intercourse when you are feeling symptoms or pain in the genitals.

IMPORTANT POINTS ON THE USE OF MEDICATION
- Only use medication on the genital area that we have prescribed.
- If a flare up of symptoms occurs, a swab for culture should be undertaken before any medication is prescribed or used.
- Go to a doctor if you feel any symptoms, see any rashes or other changes. Ask your doctor to carry out the appropriate tests before changing treatment.
- Do not treat any symptoms yourself without seeing a doctor.

Genital skin is very sensitive. It needs protection from chemical and physical damage

The genital area is also affected by the way you feel and symptoms can appear worse when you are stressed.

Further Reading

Broom B. Somatic illness and the patient's other story. Free Association Books. London. 1997

Cullari S. Treatment Resistance: A guide for practitioners. Allyn and Bacon. U.S.A. 1996.

Dains B and Perrett A. Psychodynamic Approaches to Sexual Problems. Open University Press. Great Britain. 2000

Leiblum S R and Rosen R C. (Eds) Sexual Desire Disorders. Guilford Publications. N.Y. 1988

Marin MG, King R, Dennerstein G, Sfameni S. Adverse behavioral and sexual factors in chronic vulvar disease. Am J Obstet Gynecol 2000; 183:34-38.

Marin MG, King R, Dennerstein G, Sfameni S. Dyspareunia and Vulvar disease. JReprod Med 1998:43L 952-958

Matsakis A. Managing Client Anger: What to do when a client is angry with you. New Harbinger Publications. Canada. 1998

McDougall, Theatres of the Body: A psychoanalytical approach to psychosomatic illness. Free Association Books. London 1989.

Pilowsky I. Abnormal Illness Behaviour. John Wiley and Sons. England. 1997

Skrine R. Blocks and Freedoms in Sexual Life: A handbook of psychosexual medicine. Radcliff Medical Press.UK. 1997

Taylor S E. Health Psychology. McGraw-Hill, Inc. 1995

Chapter 5

THE PATHOLOGIST'S PERSPECTIVE

Good pathology is crucial to the clinician managing vulvovaginal disease, but how is good pathology obtained? There are two clinical situations in which a tissue sample is sent for pathology: rashes and discrete lesions. Rashes are sent for accurate pathological diagnosis, margins not being relevant. Specimens of lesions require, in addition to confirmation of clinical diagnosis, pathological assessment of prognostic factors and margins.

Clinical Aspects Relevant to the Pathologist

It is particularly important that the following clinical information accompanies the biopsy of a rash: its duration, distribution and appearance (macular, papular, vasculitic or vesicular). The pathologist also needs to know the specific site and type of biopsy and will be assisted by a clinical diagnosis.

Clinical history and diagnosis

The first and most important step is the clinical assessment. The clinician needs to take a good history, perform an examination, reach the best clinical diagnosis possible and communicate this information to the pathologist. The importance of the clinical diagnosis is based on two tenets: Firstly, the clinical appearance of the rash is equivalent to macroscopic pathological examination, a crucial step to pathological diagnosis in all organs and one that, in the skin, only the clinician can perform. Secondly, while there are many diseases, the skin has relatively few reaction patterns. Furthermore, the pathological features of different diseases may overlap, making it impossible in many situations for the pathologist to reach an unequivocal diagnosis.

Clinical diagnosis is not easy in vulvar conditions. Late presentation and disguise by the effects of irritation and treatment are very frequent. Vulvar skin is more easily irritated than skin elsewhere on the body. The rashes look different as the vulva is an intertriginous area where friction, moisture and microbiological overgrowth abound. Extragenital manifestations should always be sought as rashes usually are easier to diagnose outside the vulva. The eyes and mouth can occasionally be affected in several types of unusual vulvovaginal disease and may offer important clues.

Site of biopsy

Knowing the specific site of the biopsy is very helpful to the pathologist. An assessment of what is abnormal requires a comparison with what is normal - and the normal varies so much depending on the site on the vulva.

Type of biopsy

A biopsy may be taken by excision, incision, punch, shave and curettage. For vulvar rashes, the punch biopsy is, by far, the most commonly used. While an incisional biopsy will provide more diagnostic material, for ease of performance and minimisation of patient's symptoms, punch biopsy is preferable. However, even a punch biopsy of the vulva may cause significant discomfort and may preclude sexual activity for some days. It is therefore crucial that any vulvar biopsy yield the maximum amount of information. A minimum 3mm diameter punch biopsy should be used. Anything smaller (such as 1 or 2mm punches) risks significant sampling error.

The appearance of the rash dictates how the biopsy should be taken. Vulvar rashes can be divided into two main types: maculopapular and erosive/ulcerative.

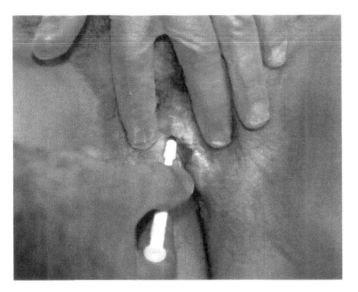

Figure 4.1. Taking a biopsy with a 4mm punch. The surrounding area has been infiltrated with 2% lignocaine. It will be closed with a single, atraumatic 5/0 absorbable suture.

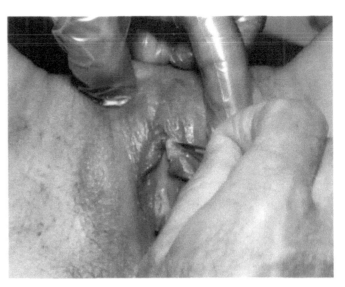

Figure 4.2. Taking scrapings from the vulva for cytology or the investigation of suspected fungal infection of the skin.

Maculopapular rashes

Small lesions can be removed entirely with a cuff of normal skin with a punch or incisional biopsy. However, many vulvar rashes are large and diffuse. Ideally, a radial incision biopsy from the edge of the lesion, including about 1mm of normal skin, is best. A punch biopsy from the centre of the lesion is next best.

Consider sending scrapings for culture if fungus or yeast infection is being considered. Culture doubles the yield for fungal infections compared to histology - and has the added advantage that it can be used to type and speciate the fungus.

Erosive/ulcerative rashes

Vulvar ulcers may be infective (particularly when sexually transmitted) or non-infective. Often the histology is non-specific. Samples for culture and serological tests are better methods of diagnosing vulvar infections. If biopsy is performed, the best diagnostic yield will be from a small, fresh lesion excised with a rim of normal skin by punch biopsy, or an incisional biopsy including the ulcer, edge and adjacent normal skin of a larger lesion.

Ulcers often have a pale slough on the surface. Red, raw and glistening skin suggests erosion. Erosive lichen planus is the classic cause of erosion in the medial vulva. The diagnostic basal layer vacuolar change of lichen planus is more frequently seen in keratinised skin than mucosa.

Vegetative (thickened) erosive lesions are the characteristic presentation of vulvar vesicobullous disease. Blisters may be entirely absent but, when they are present, they are usually found at the edge of the erosive area. A fresh lesion is best for diagnosis, as secondary changes may obscure diagnostic changes in older lesions. A small fresh vesicle is ideal if it can be removed intact with a cuff of normal skin. A punch or excision biopsy may achieve this. If there are only larger lesions present, a radial incision biopsy through the edge of the vesicle is next best. A separate biopsy of perilesional skin for immunofluorescence will greatly help in the diagnosis and subclassification of immunobullous disorders.

Lesions

Lesions such as Paget's disease and vulvar intraepithelial neoplasia (VIN - squamous dysplasia) may be diagnosed on punch biopsy. Excision should follow. Assessment for invasion and margins are crucial on excision specimens. The margins are often positive as the histological lesion often extends beyond the clinical abnormality. Vulvar excision specimens often contain anatomical folds and are particularly liable to distort if placed in formalin without being pinned out. We have seen superficial invasion mistakenly reported as deep invasion because nests of tumor appear to be deeply placed in very folded, distorted specimens. The specimen needs to be pinned out on cork or foam board and orientated with a marking suture or pin by the clinician.

The Pathologist's Report

After examining the biopsy, the pathologist should provide the following information: site of the biopsy, a list of abnormalities, a summary of the abnormalities expressed as tissue reaction patterns and the differential diagnosis.

Siting the biopsy

While the clinician should give the site on the vulva of the biopsy on the request slip, the first step for the pathologist is to site the biopsy independently. This requires a good knowledge of normal histology of the vulva. Site is always important and may be crucial for the following reasons: Only by reference to the normal can the pathologist determine what is abnormal. Secondly, certain diseases have a propensity to occur in certain areas of the vulva. Finally, the clinician may have not stated the site, or, if the vulvar anatomy has been distorted by disease or previous surgery, the site may be difficult to identify.

Listing abnormal features

The abnormal features are noted in the 'Microscopic Description' section of the report. Generally, the pathologist begins at the top, that is, the stratum corneum and works down to the deepest tissue layer in the biopsy.

In biopsies for non-neoplastic conditions, the pathologist usually begins with examination of 3 levels and a PAS stain for fungi. Reaching the most diagnostic material may require several requests by the pathologist to the laboratory technical staff for deeper levels. The pathologist should not short cut the procedure and request levels through the block if the first slides are not diagnostic because this risks wasting valuable tissue that could be used for immunoperoxidase or special stains. The clinician should understand that the best pathological opinion may be reached only after several days of going back to the block for more levels and special stains. Rapid turnaround time is not always a good indicator of quality in vulvar pathology.

The pathologist's observations about what is abnormal must be kept separate from any interpretation. The observations should be objective and immutable, but how these observations are interpreted may be very much open to opinion

Summarizing the abnormalities into patterns

Pathologists work by pattern recognition. After the individual pathologic features have been noted, the next step is to try and slot the changes into one of the major tissue reaction patterns. These are spongiotic, psoriasiform, lichenoid, vesicobullous, granulomatous and vasculopathic. Each tissue reaction pattern has a list of causes whose pathological features may overlap to a varying degree. In difficult cases, a 'Comments' section in the report is a convenient place for the pathologist to state his interpretation of the pathological findings.

Pathological Diagnosis

Depending on the difficulty of the case, the pathologist may provide a specific diagnosis, a tissue reaction pattern with differential diagnosis, or in very difficult cases, merely a summary of the pathological findings and some diagnostic suggestions.

Limitations of pathological diagnosis

Infectious and non-infectious diseases are often not distinguishable histopathologically. A classic example is pyoderma gangrenosum, which is basically a diagnosis of exclusion of infection. Histopathology is seldom a good way to identify infectious organisms. Other means are more reliable, such as culture or serology. On the other hand, supersensitive tests that may be performed on histological tissue, such as the polymerase chain reaction, may be difficult to interpret because of false positives due to contamination.

Non-infectious inflammatory disorders provide their own peculiar difficulties in diagnosis. In the case of spongiotic tissue reaction, as well as spongiosis, these biopsies also often show psoriasiform hyperplasia, parakeratosis, a superficial perivascular lymphohistiocytic infiltrate and, when there is excoriation, polymorphs within the parakeratosis. The histological differential diagnosis is spongiotic dermatitis, psoriasis, fungal infection and excoriated lichen simplex chronicus.

Spongiosis is subtle in chronic dermatitis, which merges with lichen simplex chronicus. One should look for lymphocyte exocytosis to confirm that increased prominence of intercellular prickles is due to spongiosis.

Psoriasis shows dry parakeratosis rather than wet (with serum, seen on the PAS stain) parakeratosis. Helpful signs in psoriasis are increased mitotic activity, neutrophils on the summits of parakeratotic mounds and a lack of eosinophils in the dermal infiltrate.

Fungal infection can mimic the changes of all stages of psoriasis and spongiotic dermatitis. A PAS stain for fungal elements is mandatory. However, only about a half of the cases with positive fungal culture show histological fungal infection.

The features of lichen simplex chronicus are orthokeratosis, hypergranulosis, regular acanthosis and dermal papillary fibrosis aligned parallel to the rete ridges. These changes will be best seen away from any area of excoriation. Clues to excoriation are serum and polymorphs within parakeratosis (parakeratotic scale crust), dermal fibrin and extravasated red blood cells. To report 'lichen simplex chronicus' may be considered a diagnostic failure and efforts to diagnose the primary dermal condition should be made. In particular, features of chronic spongiotic dermatitis, lichen sclerosus and lichen planus should be sought.

There are also some peculiarities to vulvar lichenoid tissue reactions. Vulvar lichen sclerosus, unlike extraanogenital lichen sclerosus, is nearly always associated with lichen simplex chronicus. Lichen sclerosus may be associated with lichen planus. In such cases, the sclerosus appears on keratinised skin and the planus on the mucosal vulva. A lichenoid tissue reaction without diagnostic features of either lichen sclerosus or planus may be seen. Patients usually present with pruritus. The significance of these changes is not known. Lichen sclerosus may show superimposed spongiotic dermatitis and lichen planus. Chronic lichen sclerosus may lose its homogenised zone of edema/hyalinisation and appear as lichen simplex chronicus. Clues to the presence of an old lichenoid tissue reaction are flattened or irregular rete ridges, squamatisation, loss of pigmentation of the basal layer, pigment incontinence and a diffuse smattering of chronic inflammatory cells. Lichen planus may be particularly difficult to diagnose in the vestibule and vagina. In this situation, basal layer vacuolar changes may be absent.

The pathology of trauma is essentially non-specific.

Difficulties with neoplasia include the following: The warty lesion in the older woman is particularly difficult to diagnose accurately. The differential diagnosis includes verrucous carcinoma, invasive squamous cell carcinoma, and squamous cell hyperplasia and differentiated vulvar intraepithelial neoplasia (VIN). Condyloma is less likely. Pathologists should be aware of the criteria for the diagnosis of differentiated VIN, in particular, that 'atypia' as usually understood is a minor feature. Other changes, for example, parakeratosis, enlarged squamous cells with eosinophilic cytoplasm, enlarged vesicular nuclei and prominent nucleoli and intraepidermal pearls need to be looked for. The pathologist should also be very clear on the criteria of invasion. Tentacles or separated nests of atypical eosinophilic squamous cells beneath rete ridges should be sought. However, pseudoepitheliomatous hyperplasia, which has been described in lichen sclerosus and lichen planus, may produce a similar appearance.

Clinicopathological Diagnosis

The final diagnosis of rashes is usually clinocopathological and the clinician must evaluate the pathologist's observations and comments in the light of clinical information and other test results. If, for example, the pathologist diagnoses spongiotic dermatitis, atopic, irritant and allergic contact dermatitis may have identical histopathology and the patient may have two or more spongiotic diseases coincidentally. The clinical evaluation of spongiotic dermatitis requires consideration of: whether the patient is atopic, the treatment history, examination of the vulvovaginal area and skin elsewhere, together with microbiological and patch testing.

Communication

There are two aspects to communication between pathologist and clinician: terminology and classification. Of these, terminology is the most important. There has been great confusion in terminology in vulvar disease in the past. Face to face discussion between the clinician and pathologist is the most effective method of ironing out terminology problems. Consensus may not always be possible

The names given to conditions reflect current knowledge and are in a constant state of evolution. The vulva is specialized skin and the terminology of vulvar disease should, where possible, follow the terminology of skin conditions elsewhere on the body. In the past, numerous terms invented specifically for the vulva and vagina have been used. Many of these have been relegated to antiquity, but others remain in current practice. We have a natural aversion to specific vulvar terminology on the grounds that the pathological processes are in skin and not usually confined to one site. The following terms continue to cause confusion.

Acute vulvar ulcer (Lipschutz ulcer)

There have been occasional reports of ulcers, often larger than typical aphthous ulcers, occurring within a day or two of intercourse, perhaps with a different partner. It has not been determined whether these are non-infectious inflammatory (usually aphthous), infectious (particularly herpes) or the result of sexual trauma. The problem is that a term like Lipschutz ulcer is not helpful.

Desquamative inflammatory vaginitis (DIV)

Also known as non-infectious vaginitis, the question here is whether DIV is a disease in its own right or a clinical variant of erosive lichen planus. Proponents differentiate DIV from erosive lichen planus by the lack of synechiae and hence, better prognosis. However, this difference begs the question.

Squamous cell hyperplasia

This term was invented by the International Society for the Study of Vulvar Disease (ISSVD) in 1986 to replace 'vulvar dystrophy'. Squamous cell hyperplasia (SCH) is in the category of the 'non-neoplastic epithelial diseases' and is defined as 'hyperplasia not due to any known cause'. It may occur alone or with lichen sclerosus. It is a pathological diagnosis, yet there are no positively identifiable pathological features. Few photomicrographs of what investigators are prepared to call 'SCH' exist. Dermatologists do not like the term because it does not occur on skin elsewhere on the body. Vulvar conditions are frequently itchy, particularly lichen sclerosus. Chronic, pruritic conditions can be expected to show the effects of scratching and rubbing. How can 'SCH' be anything else except lichen simplex chronicus? The term is disappearing from use.

Plasma cell vulvitis of Zoon (vulvitis circumscripta plasmacellularis)

These lesions have many clinical and pathological similarities with erosive lichen planus. However, the lesions have an orange hue due to hemosiderin containing macrophages. It is not known whether plasma cell vulvitis is a disease in its own right or a variant of erosive lichen planus with 'capillaritis'. Capillaritis is another term for pigmented purpuric dermatosis (PPD), a diverse group of inflammatory conditions that occur elsewhere on the skin. PPD may be associated with hemorrhages and hemosiderin deposition in skin elsewhere, where it is known as 'lichen aureus'.

Vulvar intraepithelial neoplasia (VIN)

The term VIN followed cervical intraepithelial neoplasia (CIN). The 'IN' terminology is spreading with VAIN, AIN, PAIN, PIN, TIN and KIN also being used. VIN is nothing more than squamous dysplasia. Yet this vague term does not indicate whether or not the abnormality is confined to squamous epithelium or is premalignant rather than benign (as with seborrheic keratosis). The ingrained use of this catchy, but illogical acronym makes it difficult to avoid. The problem is that the term is confusing to the uninitiated. When dealing with clinicians who are not familiar with vulvar terminology, the premalignant potential of any vulvar lesion should be explained in plain language.

Vulvar vestibulitis syndrome

This term is not in the Systematized Nomenclature of Medicine (SNOMED) and seems to dropping out of favor. When the functional cause of vulvar pain (now referred to as vulvodynia or vulvar dysesthesia) is removed, it would appear that there is no organic inflammatory disease of inflammation of the vestibule that fits the clinical syndrome of 'vulvar vestibulitis syndrome'. The term is not advocated.

Papular acantholytic genitocrural dermatosis

Is there a primary acantholytic dermatosis, confined to the groin and genitals, separate to Hailey-Hailey and Darier's disease? Since Hailey-Hailey and Darier's disease have a predilection for, and may be confined to, the genitocrural area, this is a hard question to answer. However, the onus should be on the proponents to demonstrate a different pathogenetic mechanism before this entity is accepted as a new disease.

Granulomatous vulvitis (Melkersson-Rosenthal syndrome)

Granulomatous vulvitis is analogous clinically and pathologically with granulomatous cheilitis, with which it is associated. Either may precede or follow Crohn's disease by a period of years. The question is whether granulomatous vulvitis is Crohn's disease or a disease in its own right. The burden of proof should be on proponents of the term to convince the rest of us that it is a separate disease with its own pathogenesis.

Classification

A classification is the orderly listing of different entities of the subject. Classifications of biological subjects are, a) never perfect because of continuums and overlaps, b) change with the acquisition of new knowledge and, c) may always be done in different ways. The vulva is specialized skin and, where possible, the classification of vulvar disease should follow the classification of skin diseases elsewhere on the body. The two main ways of classifying skin diseases are clinical and pathological. Examples of entities in a clinical classification are maculopapular and vesiculobullous conditions. While the clinician must have a differential diagnosis in mind when considering an abnormality in the course of examining a patient, for the purposes of systematic study, the pathological classification is better. The main problem with the clinical classification is lack of specificity. Diseases overlap in their clinical appearance and some entities have many different appearances. An example is the pathological entity of VIN, warty-basaloid type, which may occur as red, white, pink or brown lesions, which may be eroded, macular, papular or warty and so fit virtually every category of a clinical classification.

If vulvar diseases are to follow dermatological classification systems, a question that is often asked is whether or not a separate classification of vulvar diseases is needed. We believe there is such a need. The vulva is too specialized for a general dermatological classification to provide anything more than the framework and terminology for disease classification.

The vulva has its own developmental diseases related to its anatomy, development and function. Vulvar infections include sexually transmitted diseases not seen outside the genitalia. Common non-infectious inflammatory disorders in the vulva include lichen sclerosus, lichen simplex and spongiotic dermatitis. While these diseases occur elsewhere on the body, these appear differently on the vulva. For example, vulvar lichen sclerosus is usually an itchy disorder and associated with lichen simplex chronicus, dermal scarring and malignancy. Away from the vulva, it is an unusual and scarcely symptomatic disease, without propensity for architectural alterations and malignancy and is not nearly so important.

The mucosa covered vulva and vagina are subject to many causes of erosions and ulcerations akin to oral or even conjunctival disease. The hormone receptors in the vulva and vagina mean that deficiencies and excess of estrogen and androgens lead to changes not seen elsewhere on skin. Specific vulvar traumatic injuries include obstetric and sexual injury, child abuse and female circumcision. Some benign tumors appear peculiar, or virtually peculiar, to the vulvovaginal region, for example, aggressive angiomyxoma, angiomyofibroblastoma and cellular angiofibroma. By contrast, malignancies such as squamous cell carcinoma share histological similarities to extragenital tumors. However, on the vulva they have a different etiology, pathogenesis and prognosis. Functional disorders and psychological aspects form a subject on their own when applied to the vulva. Finally, many aspects of the normal and diseased vagina are unique. Examples are the complex interdependent roles of sex hormone levels, vaginal microbiological flora and the pathophysiology of sexual dysfunction.

We have found that the classification of vulvar diseases used in this book to be of great benefit in communication between pathologists and clinicians. This classification uses only SNOMED terminology as suggested by the ISSVD. The classification uses etiological broad headings of developmental diseases, infections, non-infectious inflammations, trauma, hormone, neoplasms, non-neoplastic lesions, and functional disorders. A short classification of the 25 most common and/or important diseases accounts for the great majority of conditions seen in day-to-day practice. The full classification of more than 250 entities is of great use in considering the differential diagnosis of unusual or difficult cases.

Important points to remember

- Vulvar pathology is frequently difficult and open to interpretation.
- The pathologist's observations and interpretations should be clearly distinguished in different sections of the pathology report.
- As in all specialties, the pathologist requires a regular case load to become familiar with the range of histological appearances of vulvar conditions.
- Knowledge of normal histology, terminology and classification of vulvar diseases is a great aid to the pathologist.
- A regular multidisciplinary meeting allows clinicians and pathologists to agree on terminology, learn and become aware of the limitations of each other's disciplines.

REFERENCES

Lynch PJ, Edwards L. Genital Dermatology, Churchill-Livingstone. London. 1994

Ridley CM. The Vulva. Churchill-Livingstone. London 1988.

Weedon D. Skin Pathology. Churchill-Livingstone. London 2002

Chapter 6

THE BASICS

EMBRYOLOGY

Gonadal development

Normal gonadal development depends on having a normal complement of X and Y genes. Male sexual development ultimately depends on the presence of a number of genes on the Y chromosome. The most important of these is the master regulatory gene, the SRY gene. The Y chromosome genes program the primitive indifferent gonad to develop into a testis. Gonadal dysgenesis is the development of abnormal ovaries and testes and is a consequence of an abnormal component of X or Y genes.

Genital tract development

The development of the genital tract begins in the 4th week of post-conceptual life. Two pairs of ducts develop. These are the mesonephric (wolffian) and paramesonephric (mullerian) ducts. Both run from near the primitive gonad towards the cloaca. For the next four weeks of intrauterine life, the embryo is in an indifferent stage. Then, under the influence of testosterone produced by the newly formed testis, the mesonephric ducts form the epididymis and vas and the paramesonephric ducts regress. The female phenotype is the default type of genitalia. In the absence of testosterone, the paramesonephric ducts form the fallopian tubes and then fuse to form the body and cervix of the uterus and the upper two thirds of the vagina.

Indifferent stage of external genital development

External genital development has an initial indifferent stage where the female and male embryo appear identical. This begins during the 6th or 7th week of embryonic life with the transverse subdivision of the primitive cloaca into the rectum and urogenital sinus by the urosacral septum. Mesenchymal proliferations of the anterior and lateral regions of cloaca form the genital tubercle (eventually the clitoris or penis) and labioscrotal folds respectively. As the genital tubercle is formed, the endoderm lining the cloaca expands towards it. A plate of endoderm cells (urethral plate) derived from this expansion, grows into the tubercle lying next to its ventral surface. Upon completion of the partitioning of the cloaca, the membranes covering its two subdivisions break down and expose the primitive urethral groove in the floor of the urogenital sinus. A recess, the definitive urethral groove, then forms in the urethral plate.

Definitive female external genitalia development

At the 10-11th week, the female follows a different course to that of the male. Urethral folds bordering the definitive urethral groove remain unfused and become the labia minora. The labioscrotal folds continue to enlarge and become the labia majora and are continuous with the future mons pubis. The genital tubercle turns caudally and becomes the clitoris. The urogenital sinus, now called the vestibule, remains open to the exterior and contains the external urethral orifice and the future opening of the vagina in its floor. By 13 weeks, the basic female structure is complete. By about 20 weeks, the development of the vagina is complete. It is formed by two components. The upper portion is formed by the hollowing out of the fused mullerian ducts. The lower portion is formed by the upward expansion of vestibule into the vaginal plate. The vaginal plate is the solid plate of tissue separating the two components. The vaginal plate is reduced to only a thin membrane, the hymen, between the two portions. The hymen consists of a thin layer of connective tissue with squamous epithelium on both sides and, normally, a central deficiency allowing communication between the vagina and vestibule.

Urinary tract development

The mesonephric ducts grow caudally from the mesonephros (a primitive kidney) to the urogenital sinus, where they open posteriorly. When the ducts reach the sinus, they immediately give rise to the ureteric buds, which grow back cranially to form the ureters. The cranial portion of the urogenital sinus is now termed the vesico-urethral canal. It forms the bladder and all the urethra in the female and bladder and prostatic urethra in the male.

ANATOMY OF THE VULVA

The vulva is bounded anteriorly by the superior border of the mons pubis, laterally by the genitocrural folds, posteriorly by the anus, and medially by the hymenal ring. The surface anatomical structures of the vulva are the mons pubis, labia majora, labia minora, clitoris, vestibule, urethral meatus and perineum.

1 Mons pubis

2 Interlabial sulcus

3 Labium majus

4 Labium minus

5 Posterior fourchette

6 Clitoris and clitoral prepuce

7 Urethral meatus

8 Vaginal introitus

9 Genito-femoral fold

10 Perineum

11 Anus

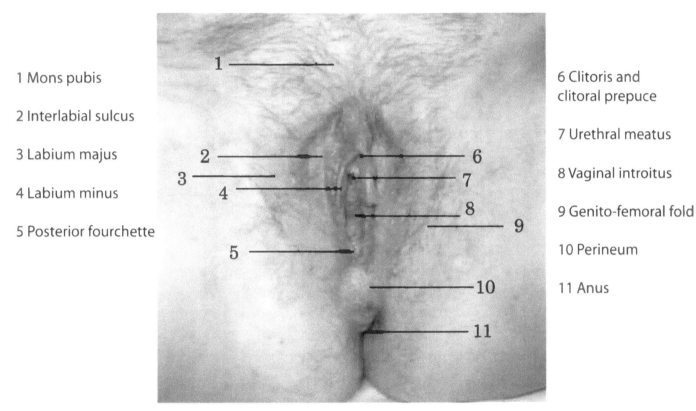

Figure 6.1. The normal vulva. The woman is multiparous and has a minor degree of vaginal prolapse showing healthy, estrogenized, rugose vaginal epithelium.

Mons pubis
The mons pubis is a rounded mass of subcutaneous fibrofatty tissue in front of the symphysis pubis. The mons becomes covered by coarse hair at puberty. The horizontal upper limit of the mons is the anterior boundary of the vulva.

Labia majora
The labia majora are symmetrical, large, lateral folds of subcutaneous fibrofatty tissue. They fuse anteriorly at the anterior commissure at the base of the mons pubis and posteriorly at the posterior commissures 3-4cm in front of the anus. They flatten posteriorly before fusing. The lateral (outer) surfaces become covered by coarse hair at puberty. The medial (inner) surfaces are hairless, but contain small yellow granules, Fordyce spots. These spots are superficially located sebaceous glands.

Labia minora

The labia minora (nymphae) are markedly variable, but usually symmetrical, thin folds of skin covered connective tissue without fat. They lie medial to the labia majora. The lateral boundaries of the labia minora are the interlabial sulci and the medial boundaries are Hart's lines. Hart's lines form the visible boundary between skin and mucosa of the vestibule. Each labium minus splits anteriorly approaching the clitoris. The right and left labia minora then fuse in the midline to form the prepuce anteriorly and the frenulum of the clitoris posteriorly. The labia minora also fuse posteriorly to form the fourchette. The labia minora are covered by thin, hairless, pigmented skin and, like the medial aspect of the labia majora (see above), may show Fordyce spots.

Vestibule

The vestibule is the central, pink mucosa-covered area of the vulva bounded laterally by Hart's line, medially by the hymenal ring, anteriorly by the frenulum of the clitoris, and, posteriorly by the fossa navicularis. The urethral meatus and vaginal opening lie in the midline within the vestibule. Minute, soft projections, the vestibular papillae, are a normal finding in the vestibule of some women. Bartholin's ducts open posterolaterally into the vestibule just superficial to the hymenal ring at positions 5 and 7 o'clock.

Hymen

The hymen is a thin diaphragm of squamous mucosa covered connective tissue that marks the border between the vulva and vagina. It is the residuum of the urogenital plate. The hymen normally contains one or two deficiencies, but is occasionally imperforate. At first intercourse, the remainder of the hymen breaks leaving a ring of small membranous remnants, the carunculae myrtiformes.

Urethral meatus

The urethral meatus lies in the midline between the clitoris and vaginal opening but its relationship to them is variable. The meatus may be everted and show some urethral mucosa. Skene's ducts open into the urethral canal just within, or external to the meatus.

Clitoral glans

The clitoris consists of a body and glans. The terminal portion of the clitoris is the glans, which appears as a pink nodule of skin-covered erectile tissue protected by its prepuce and frenulum, in the midline, anterior to the urethra.

Fossa navicularis

The fossa navicularis is a shallow depression in the vestibule posteriorly, bounded by the fourchette and labia minora.

Perineum

The perineum, the region between the vaginal opening and the anus, is covered with hair-bearing skin.

Deep anatomy

The vulva is subdivided into superficial and deep compartments by a fascia, the superficial or Colles' fascia. The superficial compartment consists of skin, skin appendages and subcutaneous fat. The deep compartment, also known as the superficial perineal pouch, contains the body of the clitoris, membranous urethra, vestibular bulbs, Bartholin's glands, three pairs of skeletal muscles and the perineal body. These structures are nestled in fatty connective tissue. The deep boundary of the vulva is the perineal membrane, also known as the inferior fascia of the urogenital diaphragm, or urogenital diaphragm.

Clitoris

The clitoris is the female homologue of the penis. Unlike the penis, it lacks a corpus spongiosus and the urethra. The body is formed by the fusion of two cylindrical masses of erectile tissue, the corpora cavernosa. The corpora cavernosa separate posteriorly to form the crus of the clitoris. The right and left arms of the crus insert onto the inferior border of the pubic arch and are covered by the ischiocavernosus muscles. The size of the clitoris varies with age and hormonal status. In normal women in the reproductive age, the mean clitoral size is 19mm^2 (length multiplied by width) and the upper limit is 35mm.

Urethra (membranous)

The female urethra is only 25-30mm long, compared to the 180-200mm of the male. Its mucosa shows longitudinal grooves, allowing dilatation.

Vestibular bulbs

The vestibular bulbs are paired masses of erectile tissue that lie in the superficial perineal pouch lateral to the vagina. They lie between skeletal muscle and perineal membrane, being covered superficially by the bulbospongiosus muscles and resting on the perineal membrane (urogenital diaphragm). They are attached to the perineal membrane and run anteriorly between each clitoral crus where they narrow and fuse on the posterior surface of the clitoris.

Bartholin's glands

Bartholin's glands are the major mucinous glands of the vulva. They are paired, lobulated glands about one centimetre in diameter, nestled in fat in the superficial perineal pouch. The surface anatomical landmark is the posterior limit of the labia, but the glands are normally not palpable. Bartholin's cysts and abscesses occur in the ducts rather than the glands themselves. A Bartholin's cyst or abscess therefore presents as a lump bulging the posterior limit of a labium minus.

Skene's glands

Skene's glands are pea-sized mucinous glands on the left and right sides of the urethra and open through ducts. Skene's ducts open into the urethral canal just within or external to the meatus.

Skeletal muscles.

Three pairs of skeletal muscles form an incomplete muscular sheet beneath the superficial (Colles') fascia and perineal membrane. These muscles form a triangle with the clitoris, perineal body and ischium. The ischiocavernosus muscles run anteromedially from their posterior attachment to the medial surface of the ischial bones to overlie the arms of the clitoral crus and join anteriorly to the clitoris. The bulbospongiosus muscles run from the perineal body bordering the deep aspect of the introitus to fuse just posterior to the clitoris. The ischiocavernosus and bulbospongiosus both overlie erectile tissue and their contraction helps with female erection. The superficial transversus perinei each run from the medial surface of the ischial bones to the perineal body.

Perineal body

The perineal body is a mass of deep fibrous tissue deep to the perineum between the vulva and the anus and functions as a point of attachment for muscles. The bulbospongiosus, superficial transversus perinei and anal muscles attach to the perineal body.

Arterial supply

The arterial supply comes from branches of the internal iliac and femoral arteries. The internal iliac artery gives off the internal pudendal artery, which supplies the perineum, and the tissues involved in female erection, the vestibule and clitoris. The femoral artery gives off the superficial and deep external pudendal arteries to supply the mons and labia.

Venous drainage

The venous drainage to the vulva follows the arterial supply and eventually reaches the internal iliac and femoral veins. While any cause of widespread blockage of the venous system in the pelvis, such as thrombosis or cancer, may produce vulvar edema and varicose veins, the common cause is pregnancy. The vulva is also involved with the porto-systemic anastomosis at the lower end of the gastrointestinal tract and portal hypertension is another predisposing cause to vulvar varicose veins.

Lymphatic drainage

The vulva is richly supplied by lymphatics and this is one possible reason why vulvar carcinomas have a much higher incidence of metastases compared to skin elsewhere. Despite its rich lymphatic drainage, the vulva is prone to the effects of lymphatic obstruction, lymphedema.

The lymphatic drainage of the vulva is to the inguinal (groin) lymph nodes. From there, the drainage is superiorly along the external iliac, common iliac and para-aortic groups. Any midline structure, defined as anterior to urethra and posterior to the fourchette, including all the perineum, has bilateral lymphatic drainage. The groin lymph nodes consist of superficial and deep groups, depending on whether they are superficial or deep to the femoral fascia. The superficial group is further divided into upper and lower groups. The upper superficial group appear along the line of the inguinal ligament and the lower group along the terminal part of the great saphenous vein. The deep nodes, 1-3 in number, lie in the fossa ovalis, medial to the femoral vein. The superficial group of nodes are the most likely to harbor the sentinel nodes.

Nerve supply

The nerve supply, which includes somatic (motor and sensory) and autonomic (both sympathetic and parasympathetic), is derived from L1-S4.

Histology of the Vulva

Six different histological regions can be identified on the vulva comprising 3 concentric rings around the vaginal opening, clitoris, mucous glands and urethra. The outermost concentric ring is the hair bearing, pigmented skin of the lateral aspects of the labia majora, mons pubis and perineal skin. The middle ring of the vulva is the hairless, pigmented skin of medial aspects of the labia majora and the entire labia minora and structures derived from the minora, that is, the prepuce and frenulum of the clitoris and fourchette. The inner ring of the vulva is the non-pigmented mucosa-covered vestibule. The clitoris is sufficiently specialized to be able to be recognised as a separate histological region. The mucous glands consist of Bartholin's, Skene's and the minor vestibular glands.

Hair bearing skin of the outer aspect of the labia majora, mons and perineum

The epidermis resembles non-genital skin with a well-developed stratum corneum, prickle cell and basal layers. Well-formed rete ridges are present. The basal layer shows a variable degree of hyperpigmentation. The dermis is divided into well-demarcated papillary and reticular dermal components, composed of fine and coarse collagen respectively. There is a full range of skin appendages, namely, hair follicles and sebaceous, apocrine and eccrine glands. Sebaceous glands are situated at the mid-dermal level and open into hair follicles. The hair-bearing skin of the vulva is one of the few sites on the body where apocrine glands occur (the others are perianal skin, axilla, breast, ear, scalp, eyelid). Blood vessels, lymphatics and nerves are prominent. The subcutaneous fat is thick. Skeletal muscle may be observed in deep biopsies.

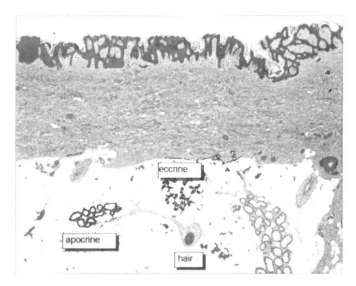

Figure 6.2. Labium majus. There is a well-developed subcutis and a full range of skin appendages.

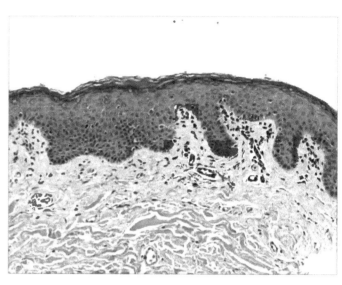

Figure 6.3. Labium majus. Keratinized skin, with a pigmented basal layer and two layers of dermis: a loose papillary (superficial) dermis and a dense reticular layer (deep).

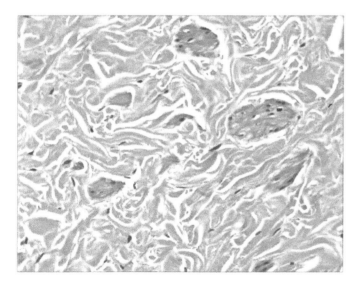

Figure 6.4. Labium majus. Bundles of smooth muscle are seen in the dermis, a finding peculiar to the labium majus and mons.

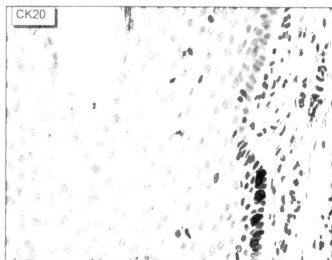

Figure 6.5. Labium majus. Cytokeratin 20 (brown) marks a row of Merkel cells in the basal layer of a hair follicle.

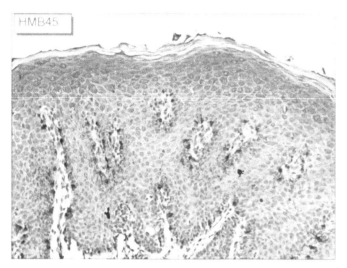

Figure 6.6. Labium majus. HMB45 marks scattered melanocytes in the basal layer.

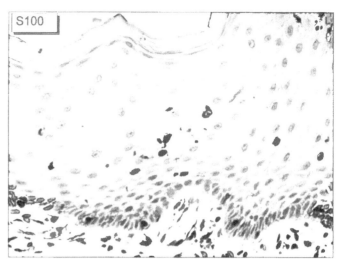

Figure 6.7. Labium majus. S100 marks both Langerhans' cells, scattered dendritic cells within the prickle cell layer and scattered basal melanocytes.

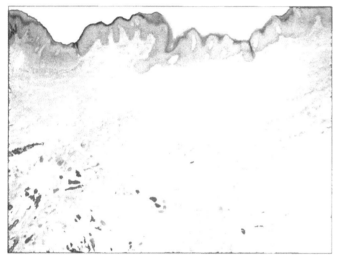

Figure 6.8. Vulva, deep structures. Skeletal muscle is seen in the deep plane. Such muscle is most frequently seen in anterior vulvectomy specimens (usually done for clitoral and paraclitoral carcinomas).

Hairless skin of the medial aspect of the labia majora, the labia minora, prepuce and frenulum of the clitoris and fourchette

The epidermis is thinner than the labium majus but is keratinized, although the stratum corneum is thin. The basal layer is variably pigmented. Small rete ridges may be present. The dermis is composed of thin collagen and elastic fibres and the papillary and reticular dermis are poorly defined. Prominent blood vessels and nerves are present. More deeply, there are large masses of elastic tissue in the deep dermis. Sebaceous glands are located superficially in the dermis and open directly onto the surface. They form the Fordyce spots seen with the naked eye or colposcope. There are no hair follicles, eccrine glands or apocrine glands. Subcutaneous fat is not seen in the labia minora or its derivatives.

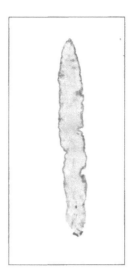

Figure 6.9. Labium minus. A transverse section of the full thickness of the leaf-like labium minus.

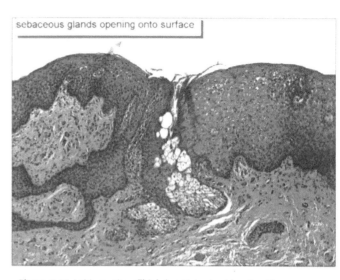

Figure 6.10. Labium minus. Thinly keratinised epidermis with a sebaceous gland which opens directly only to the epidermal surface and loose dermis.

Vestibule

The mucosa of the vestibule consists of non-keratinized stratified squamous epithelium without rete ridges. No basal pigmentation is seen. The lamina propria consists of delicate collagen and elastic fibres. A few chronic inflammatory cells, including plasma cells, may be present in many asymptomatic women and should be regarded as within normal limits. There are large spindle and stellate myofibroblastic cells in the superficial lamina propria as also seen in the vagina and lower urinary tract. There is usually an absence of all appendages. Rarely, however, sebaceous glands may be found. There is no fat. Smooth muscle is seen more deeply, particularly surrounding the introitus.

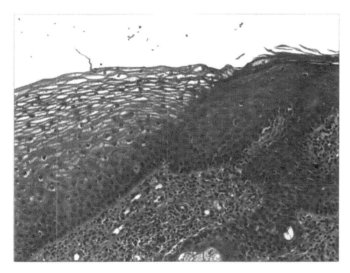

Figure 6.11. The junction between the non-keratinized squamous epithelium of the vestibule and the keratinized epithelium of the labium minus.

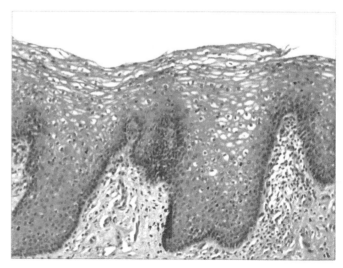

Figure 6.12. Non-keratinized squamous epithelium of the vestibule overlying the lamina propria. A lymphocytic collection is seen just beneath the mucosa in this patient who had no symptoms of vestibulitis.

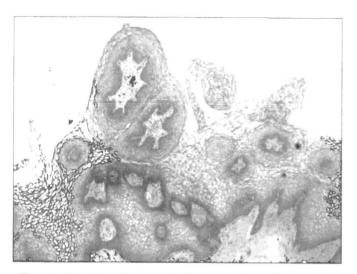

Figure 6.13. Vestibule. The normal finding of vestibular papillomatosis appears as a stromal core of loose fibrous tissue covered by normal squamous epithelium.

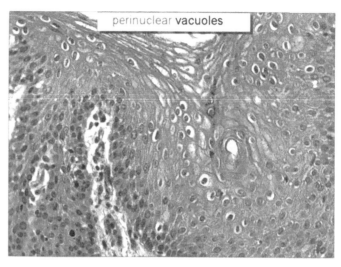

perinuclear **vacuoles**

Figure 6.14. The "HPV vulvitis" of old. This biopsy of the normal vestibule shows non-specific perinuclear haloes that have been confused with koilocytosis in the past.

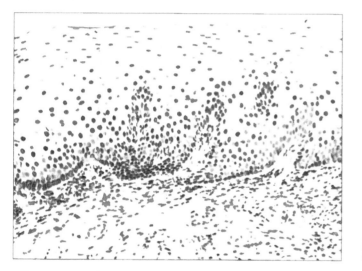

Figure 6.15. Vestibule. Estrogen receptor positive nuclei are seen in the squamous epithelial basal layers and also in the subepithelial stroma.

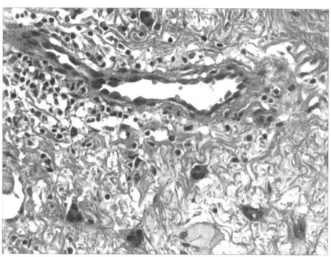

Figure 6.16. Vestibule. The lamina propria of the lower genital and urinary tract and vestibule shows multinucleated stromal myofibroblastic cells.

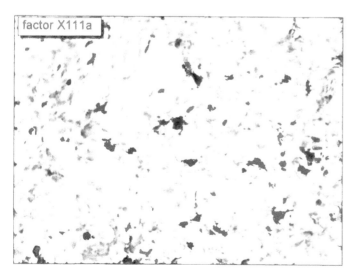

factor X111a

Figure 6.17. Vestibule. The myofibroblastic cells are factor XIIIa (shown here) and estrogen receptor positive.

Clitoris

The epidermis is thinly keratinized and, unlike the labia majora and minora, the basal layer is not hyperpigmented. The lamina propria of the glans is characteristic with numerous nerves, large blood vessels and bundles of smooth muscle separated by collagen. The corpora cavernosa consists of typical erectile tissue with numerous, gaping thin walled vessels, separated by a small amount of fibrous stroma. Skeletal muscle is lateral to and also covers the crura of the clitoris.

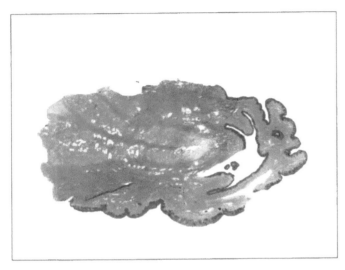

Figure 6.18. Clitoris. Panoramic view of the clitoral body with a covering of prepuce, a small portion of which is missing due to an artefact. The two corpora cavernosa are seen.

Mucous glands.

There are three types of vulvovaginal mucinous glands. All are exocrine and consist of mucinous acini that drain into a duct system lined by transitional epithelium. The largest are Bartholin's glands, located beneath the labia minora posteriorly. Skene's (paraurethral) glands lie in the lateral urethral wall. They are the homologue of the prostate and mark with prostate specific antigen and may give rise to prostatic-like adenocarcinomas. The minor vestibular glands are variable in number (1 to 100) and are found in a ring around the introitus. They are often seen incidentally in vulvovaginal biopsies taken at the level of the hymenal ring.

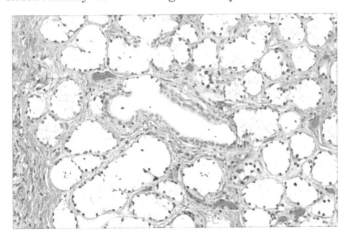

Figure 6.19. Bartholin's gland. A lobule of Bartholin's gland is composed of mucinous acini arranged around a ductule.

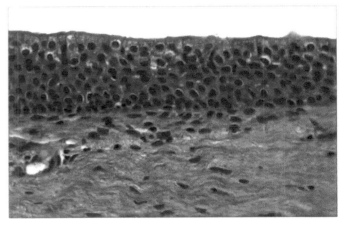

Figure 6.20. Bartholin's gland duct lined by transitional epithelium.

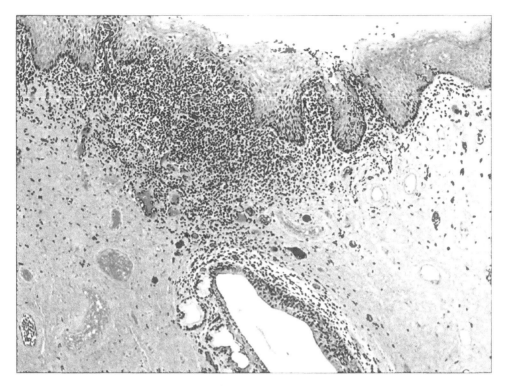

Figure 6.21. Vestibular gland showing a moderate lymphocytic infiltrate at its neck. The patient had no symptoms of vestibulitis.

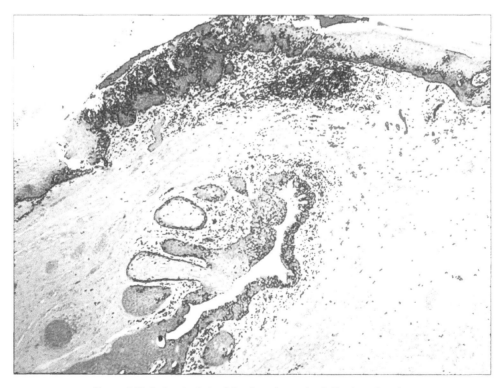

Figure 6.22. Periurethral gland. Small mucinous glands, like those found in the vestibule, may also be found in out-pouchings of the distal urethra. These microscopic glands are not to be confused with the pea- sized paraurethral (Skene's) glands.

Non-Epithelial Cells and Hormone Receptors of the Vulva

There are a number of non-epithelial cells in the epidermis and mucosa, comprising lymphocytes, Langerhans' cells, melanocytes, Merkel and Toker cells. Hormone receptors are also present in some vulvar cells.

a) Lymphocytes.

As part of immune surveillance, intraepithelial lymphocytes occur in the intestinal, respiratory and genitourinary tracts (vagina and urethra), where they are known as mucosa associated lymphoid tissue (MALT). In the skin (vulva) they are known as skin associated lymphoid tissue (SALT). Intraepithelial lymphocytes exhibit various cytotoxic activities, including alloreactive and virus specific activity, secrete cytokines, provide B-cell help, play a role in tolerance and regulate epithelial cell function, including growth. Intraepithelial lymphocytes are predominately T cells (Cluster Designation - CD3+)). T suppressor cells (CD8+) form the majority at most sites, with T-helper cells (CD4+) forming the remainder. T-cells have either alpha-beta or gamma-delta receptors and both types are present in the skin.

b) Langerhans' cells

Langerhans' cells are dendritic cells efficient at the uptake and presentation of antigen in epithelium. They possess human leukocyte antigen (HLA DR), which is necessary for the presentation of antigen to lymphocytes. Langerhans' cells become loaded with antigen, then further differentiate into matrix dendritic cells as they move towards lymph nodes. They are derived from the bone marrow via the monocyte and number about one Langerhans' cell to ten basal squamous cells. They communicate with vascular endothelium and keratinocytes through long dendritic processes. They are most reliably detected by electron microscopy and the presence of characteristic tennis racket shaped Birbeck granules, but can be more easily identified immunohistochemically by showing CD1a (HLA DR receptor) and S100 positivity.

c) Merkel cells

Merkel cells are believed to be keratinocyte-derived cells. They appear as single and clustered, sub-basal, round and angular cells with clear cytoplasm in the epidermis, hair follicles and squamous mucosa. Long cytoplasmic processes keep them in contact with keratinocytes and contiguous nerve fibres in the dermis. Their precise role is not clear, but they are involved in the perception of mechanical stimuli. They also exert trophic and attractant effects on nerves and stimulate keratin production and differentiation. They play a role in the spatial organization of the epidermis and appendages. They usually number about 1 per 10 basal cells. Merkel cells are epidermal neuroendocrine cells and are identified by finding neurosecretory granules on electron microscopy, which contain vasoactive intestinal peptide (VIP). Immunohistochemical markers include CK20, synpatophysin, chromogranin, neurone specific enolase, neurofilament, CK 7, 8 and 18, and S100.

d) Toker cells.

Toker cells are benign pagetoid cells of the nipple. In one hypothesis, they are the putative cells of origin of Paget's disease. If this hypothesis is correct, the distribution of Toker cells, which have been reported in the milk line from the nipple to the vulva and root of the penis, helps explain the distribution of Paget's disease. Toker cells are difficult to detect in routine H and E stained slides, where they are described as occasional suprabasilar cells with clear cytoplasm. They are reported to mark with CK7, which also marks the cells of Paget's disease. However, there has been no formal study of their frequency and distribution in the vulva. This observer has never encountered them in the vulva.

e) Hormone receptors:

Vulvovaginal squamous epithelium, dermal fibroblasts and vulvar subcutaneous fat are hormone sensitive tissues. Estrogen and androgen receptors show reciprocal sensitivity. Estrogen receptors (ER) are strongest medially in the mucosa-covered tissues and androgen receptors are strongest laterally in the hair-bearing vulvar skin. Estrogen and progesterone receptors (PR) are found in the squamous epithelium of the vagina and vestibule, where they are expressed in virtually all squamous cells, but most strongly in the basal layers. ER and PR abruptly disappear at the junction with keratinized skin at the origin of the labium minus (Hart's line). ER and PR are also expressed by myofibroblastic cells of the lamina propria, including the multinucleate myofibroblastic cells of the vagina, urethra and vulva. There is no sharp cut-off of stromal expression at the junction of non-keratinized epithelium with keratinized epidermis. Vaginal and vestibular epithelium responds rapidly to estrogen stimulation with an increase in thickness due to the formation of more layers and more cytoplasm of squamous cells. The rest of the vulva does not respond to any degree. The increased cytoplasm is partly due to glycogen storage. Glycogen provides a substrate for lactobacilli and corynebacteria, the normal vaginal flora during reproductive years.

Urethral Histology

The distal 2/3 of the urethra is covered by squamous epithelium, while the upper 1/3 shows transitional epithelium, similar to that seen elsewhere in the urinary tract. Numerous invaginations (analogous to the lacunae of Morgagni in the male urethra) into the lamina propria are lined by transitional epithelium. They show outpocketings of clear mucinous cells forming small glands (analogous to the urethral 'glands of Littre' in the male). The epithelium overlies a loose lamina propria. Beneath this layer, there are inner longitudinal and outer circular layers of smooth muscle. Proximally, a sphincter of skeletal muscle surrounds the layers of smooth muscle.

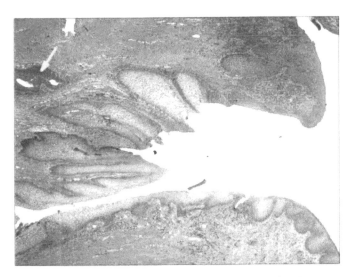

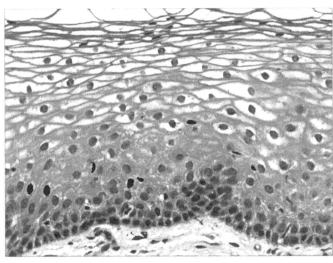

Figure 6.23. Urethra, distal. Panoramic view of the distal urethra shows non-keratinized squamous epithelium, lamina propria and a paraurethral mucous gland (arrow).

Figure 6.24. Urethra, distal. Non-keratinized squamous epithelium lines the distal urethra and meatus.

Vaginal Histology

The vagina shows 3 layers forming its wall: the mucosa, muscular coat and adventitia. The mucosa is composed of non-keratinized squamous epithelium and lamina propria. The lamina propria is denser towards the surface and looser towards the muscular layer. In the anterior vagina, lamina propria papillae are scarce, but in the posterior wall they are prominent and deep. Numerous elastic fibres are found in the lamina propria. The deeper layers of the lamina propria contain a dense plexus of small veins. There are no glands in the vagina.

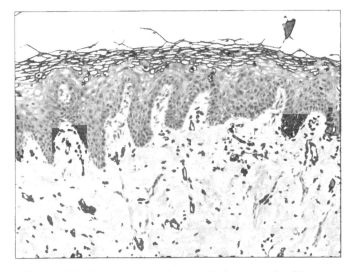

Figure 6.25. Vaginal mucosa: non-keratinized, glycogenated (pale) squamous epithelium with prominent rete ridges and thin lamina propria.

Vaginal Ecology

The vaginal squamous epithelium is sensitive to estrogen and, to a lesser extent, progestagen. Estrogen stimulates growth and maturation of the epithelium which becomes thicker and differentiated into three distinct layers: basal, intermediate and superficial. The superficial cells have abundant glycogenated cytoplasm. By contrast, progestagens tend to cause the opposite effects with thinning and a loss of maturation. The superficial layer disappears and intermediate cells are seen on the surface. A maturation index (which is simply the counting and expressing in percentage, the numbers of parabasal, intermediate and superficial cells) is a good guide to the hormonal status of the woman. Physiological estrogen deficiency occurs in children, lactating and post-menopausal women. It is associated with marked thinning and loss of maturation. Parabasal cells predominate.

For its resident flora, the vagina provides a continually changing environment which results in marked variations in the species identified, as well as variations in the concentration of the species themselves. Many suggested causes of these environmental changes are conjectural or anecdotal. They include hygiene, clothing, douching and the use of tampons. Considerable evidence exists, however, for the effects of changes in estrogen levels and sexual activity. Glycogen production with estrogenization (see above) provides a substrate, particularly for lactobacilli, the metabolism of which produces lactic acid and a marked lowering of pH. Semen, on the other hand, produces a rise in vaginal pH. Many organisms are sensitive to these pH alterations, which may range from below 4.5 to above 7.

The list of organisms isolated from the vaginas of disease-free women is long indeed. Anaerobes predominate in the prepubescent vagina, commonly *Bacteroides spp.*, which are found in conjunction with others including *Staphylococcus epidermidis* and *Gardnerella vaginalis*. With estrogenization, *Lactobacillus spp.* predominate. Also found are *Streptococcus viridans* and *Staphylococcus epidermidis*, *Bacteroides spp.*, *Gardnerella vaginalis, Staphylococcus aureus*, Group B streptococci, mycoplasmas, ureaplasmas, Mobiluncus, Corynebacteria, enteric organisms, including Enterococcus, and yeasts.

Because of their pathogenicity elsewhere in the body, staphylococci, streptococci and coliforms are frequently reported from vaginal swabs but their presence in the vagina is of no clinical significance (apart from their potential pathogenicity in pregnancy complications). On the other hand, although *Candida albicans* may be found in swabs from asymptomatic women, it is the commonest potential pathogen of the vagina.

There are no glands in the vagina. Cervical mucus, vaginal transudate, vulvovestibular gland secretions, epithelial desquamation, menstrual flow and ejaculate contribute to vaginal secretions. The vagina is kept moist partly by cervical mucus. High levels of estrogen and progesterone cause a change in the quantity and consistency of cervical mucus. Increased mid-cycle mucus (ovulation cascade) may produce a sensation of vaginal wetness. Vaginal transudate occurs during sexual arousal. Vascular congestion mediated by the parasympathetic nervous system induces engorgement and vaginal transudate, a watery, alkaline fluid. Vestibular mucus gland secretions are also part of the female sexual response. Coitus may raise the pH of the vagina because ejaculate is alkaline.

The female genital tract has specialized immunological needs. It must allow fertilization by invading sperm and growth of the embryo, yet retain immune surveillance. Local and systemic, humeral and cell mediated immunity are all present. It is part of the MALT and SALT systems (see above under lymphocytes). Recent studies provide evidence that an immunosuppressive function of sperm may limit immune surveillance of the female genital tract, although spermatozoa that invade tissue are destroyed by cytolytic T-cells. Seminal fluid may limit the response to viral infection. The conceptus expresses paternal alloantigens. Why these are not subjected to immune attack is still not understood.

References

Elsner P, Maibach HI. Microbiology of specialised skin: the vulva. Semin Dermatol 1990; 9: 300-4

Eva LJ, MacLean AB, Reid WMN, Rolfe KJ, Perrett CW Estrogen receptor expression in the vulvar vestibulitis syndrome Am J Obstet Gynecol 2003; 189: 458-461

Kurman RJ (ed) Blausteins pathology of the female genital tract, 5th edn., Springer NewYork 2002

Lepargneur JP, Rousseau V Protective role of the Doderlein flora J Gynecol Obste Biol Reprod (Paris) 2002; 31: 485-94

Lundquist K, Kohler S, Rouse RV Intraepidermal cytokeratin 7 expression is not restricted to Paget cells but is also seen in Toker cells and Merkel cells. Am J Surg Pathol 1999; 23: 212-9

Mandel G, Bennet JE, Dolin R. Principles and Practice of Infectious Diseases. 5th edn. Churchill Livingston, 2000.

Micheletti L, Prei M, Bogliatto F, Chieppa P Vestibular papillomatosis. Minerva Ginecol 2000; 52 Suppl 87-91

Murray PR, Baron EJ, Pfaller MA, Tenover FC, Yolken RH. Manual of Clinical Microbiology. 7th edn. American Society for Microbiology, 1999.

Ridley CM (ed) The vulva, Churchill-Livingstone, Edinburgh 1987

Simpson JL Genetics of the female reproductive ducts. Am J Genet 1999; 89: 224-39

Van der Putte SC Anogenital "sweat" glands. Histology and pathology of a gland that may mimic mammary glands Am J Dermatopathol 1991; 13: 557-67

Van der Putte SC Mammary-like glands of the vulva and their disorders. Int J Gunecol Pathol 1994; 13: 150-60

Wiener JS, Marcelli M, Lamb DJ Molecular determinants of sexual differentiation. World J Urol 1996; 14: 278-94

MODES OF PRESENTATION

1. Pruritus

2. Discharge

3. Dyspareunia/'vestibulitis syndrome' *

4. Lump/swelling/papules

5. Burning/pain/stinging/discomfort other than pruritus. 'Vulvodynia'

6. Ulceration/erosion/blisters

7. Odor

8. Dysuria

9. Splitting (fissuring)

10. Bleeding

11. Primarily extragenital

12. Asymptomatic. Incidental finding by doctor or other. Concern about color or change in appearance. Macules.

13. Pediatric

Friedrich in 1987 introduced the term "vulvar vestibulitis syndrome" to encompass the following clinical features: vestibular pain on touch or attempted entry; localized vestibular tenderness; vestibular erythema.

	1. PRURITUS	2. DISCHARGE	3. DYSPAREUNIA ETC.	4. LUMP ETC.	5. BURNING ETC.	6. ULCERATION ETC.	7. ODOR	8. DYSURIA	9. FISSURING	10. BLEEDING	11. EXTRAGENITAL	12. INCIDENTAL	13. PEDIATRIC
1. Fordyce spots												•	
2. Large labia minora												•	
3. Vestibular papillomatosis												•	
4. Labial adhesions in infancy												•	•
5. Physiological discharge		•											
6. Estrogen deficiency – atrophy			•										
7. Double vulva													•
8. Cyst of canal of Nuck				•									
9. Dermoid cyst				•									
10. Vascular malformations				•								•	•
11. Congenital lymphedema (Milroy's disease)				•									
12. Imperforate hymen				•									
13. Vaginal septa				•								•	
14. Double vagina												•	•
15. Vaginal hypoplasia												•	•
16. Vaginal atresia												•	
17. Vaginal agenesis			•									•	
18. DES associated abnormalities		•										•	
19. Cyst of Gartner's duct (cyst of mesonephric duct)				•								•	
20. Ectopic ureter draining into vagina		•											•
21. Epispadias												•	•
22. Hypospadias												•	•
23. Imperforate anus with vulvar or vaginal fistula												•	•
24. Turner's syndrome												•	•
25. Klinefelter's syndrome												•	•
26. True hermaphroditism												•	•

	1. PRURITUS	2. DISCHARGE	3. DYSPAREUNIA ETC.	4. LUMP ETC.	5. BURNING ETC.	6. ULCERATION ETC.	7. ODOR	8. DYSURIA	9. FISSURING	10. BLEEDING	11. EXTRAGENITAL	12. INCIDENTAL	13. PEDIATRIC
27. Gonadal agenesis												•	•
28. Pediculosis pubis	•												
29. Scabies	•										•		
30. Oxyuriasis	•												•
31. Schistosomiasis				•		•					•		
32. Filariasis				•									
33. Hydatid disease				•									
34. Trichomoniasis		•			•			•					
35. Amebiasis						•							
36. Leishmaniasis						•					•		
37. Candida albicans infection	•	•	•		•	•		•	•				•
38. Non-albicans yeast infection	•												
39. Tinea cruris	•												•
40 Pityriasis versicolor	•											•	•
41. White piedra											•		
42. Impetigo	•			•	•	•							•
43. Folliculitis				•	•								•
44. Abscess				•	•								•
45. Cellulitis				•	•								•
46. Necrotizing fasciitis				•	•	•							•
47. Toxic shock syndrome											•		
48. Infected Bartholin's duct cyst				•	•								
49. Gonorrhea		•						•					
50. Actinomycosis		•											
51. Erythrasma												•	
52. Trichomycosis												•	

	1. PRURITUS	2. DISCHARGE	3. DYSPAREUNIA ETC.	4. LUMP ETC.	5. BURNING ETC.	6. ULCERATION ETC.	7. ODOR	8. DYSURIA	9. FISSURING	10. BLEEDING	11. EXTRAGENITAL	12. INCIDENTAL	13. PEDIATRIC
53. Diphtheria						•							
54. Chancroid				•		•							
55. Donovanosis (granuloma inguinale)				•		•							
56. Malakoplakia				•									
57 Tuberculosis						•					•		
58. Syphilis				•		•					•		
59. Chlamydial oculogenital infection		•						•					
60. Lymphogranuloma venereum						•							
61. Bacterial vaginosis		•					•						
62. Herpes simplex					•	•							
63. Herpes zoster					•	•							
64. Cytomegalovirus infection						•							
65. Infectious mononucleosis					•						•		
66. Human papillomavirus infection				•									•
67. Molluscum contagiosum				•									•
68. HIV infection				•	•	•					•		
69. Irritant contact dermatitis	•		•		•				•	•			•
70. Allergic contact dermatitis	•				•	•			•	•			•
71. Atopic dermatitis	•										•		•
72. Lichen simplex chronicus	•			•									
73. Intertrigo	•								•				
74. Psoriasis	•				•				•		•		•
75. Seborrheic dermatitis	•					•					•		
76. Reiter's syndrome (circinate vulvitis)					•	•							
77. Lichen sclerosus	•		•			•							•
78. Lichen planus	•	•	•		•	•		•			•		

	1. PRURITUS	2. DISCHARGE	3. DYSPAREUNIA ETC.	4. LUMP ETC.	5. BURNING ETC.	6. ULCERATION ETC.	7. ODOR	8. DYSURIA	9. FISSURING	10. BLEEDING	11. EXTRAGENITAL	12. INCIDENTAL	13. PEDIATRIC
79. Desquamative inflammatory vaginitis		•	•					•					
80. Vulvitis circumscripta plasmacellularis (Zoon's vulvitis)			•		•			•					•
81. Lupus erythematosus	•				•	•					•		
82. Graft versus host disease		•	•		•	•		•			•		
83. Fixed drug eruption	•			•									
84. Pemphigus and variants		•	•		•	•	•			•	•		
85. Bullous pemphigoid		•			•	•				•	•		
86. Cicatricial pemphigoid		•	•		•	•					•		
87. Linear IgA disease of childhood	•				•	•					•		•
88. Stevens-Johnson disease (Erythema multiforme)	•				•	•					•		•
89. Toxic epidermal necrolysis (Erythema multiforme)					•	•					•		
90. Darier's disease	•				•	•					•		•
91. Papular acantholytic genitocrural acantholysis	•				•	•			•		•		
92. Benign familial chronic pemphigus	•				•	•			•		•		
93. Epidermolysis bullosa					•	•					•		•
94. Sarcoidosis				•							•		
95. Anogenital granulomatosis				•	•								
96. Crohn's disease					•	•			•				
97. Foreign body granuloma					•	•							
98. Urticaria	•			•							•		•
99. Leukocytoclastic vasculitis: Henoch-Schonlein purpura					•	•					•		•
100. Neutrophilic dermatosis: Pyoderma gangrenosum				•	•	•							•
101. Aphthous ulcers			•		•	•	•						•
102. Behcet's disease			•		•	•	•				•		
103. Fox Fordyce disease	•				•								
104. Hidradenitis suppurativa (acne inversa)				•	•		•						

	1. PRURITUS	2. DISCHARGE	3. DYSPAREUNIA ETC.	4. LUMP ETC.	5. BURNING ETC.	6. ULCERATION ETC.	7. ODOR	8. DYSURIA	9. FISSURING	10. BLEEDING	11. EXTRAGENITAL	12. INCIDENTAL	13. PEDIATRIC
105. Pilonidal sinus complex				•	•								
106. Estrogen therapy	•	•											
107. Precocious puberty		•								•			
108. Estrogen deficiency – sequelae		•	•										
109. Adrenocortical syndromes												•	•
110. Topical testosterone induced virilization					•								
111. Glucagonoma syndrome					•	•					•		
112. Acanthosis nigricans											•	•	•
113. Zinc deficiency (Acrodermatitis enteropathica)						•							•
114. Amyloidosis	•			•							•		
115. Ligneous vaginitis				•									
116. Calcinosis				•									
117. Verruciform xanthoma				•									
118. Vitiligo												•	
119. Hyperpigmentation												•	
120. Obstetric trauma			•		•					•			
121. Sexual trauma			•						•	•			
122. Accidental trauma					•					•			
123. Self-induced trauma	•	•								•			
124. Surgical trauma			•		•					•			
125. Chemical trauma			•		•	•							
126. Radiation trauma			•		•								
127. Female circumcision and related procedures			•		•								
128. Foreign body		•				•	•			•			•
129. Seborrheic keratosis				•									
130. Vulvar intraepithelial neoplasia	•											•	

	1. PRURITUS	2. DISCHARGE	3. DYSPAREUNIA ETC.	4. LUMP ETC.	5. BURNING ETC.	6. ULCERATION ETC.	7. ODOR	8. DYSURIA	9. FISSURING	10. BLEEDING	11. EXTRAGENITAL	12. INCIDENTAL	13. PEDIATRIC
131. Differentiated VIN	•											•	
132. Squamous cell carcinoma (SCC) – common type	•			•		•	•						
133. Verrucous carcinoma	•			•		•	•						
134. Keratoacanthoma				•									
135. Basal cell carcinoma	•			•		•							
136. Merkel cell tumor	•			•		•							
137. Syringoma	•			•								•	
138. Pleomorphic adnemoa				•									
139. Microcystic adnexal carcinoma	•			•		•							
140. Hidradenoma papilliferum				•									
141. Fibroadenoma (Benign)				•									
142. Cystosarcoma phyllodes (Benign)				•									
143. Extramammary Paget's (EMPD – Premalignant)	•												
144. Adenocarcinoma ex EMPD (Malignant)	•			•		•							
145. Primary breast-like carcinoma (Malignant)	•			•		•							
146. Trichofolliculoma	•			•		•							
147. Sebaceous carcinoma	•			•		•							
148. Endometrioid carcinoma	•			•		•							
149. Clear cell carcinoma	•			•		•							
150. Pleomorphic adenoma (Benign mixed tumor)				•									
151. Squamous cell carcinoma				•		•	•			•			
152. Adenosquamous carcinoma				•		•	•			•			
153. Mucinous adenocarcinoma				•		•	•			•			
154. Salivary gland types adenocarcinoma				•		•	•			•			
155. Prostatic type carcinoma				•		•	•			•			
156. Transitional cell carcinoma				•		•	•			•			

	1. PRURITUS	2. DISCHARGE	3. DYSPAREUNIA ETC.	4. LUMP ETC.	5. BURNING ETC.	6. ULCERATION ETC.	7. ODOR	8. DYSURIA	9. FISSURING	10. BLEEDING	11. EXTRAGENITAL	12. INCIDENTAL	13. PEDIATRIC
157. Genital melanocytic macule (melanosis)												•	
158. Lentigo												•	
159. Nevus (Mole) – common type				•								•	
160. Atypical melanotic nevus of genital tract				•								•	
161. Melanoma in situ												•	
162. Melanoma				•		•				•			
163. Superficial angiomyxoma				•									
164. Cellular angiofibroma				•									
165. Angiomyofibroblastoma				•									
166. Aggressive angiomyxoma				•									
167. Dermatofibrosarcoma protruberans				•									
168. Fibrosarcoma				•									
169. Kaposi's sarcoma				•								•	
170. Angiosarcoma				•									
171. Leiomyoma (myxoid and epithelioid)				•									
172. Smooth muscle tumor of intermediate differentiation				•									
173. Leiomyosarcoma				•									
174. Rhabdomyosarcoma (sarcoma botryoides)				•									
175. Neurofibroma – Neurofibromatosis				•									
176. Schwannoma				•									
177. Granular cell tumor				•		•							
178. Malignant peripheral nerve sheath tumor				•									
179. Malignant granular cell tumor				•									
180. Spindle cell lipoma				•									
181. Fibrolipoma				•									
182. Liposarcoma				•									

	1. PRURITUS	2. DISCHARGE	3. DYSPAREUNIA ETC.	4. LUMP ETC.	5. BURNING ETC.	6. ULCERATION ETC.	7. ODOR	8. DYSURIA	9. FISSURING	10. BLEEDING	11. EXTRAGENITAL	12. INCIDENTAL	13. PEDIATRIC
183. Synovial sarcoma				•									
184. Rhabdoid tumor				•									
185. Epithelioid sarcoma				•									
186. Alveolar soft parts sarcoma				•									
187. Langerhans' histiocytosis						•	•				•		•
188. Myeloid/monocytic leukemia											•		
189. Non-Hodgkins's lymphoma				•									
190. Diffuse large cell B cell lymphoma				•									
191. Diffuse small cell B cell lymphoma				•									
192. Peripheral T cell lymphoma				•									
193. Cutaneous T cell lymphoma	•			•							•	•	
194. Gynecological secondary tumors				•									
195. Non-gynecological secondary tumors				•									
196. Vaginal intraepithelial neoplasia												•	
197. Papillary squamotransitional squamous cell carcinoma				•		•	•			•			
198. Verrucous squamous cell carcinoma				•		•	•			•			
199. Mullerian papilloma				•									•
200. Pleomorphic adenoma (benign mixed tumor)				•									
201. Adenocarcinoma in situ (cervix-like) occurring in vaginal adenosis												•	
202. Clear cell adenocarcinoma				•						•			
203. Endometrioid adenocarcinoma				•		•	•			•			
204. Mucinous carcinoma				•		•	•			•			
205. Adenosquamous carcinoma				•		•							
206. Carcinosarcoma (MMMT)				•						•			

	1. PRURITUS	2. DISCHARGE	3. DYSPAREUNIA ETC.	4. LUMP ETC.	5. BURNING ETC.	6. ULCERATION ETC.	7. ODOR	8. DYSURIA	9. FISSURING	10. BLEEDING	11. EXTRAGENITAL	12. INCIDENTAL	13. PEDIATRIC
207. Small cell undifferentiated/neuroendocrine carcinoma				•						•			
208 Genital melanocytic macule (melanosis)												•	
209. Melanoma in situ												•	
210. Malignant melanoma				•						•			
211. Cellular angiofibroma				•									
212. Angiomyofibroblastoma				•									
213. Aggressive angiomyxoma				•									
214. Kaposi's sarcoma				•									
215. Angiosarcoma				•									
216. Leiomyoma				•									
217. Smooth muscle tumor, intermediate differentiation				•									
218. Leiomyosarcoma				•									
219. Rhabdomyoma				•									
220. Rhabdomyosarcoma				•									
221. Neurofibroma				•									
222. Schwannoma				•									
223. Granular cell tumor.				•									
224. Endometrial stromal sarcoma				•						•			
225. Mullerian adenosarcoma				•						•			
226. Non-Hodgkin's lymphoma				•									
227. Yolk sac tumor		•		•						•			•
228. Secondary tumor				•									
229. Squamous dysplasia/carcinoma in situ												•	
230. Squamous cell carcinoma				•				•		•			
231. Villous adenoma				•									
232. Colonic type adenocarcinoma				•				•		•			

	1. PRURITUS	2. DISCHARGE	3. DYSPAREUNIA ETC.	4. LUMP ETC.	5. BURNING ETC.	6. ULCERATION ETC.	7. ODOR	8. DYSURIA	9. FISSURING	10. BLEEDING	11. EXTRAGENITAL	12. INCIDENTAL	13. PEDIATRIC
233. Clear cell adenocarcinoma				•				•		•			
234. Carcinoma in situ												•	
235. Transitional cell carcinoma				•				•		•			
236. Prostatic carcinoma				•				•		•			
237. Carcinoid				•									
238. Small cell undifferentiated/neuroendocrine carcinoma				•				•					
239. Melanoma in situ												•	
240. Malignant melanoma				•		•				•			
241. Leiomyoma				•									
242. Rhabdomyosarcoma (sarcoma botryoides)				•						•			•
243. Lymphoma				•						•			
244. Plasmacytoma				•									
245. Metastic and direct spread				•									
246. Epidermal inclusion cyst (implantation dermoid)				•									
247. Skin tag				•									
248. Fibroepithelial (superficial mesodermal) polyp				•									
249. Hemangioma				•									•
250. Angiokeratoma	•			•						•			
251. Pyogenic granuloma				•						•			•
252. Campbell de Morgan (cherry) angioma												•	
253. Acquired lymphangioma		•		•									
254. Varicose veins	•			•	•								
255. Angiolymophoid hyperplasia with eosinphilia	•			•									
256. Epidermoid cyst (epidermal or infundibular cyst)				•									
257. Endometriosis										•		•	
258. Ectopic breast				•									

	1. PRURITUS	2. DISCHARGE	3. DYSPAREUNIA ETC.	4. LUMP ETC.	5. BURNING ETC.	6. ULCERATION ETC.	7. ODOR	8. DYSURIA	9. FISSURING	10. BLEEDING	11. EXTRAGENITAL	12. INCIDENTAL	13. PEDIATRIC
259. Bartholin's Duct cyst				•									
260. Lobular hyperplasia				•	•								
261. Perineal hernia				•									
262. Fibroepithelial (superficial mesodermal) polyp				•									
263. Nodular fasciitis (postoperative spindle cell nodule)				•									
264. Mullerian cysts				•									
265. Caruncle			•	•	•			•		•			
266. Prolapse			•	•	•			•		•			•
267. Paraurethral cyst				•								•	•
268. Suburethral diverticulum				•	•			•					
269. Nephrogenic adenoma				•									
270. Dysesthesia (vulvodynia)			•		•								
271. Neuralgia					•								
272. Somatoform disorder	•	•	•	•	•		•	•					
273. Arousal disorder			•										
274. Vaginismus			•		•								
275. Orgasmic disorder			•		•								

Chapter 7

1. NORMAL VARIATIONS

A. Vulva

1. FORDYCE SPOTS (Sebaceous glands)

Sebaceous glands occur as part of the pilosebaceous unit with the notable exceptions of some of the vulva, nipple and mouth where they occur alone. Microscopically, the sebaceous glands in these regions are more superficially located and open directly onto the surface, compared to those of the hair-bearing skin which are more deeply placed and open into hair follicles. On the vulva these superficial sebaceous glands may be visible on the labia minora and medial aspects of the labia majora as yellow spots, usually less than a couple of millimetres in diameter, where they are referred to as Fordyce spots. When unduly prominent, the term sebaceous hyperplasia may be more appropriate.

Although only a variation of normal, Fordyce spots may attract the attention of the patient or her medical attendant and create diagnostic confusion.

2. LARGE LABIA MINORA

Wide variations of normal anatomy could be considered a feature of the vulva. This applies particularly to the labia minora which vary from relatively insignificant skin folds to the most prominent vulvar structure protruding well beyond the labia majora and sometimes asymmetrically with one side considerably larger than the other. Unduly long and prominent labia minora are referred to as hypertrophy of the labia minora. The vast majority of women exhibiting this variation are either unaware that they differ in this way or it causes them no concern and it is rare for women to seek treatment for it.

Occasionally, women may find awareness of their prominent labia a nuisance when walking, during intercourse or when wearing tight clothing and request surgical correction. Examination should exclude any pathology responsible for this enlargement and the woman's awareness of it, such as vulvitis or significant psychopathology. When no such pathology exists and the patient insists on treatment, the labia may be simply reduced in size by wedge resection of their posterior borders. Histology of the removed tissue should be performed and should be normal.

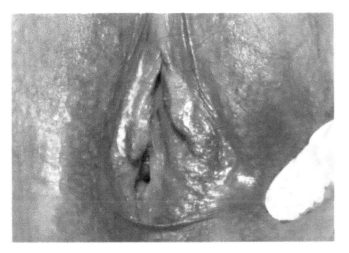

Figure 7.1. Sebaceous glands visible through the skin of the labia minora (Fordyce spots). The material in the interlabial sulcus consists of normal secretions.

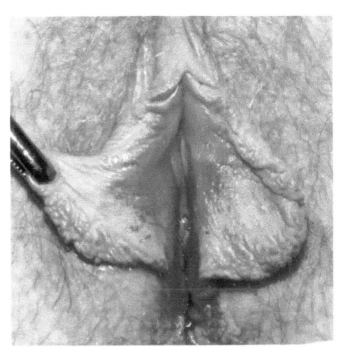

Figure 7.2. Large labia minora.

3. VESTIBULAR PAPILLOMATOSIS

It is common to find in the vestibule, usually adjacent to or on the hymenal ring, tiny, finger-like projections, several millimetres long and about 1 millimetre in diameter, the same colour and consistency as the adjacent vestibule and easily confused with condylomata acuminata. These vestibular papillomata are covered with normal epithelium. Microscopically, these vestibular papillomata are composed of a thin fibrovascular core covered by normal squamous epithelium (Fig. 6.13). Their only significance is their easy confusion with genital warts, especially when warts are also present. They can usually be distinguished by applying 5% acetic acid and examination under magnification. Vestibular papillomata do not take up acetic acid differently from their surrounds whereas condylomata become aceto-white and their verrucous surface is apparent under magnification. Occasionally, excision biopsy will be necessary to satisfy the more demanding patient.

4. LABIAL ADHESIONS IN INFANCY

Agglutination or adhesion formation affecting the labia minora can result in varying degrees of occlusion of the introitus. It is seen not uncommonly in infants and resolves with the topical application of estrogen (or at puberty) suggesting that the condition is a manifestation of estrogen lack. Inflammatory causes of adhesions also occur in children.

Clinical features

Parental concerns regarding the appearance of the vulva is the usual mode of presentation in the infant.

Treatment

Labial agglutination in the infant will resolve with the application of an estrogen cream applied with the fingertip once daily for a week or two. Under no circumstances should the adhesions be separated by force or surgery. Recent publications suggest that reassurance is all that is required because the condition usually resolves spontaneously.

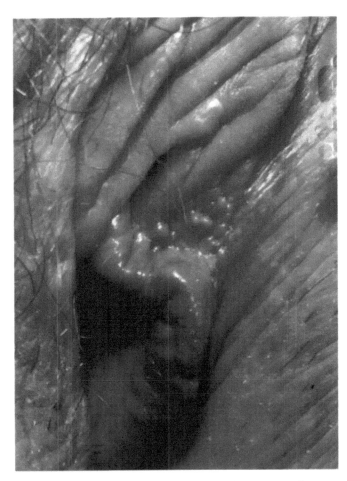

Figure 7.3. Labial papillomatosis (lateral aspect left labium minus).

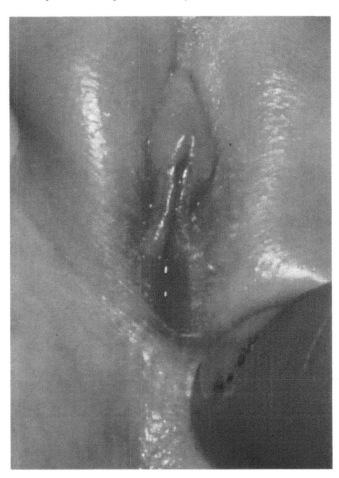

Figure 7.4. Labial adhesions partially occluding the introitus of an infant.

B. Vagina

5. PHYSIOLOGICAL DISCHARGE

Normal vaginal secretions consist of desquamated epithelial cells and bacteria, usually lactobacilli, suspended in vaginal wall transudate and cervical mucus. Bartholin's, paraurethral, vestibular and vulvar sweat glands make a variable contribution. The quantity of these secretions is thus affected by hormonal, microbiological, autonomic nervous and sexual influences. In the ovulating woman, the volume may peak with the 'ovulation cascade' of clear, egg white-like mucus resulting from the effect of the estrogen peak on the cervical columnar epithelium.

The healthy woman should not require sanitary protection for these secretions. Nevertheless, some women do perceive their normal vaginal secretions as excessive and will seek medical advice.

Clinical features

The presentation for medical advice regarding physiological discharge may be because it is at the extreme of the normal spectrum. That is, the volume is sufficient, say, to require sanitary protection. Alternatively, the presentation may have resulted from anxiety arising from a fear of sexually transmitted disease and/or cancer.

The physiological discharge is sticky, clear or white (but may appear yellow when it dries on clothing). It does not irritate unless there have been fastidious hygiene efforts causing contact dermatitis.

Examination should reveal an absence of inflammatory changes and often an outpouring of clear cervical mucus. Eversion of the cervical columnar epithelium on to the ectocervix may be seen.

Diagnosis

A negative vaginal swab and Papanicolaou smear are prerequisites for this diagnosis. The diagnosis is best made, however, on the clinical features (above) and microscopic findings (Figure 1.2).

Treatment

Appropriate counselling is required, especially when anxiety is present. This may be the only treatment required. Safe, effective reduction in the volume of these secretions, in the woman who does not wish to conceive, can be obtained with progestogen only ovulation suppression such as that produced by medroxyprogesterone acetate 150 mg intramuscularly 12 weekly.

If eversion of the cervical epithelium is resulting in a substantial contribution of mucus and the patient does not wish to have ovulation suppressed, destruction of the visible glandular epithelium may be beneficial. This may be carried out by radial cautery, diathermy loop excision or laser. Squamous epithelium (not mucus secreting) can then be expected to cover the defect.

6. ESTROGEN DEFICIENCY

Vaginal epithelium is one of the body's most estrogen responsive tissues. So much so that, prior to the introduction of radioimmunoassay for estrogens, the examination of a lateral vaginal smear for epithelial maturation was frequently used as a guide to circulating estrogen levels (exemplified in Figs. 1.1 and 1.2). Estrogen lack results in vaginal epithelial atrophy, a common cause of clinical distress even when the hypoestrogenism is physiological in origin. Thus, vaginal atrophy is normally found before puberty, during lactation and after the menopause. Pathological causes of estrogen deficiency include surgical removal of the ovaries, premature ovarian failure and suppression of pituitary gonadotrophins by GnRH analogues and sometimes by progestogen only therapy. Irrespective of the cause, the clinical features at the genital level and principles of treatment are the same. The epithelium of the bladder and urethra and, to a degree, their supporting tissues, may also be adversely affected by estrogen lack.

Atrophy may be found with or without inflammatory changes. In the latter case, the condition is referred to as atrophic vaginitis. The most likely cause of the vaginitis is sexual intercourse traumatising the relatively dry, fragile epithelium. Atrophic vaginitis is not an infective disorder. The organisms present in the condition are nearly always the usual commensals and the vaginitis resolves with estrogenisation alone. The atrophic epithelium is more sensitive to chemical trauma and contact dermatitis may complicate the picture.

Labial adhesions may be found in older women. The condition might be the result of atrophy but an erosive disorder, such as lichen planus, should be suspected. When labial adhesions are found in the elderly, it is usually unclear whether or not atrophic vaginitis alone is responsible. The older woman will present with apareunia or interference with or even obstruction of the urinary stream.

Clinical features

Superficial dyspareunia and/or discharge from the vaginitis are the commonest presenting symptoms. Soreness other than that associated with sexual activity may be present if the vaginitis is pronounced. Other presentations include postmenopausal bleeding from the easily traumatised atrophic epithelium and difficulties interpreting cervical cytology. The postmenopausal state can impair sexuality at several levels but thinness of the epithelium permitting ease of pain response will in turn impair arousal and lubrication.

The vagina demonstrates most of the changes resulting from estrogen lack. Moving outward from the vagina, the changes are progressively less apparent. Thus vestibular epithelium shows a shift in maturation similar to the vagina but not to the same degree. The labia minora and clitoris may show a small reduction in size but epithelial changes are minimal. The labia majora mainly show the ageing changes associated with hair bearing skin elsewhere.

Atrophic vaginal epithelium is pale, dry and its rugosity is diminished. In the case of atrophic vaginitis the vagina may be obviously inflamed with a thin discharge and hemorrhagic spots resembling trichomoniasis (with which it must not be confused). Shrinkage of vaginal tissue may result in urethral caruncle or prolapse (**265** and **266**).

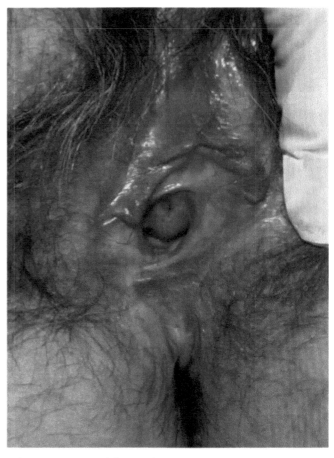

Figure 7.5. Estrogen deficient vulva demonstrating introital shrinkage.

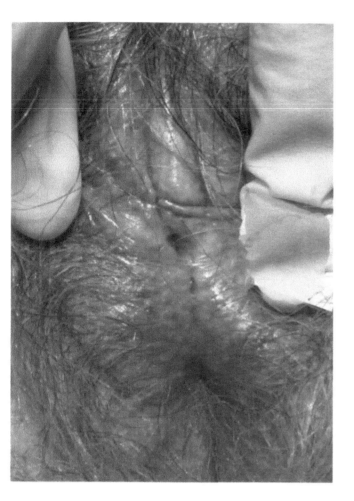

Figure 7.6. Severe atrophy in this elderly patient has resulted in labial adhesions and introital stenosis.

Diagnosis

The cytological changes characteristic of estrogen deficiency are described in Chapter 1. The serum estradiol will be in the postmenopausal range. The FSH is elevated in the natural menopause but might be normal where the estrogen deficiency is drug induced.

In cases of doubt, the vaginal swab should be cultured. If estrogen deficiency is the sole diagnosis, commensals will be grown. These may include coliforms, Streptococci and Staphylococci which are not pathogens under these circumstances and do not require treatment.

Biopsy is indicated in the post-pubertal female where a non-infectious inflammatory disorder may be responsible for the presentation.

Treatment

Estrogen is the treatment for symptomatic vaginal atrophy and atrophic vaginitis. Particularly when dyspareunia has been present for more than, say, 6 months, sexual counselling may be necessary to complete resolution.

Estrogen may be used topically or systemically. It should never be necessary to use both means of administration. Systemic estrogen is generally preferable because the vaginal response is more predictable. In addition, the woman will receive the other benefits of estrogen replacement (for example, prevention of osteoporosis), the adequacy of replacement can be monitored by estimation of serum estradiol and FSH and most women prefer systemic to vaginal medication and will use the former more reliably. One suggested regimen is estradiol 2mg and (to prevent endometrial proliferation) medroxyprogesterone acetate 5mg orally daily. This dose can generally be halved in older women, say, over 60. The progestogen may be omitted if the woman has undergone hysterectomy. Alternatively, the estrogen can be administered transdermally, by implant or intranasally.

Estrogen can be used topically by vaginal tablet, in a vaginal cream through an applicator or in cream pessary form. Examples of these are estradiol and estriol pessaries and estriol and conjugated estrogens vaginal cream. Systemic absorption of these preparations is minimal. Thus, endometrial response resulting in bleeding does occur but rarely. Vaginal tablets might not dissolve in the absence of moisture and thus prove ineffective. Conversely, an excessive response to vaginal estrogen can predispose the woman to recurrent candidiasis. Another drawback to topical estrogen replacement, when used long term, is the potential for sensitization to the estrogen vehicle resulting in contact dermatitis.

Surgery will be required in the older woman with symptomatic labial adhesions. It must be followed with estrogen therapy and/or a topical steroid, depending on the cause.

REFERENCES

Birge SJ. The use of estrogen in older women. [Review] Clinics in Geriatric Medicine. 19(3):617-27, viii, 2003 Aug.

Doren M. Urogenital ageing--creation of improved awareness. [Review] American Journal of Obstetrics & Gynecology. 178(5):S254-6, 1998 May.

Robinson D. Cardozo LD. The role of estrogens in female lower urinary tract dysfunction. [Review] Urology. 62(4 Suppl 1):45-51, 2003 Oct.

Rouzier R, Louis-Sylvestre C, Paniel BJ, Haddad B. Hypertrophy of the labia minora: experience with 163 reductions. Am J Obstet Gynecol 2000; 182: 35-40

Samsioe G. Urogenital ageing--a hidden problem. [Review] American Journal of Obstetrics & Gynecology. 178(5):S245-9, 1998 May.

Stenberg A. Heimer G. Ulmsten U. The prevalence of urogenital symptoms in postmenopausal women. [Review] Maturitas. 22 Suppl:S17-S20, 1995 Dec.

Chapter 8

2. DEVELOPMENTAL ABNORMALITIES

Most developmental abnormalities are manifest at birth but others present with delayed puberty, sexual problems, infertility or obstructed labor. They are divided into conditions where the gender of the genitalia is not in question and those where various degrees of clitoral enlargement, labial fusion and gonadal abnormality show a resemblance to one or more facets of male genitalia.

The cause of developmental abnormalities is usually not known, but they are occasionally familial and some may be associated with renal, lower gastro-intestinal tract and distant maldevelopments.

A. Malformations that do not lead to sexual ambiguity

The mullerian ducts form the fallopian tubes, then fuse, forming the uterus and, with a contribution from the urogenital plate, the vagina. The most common mullerian disorders are aplasia or atresia and incomplete fusion. Abnormalities involving the urogenital plate include an imperforate hymen and transverse vaginal septum. The wolffian ducts regress in most females but remnants may develop into cysts (Gartner's duct cysts).

7. DOUBLE VULVA

Duplication of the vulva is an extremely rare genital malformation often associated with other multiple organ abnormalities that are incompatible with survival. There may be side by side duplication of the entire vulva. The condition may be the result of imperfect twinning.

8. CYST OF THE CANAL OF NUCK (hydrocele of the vulva)

The processus vaginalis peritonei (canal of Nuck) is the extension of the peritoneal cavity into the labioscrotal swellings of the embryo. It is normally obliterated by mid-pregnancy. Its persistence may result in a cyst anywhere along a line from inguinal ring to the labium majus inclusive.

Clinical features

The patient presents with a cystic swelling in the pubic region or in the labium majus. It should not be particularly painful. Unlike inguinal hernia, it is irreducible and contains no abdominal contents. A previously undiagnosed patent processus may lead to an acute pneumatocyst during laparoscopy when a pressurised pneumoperitoneum is produced.

Pathology

The cyst wall is peritoneum and consists of mesothelial lining resting on a thin layer of fibrous connective tissue with more deeply placed fat.

Treatment

Treatment is by excision of the cyst, with or without repair of the inguinal ring. In the case of a pneumatocyst resulting from laparoscopy, simple ligation of the processus at the level of the internal inguinal ring will quickly cause the swelling to disappear, even while the pneumoperitoneum is present.

9. DERMOID CYST

A developmental cyst due to embryological inclusion during ectodermal fusion is known as a (congenital) dermoid cyst. Such developmental cysts, found along developmental fusion lines, particularly on the face, are occasionally found in the vulva. When they occur adjacent to the clitoris of the neonate, the possibility of ambiguous genitalia may arise.

Acquired epidermal cysts (246), usually resulting from traumatic implantation, are discussed in Chapter 14.

10. VASCULAR MALFORMATIONS AND DILATATIONS

Vascular malformations must be distinguished from vascular neoplasms, that is, hemangiomas. The former are present at birth and have a segmental distribution. They are much less common on the vulva than, say, the face, but are important to recognise in order to avoid confusion with inflammatory disorders. The common variety is the **nevus flammeus** (port wine stain). They appear initially as flat, dark pink, unilateral lesions that cause no discomfort. With time they may become darker with scattered small nodules.

Vascular dilatations are seen in hereditary hemorrhagic telangiectasia (Osler's disease), spider angiomas and angiokeratomas (discussed above). Osler's disease only rarely affects vulva and vagina and presents in the child or young adult with small telangiectatic vessels which may bleed easily. It is an autosomal dominant condition. Spider angiomas or nevi are commonly found in the upper half of the body in association with the increased estrogen levels of pregnancy and liver disease. They are rare on the vulva. They have a central arteriolar formation with radiating capillaries.

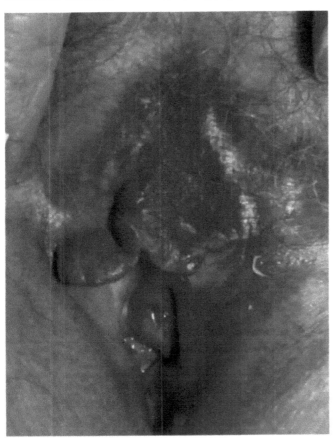

Figure 8.1. Nevus flammeus.

Pathology

The changes are in the capillaries, post-capillary venules and small veins of the superficial plexus. In infancy, the changes are a subtle telangiectasia. With time, vessels become more dilated and develop congestion. There may be an associated deeper cavernous hemangioma.

Treatment

These lesions generally require no treatment but are amenable to removal by laser.

11. CONGENITAL LYMPHEDEMA (MILROY'S DISEASE)

Congenital lymphedema is a genetic disorder of lymphangiogenesis resulting in hypoplasia of peripheral lymphatic vessels. It presents in the young with swelling, usually of the lower limbs, but occasionally the swelling is isolated to the genitals. Its early onset in otherwise healthy women should help distinguish it clinically from lymphangioma circumscriptum (253) and filariasis (32). Tissue affected with lymphedema, whether congenital or acquired, is predisposed to infection, which can be relapsing.

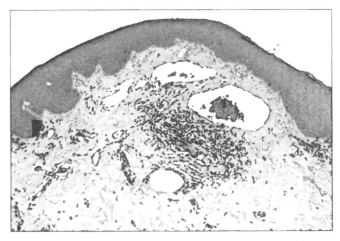

Figure 8.2. Congenital lymphedema. Dilated lymphatics in the papillary dermis and separation of dermal collagen fibres. The macrophages in the lymphatics and adjacent round cells in the stroma are evidence of chronic cellulitis, a common accompaniment of lymphedema.

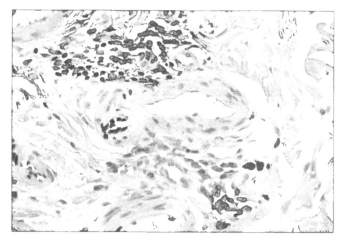

Figure 8.3. Congenital lymphedema. Deep perivascular plasma cells are further evidence of chronic cellulitis in this patient with lymphedema.

12. IMPERFORATE HYMEN

At about 20 weeks, the vaginal plate and cavity of the foetus expand into the urogenital sinus creating a membrane between the two. This membrane, the hymen, ultimately consists of a thin layer of connective tissue with squamous epithelium on both sides and a central deficiency allowing communication between the vagina and vestibule. If no opening develops, the condition is called imperforate hymen. It is a rare cause of primary amenorrhoea

Clinical features

About one in 2,000 girls are born with an imperforate hymen. Some are recognized at birth because of a mucocolpos. Most commonly, however, the diagnosis is delayed until puberty, following which the patient presents with primary amenorrhoea and abdominal pain with or without a mass arising from the pelvis. This results from the accumulation of menstrual flow behind the imperforate hymen. Untreated, hematometra, urinary retention and severe endometriosis may occur. Rarely, imperforate hymen is associated with lower urinary tract or anorectal congenital maldevelopments.

Separation of the labia reveals the vagina occluded at the level of the hymen. This may be confirmed by gentle probing with a swab stick.

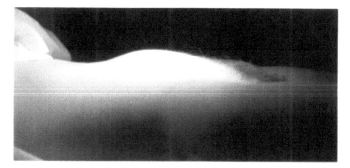

Figure 8.4. Mass arising from the pelvis of an 18 year old due to an imperforate hymen.

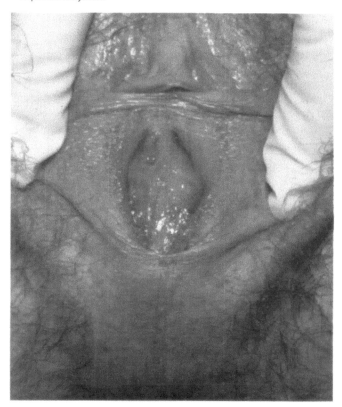

Figure 8.5. Imperforate hymen of the patient in Fig. 8.4.

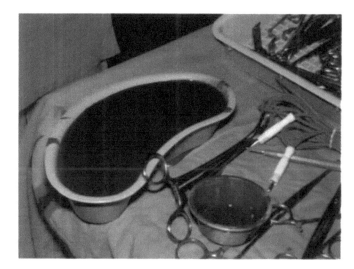

Figure 8.6. Vaginal contents obtained from incision of the hymen in Fig.8.5.

Treatment
Treatment consists of cruciate incision of the hymen.

13. VAGINAL SEPTA
Vaginal septa may be transverse, longitudinal or oblique. Their etiology, presentation and management are different so they will be discussed individually.

Transverse vaginal septa are rare and presumably arise from incomplete fusion between the mullerian duct and urogenital sinus components of the vagina. They therefore tend to involve the upper half of the vagina and characteristically demonstrate columnar epithelium on the superior surface and squamous epithelium on the inferior surface. Thickness varies from a thin membrane to tissue occluding most of the upper vagina. There is not the association with other urogenital abnormalities seen, for example, with vaginal agenesis.

A longitudinal septum, usually (but not always) extending the length of the vagina, is caused by defective lateral fusion of the mullerian ducts. It can result in division of the vagina into left and right halves. These patients commonly have a didelphic uterus with a cervix either side of the septum.

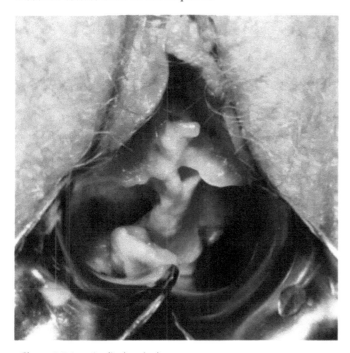

Figure 8.7. Longitudinal vaginal septum.

Non-midline, longitudinal and oblique septa result from less clear-cut embryogenesis but are not usually associated with abnormalities of the uterus

Diagnosis
The presentation of a transverse septum is similar to that of an imperforate hymen.

The patient with a longitudinal septum may be aware of difficulties with intercourse or insertion of tampons. Diagnosis may be obvious on separating the labia but the clinician might miss the diagnosis if the speculum is passed too quickly to one side of a longitudinal septum. Occasionally, the condition presents with the septum stretched over the baby's head in the second stage of labour.

Definitive diagnosis may require, in addition to vaginal examination, diagnostic imagery and laparoscopy.

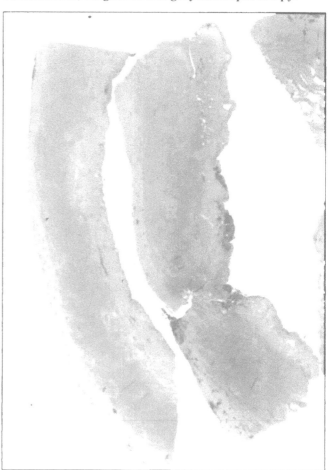

Figure 8.8. Oblique septum. A 16 year old with delayed menarche was found to have a hematocolpos due to a vaginal septum, which was excised. The septum is composed of a thick layer of smooth muscle sandwiched between two layers of normal squamous mucosa

Treatment

A thin transverse septum can be easily incised (like an imperforate hymen). However, the thicker, higher placed septa can provide a particularly difficult surgical challenge, especially when anastomosis of the vagina above and below the septum is not possible.

Longitudinal vaginal septa are usually amenable to simple excision between clamps and the cut edges are oversewn.

14. DOUBLE VAGINA

True double vagina should not be confused with septate vagina (see above). In the former, the two vaginas, in addition to separate epithelia, have a separate lamina propria and muscle coat. The condition is very rare and, like double vulva with which it may be associated, may be found in a neonate demonstrating other life threatening abnormalities as a result of imperfect twinning.

15. VAGINAL HYPOPLASIA

Vaginal hypoplasia is usually found in conjunction with other urogenital abnormalities and may present as a newborn with ambiguous genitalia. The hypoplastic vagina may open into a cloaca-like urogenital sinus or even into the urethra.

16. VAGINAL ATRESIA

Partial or complete failure of canalisation of the vaginal plate results in a vagina represented by a solid epithelial cord above which there is a structurally normal reproductive tract. Vaginal atresia is easily confused with vaginal agenesis if the lower vagina only is involved. In such a case, vaginal atresia will present with hematocolpos after puberty. Hematometra and severe endometriosis may occur if the condition is left untreated.

17. VAGINAL AGENESIS

Vaginal agenesis, a result of failure of development of the mullerian system, occurs in 1/4000 to 1/10,000 females. There is usually an absent uterus as well (Mayer-Rokitansky-Kuster-Hauser syndrome) but there may be a normal upper reproductive tract. It may be familial or sporadic. Renal tract or skeletal abnormalities are present in about a half of the cases, particularly when familial. The ovaries are present and, apart from amenorrhoea, pubertal development proceeds.

Treatment

A functioning vagina can be created with the use of vaginal dilators over a long period of time - a form of treatment requiring a high level of patient motivation. An alternative is a surgical procedure such as the McIndoe operation. In this operation, the space between the bladder and rectum is opened and a mould covered with split skin (with the dermal surface on the outside) is sutured in place. The mould is removed after a week or so. The operation must be followed by repeated dilatation of the neovagina.

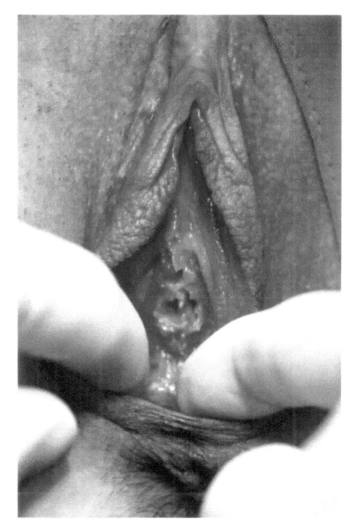

Figure 8.9. Vaginal agenesis.

18. DIETHYLSTILBESTROL (DES) ASSOCIATED ABNORMALITIES

DES is a synthetic estrogen introduced in 1946 and used for nearly 30 years (on what were shown to be empirical grounds) for a variety of pregnancy conditions including threatened and recurrent abortion. Millions of women in the United States, Australia and parts of Western Europe received the drug. The daughters of mothers who took DES went on to demonstrate fairly characteristic vaginal and cervical lesions including adenosis (replacement of squamous with columnar epithelium) of the upper vagina and transverse ridges. There is an increased chance of women so affected developing cervical or vaginal clear cell carcinoma. There is also a mildly increased incidence of HPV-related premalignant and malignant squamous cancers of the cervix and vagina, presumably related to the presence of multiple transformation zones, as the vaginal adenosis heals by squamous metaplasia.

19. GARTNER'S DUCT CYST

In the embryo, as the paramesonephric (mullerian) ducts fuse to form the female internal genitalia, the mesonephric (Gartner's) ducts lying lateral to them regress. If this regression is incomplete the remnants may form cysts arising from the lateral vaginal wall. It is possible that many so-called Gartner's ducts cysts, in fact, arise from the paramesonephric ducts.

Clinical features

Gartner's duct cysts are the commonest cause of swellings found in the vagina. Most are asymptomatic and found on routine examination. They can be found anywhere from the vaginal fornices almost to the introitus and range in size from a couple of centimetres diameter to about 10 cm diameter. They are most frequently seen as paravaginal masses at the level of the vaginal fornix and may be bilateral. Large ones occasionally present distending the introitus of the infant or tending to obstruct the vagina of the older female. Gartner's duct cysts occasionally occur with an anomalous fistulous connection to the cervix or an ectopic ureter or may be associated with renal tract abnormalities including ectopic ureter draining elsewhere, absent, hypoplastic or cystic kidney. These associated anomalies tend to be more common, the larger the cyst.

Pathology

Gartner's duct cysts are thin-walled cysts containing watery, colourless fluid. They are lined by a simple layer of cuboidal to columnar epithelium and characteristically have smooth muscle in their walls.

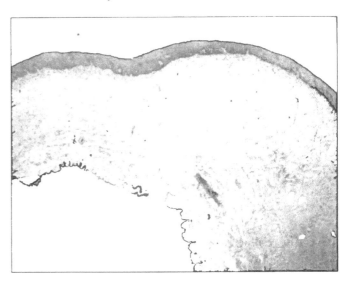

Figure 8.10. Gartner's duct cyst. A cyst is present in the wall of the vagina.

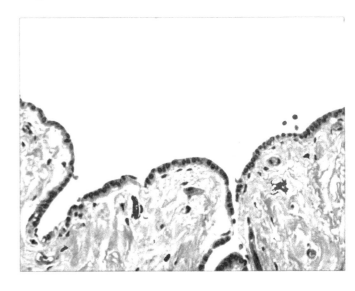

Figure 8.11. Gartner's duct cyst. The cyst is lined by a simple layer of cuboidal epithelium.

Treatment

Small asymptomatic cysts require no treatment. Larger cysts of which the woman is aware may be excised. However, they do not always have a good plane of dissection around them and may extend higher into the pelvis thereby creating a considerable surgical challenge with the risk of damage to the bladder, ureter or rectum. In such a case it is probably simplest to marsupialize the cyst by excising the superficial half of the cyst and overlying vaginal epithelium and then uniting the remaining cyst wall and adjacent vaginal cut edges with absorbable sutures.

20. ECTOPIC URETER DRAINING INTO THE VAGINA

An ectopic ureter may be the sole drainage from a kidney, part of a duplex system, unilateral or bilateral. It may open into the urinary system distal to the trigone or into the vagina.

Diagnosis

These patients void normally but are wet at other times or continually. If the urinary flow is not great, the patient may be misdiagnosed as having a vaginal discharge from some other cause. The opening of the ureter into the vagina may be very hard to find, even with dye injection. Radiographic studies with contrast medium should provide the diagnosis.

Treatment

If the ectopic ureter is the sole drainage of that kidney, then reimplantation of the ureter into the bladder is the procedure likely to be undertaken by a pediatric urologist. If it is part of a duplex system, then optimal treatment will be removal of the kidney segment drained by the ectopic ureter with removal of as much of the ureter as possible.

21. EPISPADIAS

This rare malformation, more common in males, results from failure of mesodermal invasion of the cloacal membrane. Bladder exstrophy is the condition where the invasion failure is more severe and involves the bladder.

Diagnosis

Incontinence results from urethral sphincter incompetence due to deficiency of the sphincter anteriorly. The clitoris is bifid and there is anterior separation of the labia. The urethra is short and patulous. Pubic bone separation will be seen on x-ray or will be palpable.

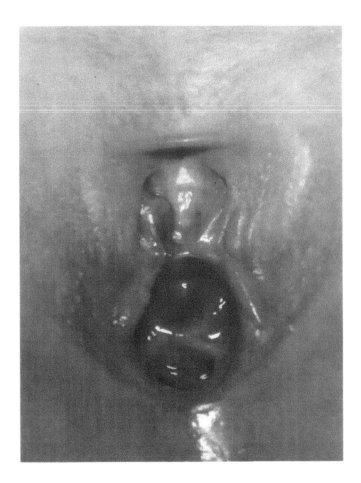

Figure 8.12. Infant demonstrating epispadias.

Treatment

Surgical correction, nowadays performed at ages 3 to 5 years, is aimed at improving continence, often using a strip of bladder mucosa. The vulvar abnormalities may require no attention and these patients are potentially able to deliver vaginally.

22. HYPOSPADIAS

There are wide variations in the normal placement of the urethral meatus in relation to the vaginal introitus. Hypospadias is said to be present when its placement is abnormally high in the vagina when there may be associated incontinence, possibly meatal stenosis, pooling of urine in the vagina and occasional vaginal and uterine abnormalities.

It is treated by urethroplasty using vaginal and sometimes labial skin.

23. IMPERFORATE ANUS WITH VULVAR OR VAGINAL FISTULA

Congenital malformation of the cloacal derivatives may present in the infant with complete obstruction of the anus which can even appear to be absent. This may be associated with a fistulous opening into the vagina or perineum, otherwise the condition will create a surgical emergency due to bowel obstruction. In the former case, the fistula may open anywhere from the lower half of the vagina to the perineum anterior to the anal pit inclusive.

B. Malformations with ambiguous external sexual organs

When genital ambiguity occurs, gender cannot be readily assigned by visual inspection of the external genitalia. Conditions leading to this are also referred to as intersex, male and female pseudohermaphroditism and true hermaphroditism. They are clinical groupings of a variety of disorders resulting from readily demonstrable abnormalities of chromosomes and/or disordered foetal endocrine function including androgen insensitivity. They form more or less a spectrum from the apparent male who is 46XX to the apparent female who is 46XY. In practice, they present within the realms of neonatal paediatrics and antenatal diagnosis.

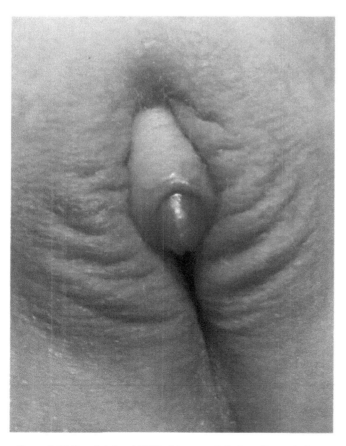

Figure 8.13. Female infant (46XX) with congenital adrenal hyperplasia and genital ambiguity.

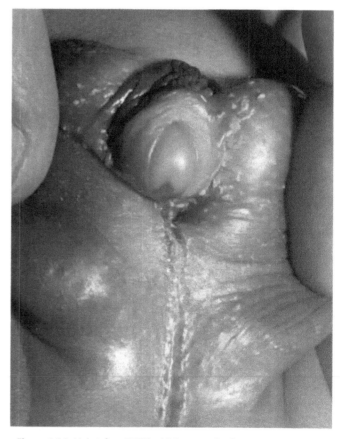

Figure 8.14. Male infant (46XY) with hypospadias for comparison with Fig.8.13 to highlight the difficulty of genital ambiguity.

These ambiguous genitalia may present with any of the following in various combinations: small phallus in the genetic male or enlarged clitoris in the genetic female, varying degrees of fusion of the labioscrotal folds, misplacement of the urethral meatus, chordee and gonads inappropriately above or below the inguinal ring. The presence of ovarian and testicular tissue in the one individual is the hallmark of true hermaphroditism.

The main causes of genital ambiguity are gonadal dysgenesis and congenital adrenal hyperplasia. The latter is discussed in Chapter 11 (endocrine and metabolic disorders).

GONADAL DYSGENESIS
Gonadal dysgenesis is the development of abnormal ovaries and testes and is a consequence of an abnormal compliment of X or Y genes.

24. OVARIAN DYSGENESIS (TURNER'S SYNDROME)
Turner's syndrome is the commonest form of ovarian dysgenesis with an incidence of 1:2,500 to 1: 10,000 live female births and is due to a 45X karyotype. 45X/46XX and 45X/46XY mosaicism are also found, the former the more common. Occasional cases have a normal chromosome number but abnormalities of X/Y.

Clinical features
The external genitalia are characteristically female but other features of the syndrome (short stature, low-set ears, webbed neck, cubitus valgus) may provide the clues. Otherwise, the condition manifests by delayed or absent pubertal development.

25. TESTICULAR DYSGENESIS (KLINEFELTER'S SYNDROME)
Testicular dysgenesis most commonly refers to Klinefelter's syndrome due to the karyotype 47XXY. Other karyotypes producing similar clinical features include XXXY, XXYX and 46XX phenotypic males. There is an association between these conditions and gonadoblastoma, dysgerminoma and yolk sac tumor.

Clinical features
These individuals are generally apparent males at birth but have small testes and a tendency to eunuchoid characteristics including obesity. The diagnosis is apparent at adolescence and they are infertile.

26. TRUE HERMAPHRODITISM
True hermaphrodites contain both ovarian and testicular tissue. The female and male gonadal tissue may be separate or a single mass, the ovotestis. Mosaicism may explain the development of the ovotestis, as the SRY gene, a product of the Y chromosome, has been found in the testicular component in XX karyotypes. Most true hermaphrodites are 46XX, but other karyotypes are found. The gonads may be situated above or below the inguinal ring. External genitalia are predominantly female but a broad spectrum of genital characteristics may be found.

27. GONADAL AGENESIS
Also known as agonadia or testicular regression syndrome, this rare syndrome is characterised by failure of development of mullerian and wolffian derivatives of unknown cause. The phallus is of female dimensions and the underdeveloped labia majora are fused with a tendency to persistence of the urogenital sinus. By definition, gonads are undetectable.

Investigation and treatment of intersex
The multidisciplinary team required in most of these cases includes a paediatrician, gynecologist, urologist, endocrinologist and psychologist. The most urgent considerations are biochemical abnormalities resulting from disordered endocrine function and urinary difficulties. Gender assignment and genital surgery are not priorities. Experience has shown that patients with congenital adrenal hyperplasia can be safely regarded as girls. Major abnormalities may be corrected early, although a relatively minor abnormality, for example enlarged clitoris, may be left until the patient makes up her own mind. In gonadal dysgenesis the situation is more difficult and counseling should be similar to that of other patients with other major congenital abnormalities.

The timing of surgery is seldom an easy decision. When surgery has not been performed in infancy, often by mid childhood the patient's psychological need for surgery may arise. This can be followed by a decision to change sex some years later. Under such circumstances, the surgical result may not match the patient's expectations.

Turner's syndrome patients will require estrogen for puberty and growth hormone for height. One other consideration in these patients is that hidden Y mosaicism is a recognised risk factor for the development of gonadal tumors.

REFERENCES

ACOG Committee on adolescent health care. ACOG committee opinion. Nonsurgical diagnosis and management of vaginal agenesis. Obstet Gynecol 2002; 100: 213-6

Bava GL. Dalmonte P. Oddone M. Rossi U. Life-threatening hemorrhage from a vulvar hemangioma. Journal of Pediatric Surgery. 37(4):E6, 2002 Apr

Blackwell AL. Gillmer MD. Vaginal atresia treated successfully with vaginal dilators. Journal of Obstetrics & Gynaecology. 22(3):326, 2002 May.

Blanton EN. Rouse DJ. Trial of labor in women with transverse vaginal septa. Obstetrics & Gynecology. 101(5 Pt 2):1110-2, 2003 May.

Carpenter S E K and Rock J A. Pediatric and Adolescent Gynecology. 2nd ed., Philadelphia. Lipincott, Williams and Wilkins, 2000.

Del Rossi C. Attanasio A. Del Curto S. D'Agostino S. De Castro R. Treatment of vaginal atresia at a missionary hospital in Bangladesh: results and follow-up of 20 cases. Journal of Urology. 170(3):864-6, 2003 Sep.

Economy KE. Barnewolt C. Laufer MR. A comparison of MRI and laparoscopy in detecting pelvic structures in cases of vaginal agenesis. Journal of Pediatric & Adolescent Gynecology. 15(2):101-4, 2002 Apr.

Emmons SL, Petty WM. Recurrent giant Gartner's duct cysts. A report of two cases. J Reprod Med 2001; 46: 773-5

Faithi K, Pinter A Paraurethral cysts in female neonates. Case reports. Acta Paediatr 2003; 92: 758-9

Fischer GO. Vulval disease in prepubertal girls. Aust J Derm 2001; 42: 225-236

Frost-Arner L. Aberg M. Jacobsson S. Split skin graft reconstruction in vaginal agenesis: a long-term follow-up. Scandinavian Journal of Plastic & Reconstructive Surgery & Hand Surgery. 38(3):151-4, 2004.

Holmes M. Upadhyay V. Pease P. Gartner's duct cyst with unilateral renal dysplasia presenting as an introital mass in a new born. [Review] [12 refs] Pediatric Surgery International. 15(3-4):277-9, 1999.

Kempinaire A. De Raeve L. Roseeuw D. Boon L. De Raeve H. Capillary-venous malformation in the labia majora in a 12-year-old girl. Dermatology. 194(4):405-7, 1997.

LappohnRE. Congenital absence of the vagina--results of conservative treatment. European Journal of Obstetrics, Gynecology, & Reproductive Biology. 59(2):183-6, 1995

Leonovicz PF 3rd. O'Connell BJ. Uehling DT. Vaginal ectopic ureter with Gartner's duct cyst. Journal of Urology. 158(6):2235, 1997 Dec.

Lim Y H, Ng S P, Jamil M A. Imperforate hymen: Report of an unusual familial occurrence. J. Obstet. Gynaecol. Res.; 29(6):399-401.

Ludwig KS. The Mayer-Rokitansky-Kuster syndrome. An analysis of its morphology and embryology. Part I: Morphology. Archives of Gynecology & Obstetrics. 262(1-2):1-26, 1998.

Minto CL. Liao KL. Conway GS. Creighton SM. Sexual function in women with complete androgen insensitivity syndrome. Fertility & Sterility. 80(1):157-64, 2003 Jul.

Moon TD. Kennedy AA. Knight KM. Vaginal discharge due to undiagnosed bilateral duplicated collecting system with ectopic ureters in a three-year-old female: an initial high index of suspicion for sexual abuse. Journal of Pediatric & Adolescent Gynecology. 15(4):213-6, 2002 Aug.

Mori Y. Takiuchi H. Nojima M. Kondoh N. Yoshimoto T. Maeda N. Kurachi M. Shima H. [Ectopic ureter in 54 children]. [Japanese] Nippon Hinyokika Gakkai Zasshi - Japanese Journal of Urology. 92(3):470-3, 2001 Mar.

Powell DM. Newman KD. Randolph J. A proposed classification of vaginal anomalies and their surgical correction. Journal of Pediatric Surgery. 30(2):271-5; discussion 275-6, 1995 Feb.

Robboy SJ, Ross JS, Prat J, Keh PC, Welch WR Urogenital sinus origin of mucinous and ciliated cysts of the vulva. Obstet Gynecol 1978; 51: 347-51

Robson S. Oliver GD. Management of vaginal agenesis: review of 10 years practice at a tertiary referral centre. Australian & New Zealand Journal of Obstetrics & Gynaecology. 40(4):430-3, 2000 Nov.

Shiraishi K, Ishizu K, Takeuchi K, Takai K, Takihara H, Koga M, Naito K. Idiopathic clitoral hypertrophy Urol Int 1999; 62: 174-6

Stallion A Vaginal obstruction. Semin Pediatr Surg 2000; 9: 128-34

Tjaden BL. Buscema J. Haller JA Jr. Rock JA. Vulvar congenital dysplastic angiopathy. Obstetrics & Gynecology. 75(3 Pt 2):552-4, 1990 Mar.

Wai CY, Zekam N, Sanz LE Septate uterus with double cervix and longitudinal vaginal septum. A case report. J Reprod Med 2001; 46: 613-7

Wang J, Ezzat W, Davidson M Transverse vaginal septum J Reprod Med 1995; 40: 163-6

Yen CF, Wang CJ, Chang PC, Lee CL, Soong YK Concomitant closure of patent canal of Nuck during laparoscopic surgery: case report Hum Reprod 2001; 16: 357-9

Chapter 9

3. INFECTIONS

Advances in diagnosis and treatment and the development of vaccines are rapidly following molecular research into infections. Drug resistance is a continuing problem. As a result, diagnostic tests and treatment guidelines are changing quickly. It is suggested that the latest information is obtained from appropriate specialist societies and public health offices through the internet (see reference section for some suggestions).

Parasites

28. PEDICULOSIS PUBIS

Pthirus pubis is the sucking louse responsible for pediculosis pubis. This condition is known colloquially as "crabs" because of the crab-like form and peculiar sideways movement of the parasite just visible to the naked eye. It is generally considered a sexually transmitted disorder because the adult louse is unable to live more than about 24 hours off the host and is transmitted by intimate contact. The pubic louse is dependent on human blood. It cements its eggs (nits) to hair - usually pubic but also axillary and eyelashes. The adult is smaller than head and body lice *(Pediculus humanus capitus and P. humanus humanus)*. Pubic lice are usually seen in the setting of the sexually transmitted disease (STD) clinic and the patient may have other sexually transmitted infections.

Clinical features

Pubic lice is one of the two common pruritic disorders (the other being scabies) seen in the setting of the STD clinic. The incubation period is about one month. Pruritus, especially of the hair bearing skin around the genitals, is the leading complaint. The woman or her partner may have seen the lice moving. Examination will reveal the effects of scratching (excoriation, possible

infection and lichenification) and the nits: minute (a loupe might be necessary to find them), white ovoids best seen attached to peripheral pubic hairs.

Diagnosis

The finding of nits confirms the diagnosis. If in doubt, removal of the hair and examination under low magnification will demonstrate the egg case attached to the hair. It may or may not have hatched (Figs. 9.2 and 9.3).

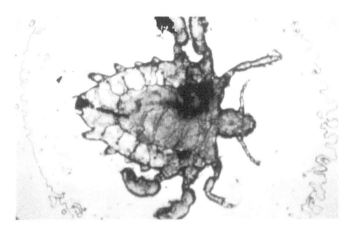

Figure 9.1. Phthirus pubis.

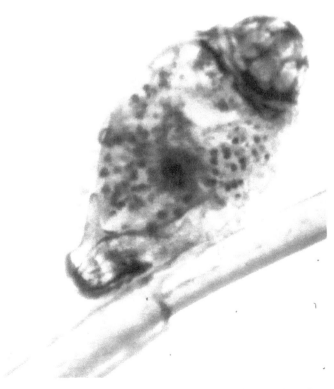

Figure 9.2. Unhatched nit on pubic hair. The louse can be seen through the wall of the case. Photo courtesy of Dorevitch Pathology.

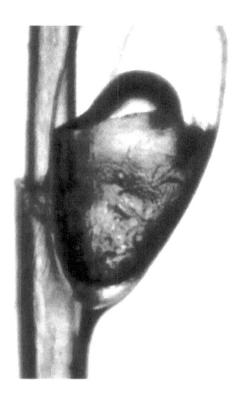

Figure 9.3. Hatched nit (empty egg case) on pubic hair. Photo courtesy of Dorevitch Pathology.

Treatment

Several pediculocides are available. Permethrin is suitable for use against *Pthirus pubis*. Pediculocides are generally effective in liquid, shampoo or cream shampoo vehicles used in a single application. However, treatment should be repeated one week later to catch hatching nits. The patient's partner must be simultaneously treated as with other sexually transmitted infections. Although the itching usually clears immediately the lice are killed, the patient should be warned about post-treatment pruritus from the infestation itself and/or the treatment in order to avoid parasitophobia and over-treatment.

29. SCABIES

Scabies is a pruritic skin disorder resulting from infestation with the human itch mite, *Sarcoptes scabiei*. The condition is found throughout the world, most commonly under low socio-economic circumstances. In developed countries, the incidence varies cyclically depending on general 'herd' immunity. Genital involvement is only part of the wider skin involvement. Any close contact can result in transmission, not only sexual intercourse. The mite burrows into the stratum corneum and the pruritus results from a subsequent immune-mediated inflammatory response.

Clinical features

Symptoms appear three to four weeks after the infestation has been acquired. Generalised itching tends to be nocturnal with accentuation of lesions in the finger webs, sides of digits, flexor surface of wrists, anterior axillary folds, areolae of breasts, abdomen, buttocks as well as genitals. This is associated with a papular eruption

Scabies may be confused with other common pruritic dermatoses. However, if a burrow can be found, this is the site to scrape to find microscopic evidence of the mite. It is a short, wavy, dirty-appearing line which often crosses skin lines. The search for the burrow should commence in the finger web.

Crusted (or Norwegian) scabies is a clinical variant found in the intellectually disabled or immunosuppressed (eg. AIDS) patient. In these cases, the mite population is massive and hyperkeratotic, fissured and crusted lesions develop, particularly on the hands and feet.

Animal scabies transferred from dogs and other animals tends to be found at the site of contact and is usually rapidly self-limiting.

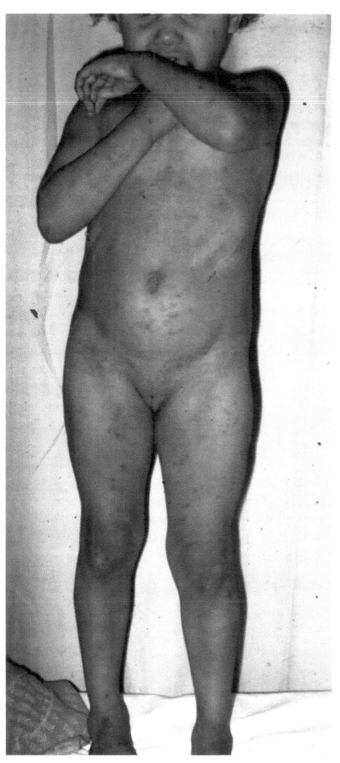

Figure 9.4. Scabies.

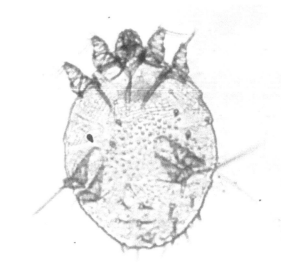

Figure 9.5. Sarcoptes scabiei.

Diagnosis

The diagnosis of scabies is made by microscopy of scrapings of burrows and looking for a trail of irregular dark blobs (feces) or the mite itself.

Biopsy of the rash usually shows a hypersensitivity reaction and not the mite or its by-products. There are non-specific findings of superficial and deep perivascular lymphocytic infiltrate with plentiful eosinophils. This pattern of inflammation may also be seen with other infestations, arthropod bites, bullous pemphigoid, Well's syndrome and the hypereosinophilic syndrome.

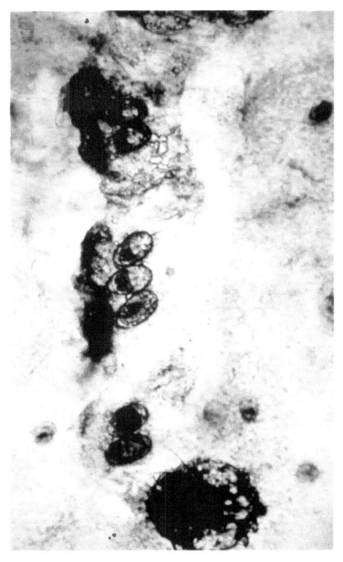

Figure 9.6. Microscopy of material scraped from a skin burrow in a patient with scabies, including a mite at the bottom of the photo.

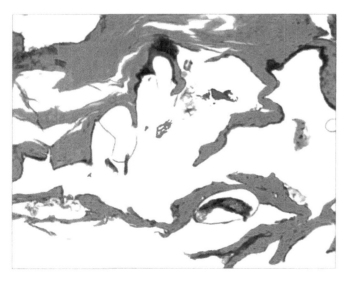

Figure 9.7. Scabies (non-genital): a number of eggs are seen within parakeratosis in this skin scraping from the finger web.

Treatment

Five percent permethrin cream is applied to the whole body below the neck and left eight hours, then washed off. This treatment should be repeated one week later. In resistant cases or crusted scabies, oral ivermectin (400microgram/kg in a single dose) may be used.

Pruritus may persist for some time after eradication of the mite. Topical corticosteroids can be used for control of the itch. Public health measures and washing of clothes and bed linen should not be overlooked.

30. OXYURIASIS

Oxyuriasis is also known as enterobiasis, threadworm, pinworm or seatworm infection. It is caused by *Enterobius vermicularis*, the commonest human intestinal worm with a world-wide distribution. The infection results from ingestion of fertile eggs which mature in the cecum eventually growing into worms 10 mm in length. These migrate out of the anus at night on to the perineum and into the vagina (occasionally higher in the genital tract) producing inflammation and pruritus.

Clinical features

More common in children, the leading symptom is anal, perineal and vulvar pruritus. The affected areas will be erythematous and there may be excoriation and urticaria. The worms themselves may be visible at night, on toilet paper or in the stools.

Diagnosis

The diagnosis is made by the traditional method of Graham's adhesive tape test or stool microscopy. A slide covered with adhesive tape is applied to the perianal region in the morning before washing then examined under the microscope for ova. At least 6 separate preparations are advisable. The worms, which are 3-12mm long, may also be directly visualised on the perianal region at night, between the labia or in the vagina.

Sometimes the eggs may be present in tissue from the genital tract, where they must be distinguished from schistosomiasis. A chronic granulomatous reaction to ova in vulvar tissue has been rarely reported.

Treatment

Sometimes, despite typical clinical circumstances, ova or worms are not identified and treatment may be presumptive. The following anthelmintic drugs are all effective against E. vermicularis: mebendazole, pyrantel, pyrvinium and piperazine. The whole family needs treatment and hand washing is essential on rising, after defecation and before eating. Likewise, hygiene of bedding will require attention.

31. SCHISTOSOMIASIS (Bilharziasis)

The tropical disease schistosomiasis is caused by the human blood flukes *Schistosoma mansoni, S. japonicum* (both produce eggs in feces), *S.haematobium* (produces eggs in the urine) and rarely *S. mekongi* and *S. intercalatum*. Certain aquatic snails are involved in the life cycle and it is the cercaria of the fluke which enters the human host by skin penetration. Free-swimming cercaria penetrate the skin of waders or swimmers on route to mesenteric (*S. mansoni and S. japonicum*) or vesical venous plexuses (*S. haematobium*), where they penetrate into tissue and lay their eggs. The manifestations of the disease occur due to the granulomatous and fibrous reaction to the ova.

Clinical features

Dermatitis results from skin penetration by the cercariae and is usually in the areas immersed in the water inhabited by the snail host. Urticaria and a febrile systemic response involving liver, spleen, joints and bowel occur one to two months later. Female genital tract schistosomiasis usually occurs on the vulva of children and young women and is due to S. *hematobium*. Vulvar schistosomiasis ranges from an incidental finding on histology in a biopsy taken for some other reason to a severe clinical disease. The labia majora are affected firstly, but the entire vulva may be involved. Ulceration and eventually much scarring and lymphedema may occur. The most dramatic vulvar manifestation of the infection is the formation of granulomatous condylomata around the perineum and vulva seen in regions of high endemicity. The lesions may demonstrate sinus and fistula formation and may extend to the groin and buttocks. A papular eruption on the trunk resulting from embolism of ova may assist clinical diagnosis. Late complications include acquired lymphangioma and carcinoma.

Diagnosis

The standard method of diagnosing schistosomiasis is serology. Enzyme linked immunoabsorbent assay (ELISA) and other newer immunoassays have near 100% sensitivity and very high specificity. Two months should have elapsed from the time of exposure.

The histopathological diagnosis of schistosomiasis depends on finding and identifying eggs and is particularly useful in unsuspected cases.

Histologically, the epidermis shows hyperkeratosis, acanthosis and pseudoepitheliomatous hyperplasia. Rarely, there are focal ulceration and drainage sinuses accompanied by acute inflammation. The dermis contains numerous ova, which may be calcified and accompanied by no reaction, a granulomatous reaction, including foreign body giant cells, or lie in microabscesses, often with eosinophils.

Treatment

Praziquantel, metrifonate, oxamniquinine and niridazole are all effective against *Schistosoma*.

32. FILARIASIS (Elephantiasis)

Filariasis is a mosquito-borne worm infection of the tropics, most commonly due to *Wuchereria bancrofti*. The larvae develop and reproduce in the lymphatics where they induce an inflammatory reaction causing chronic lymphatic obstruction.

Filariasis remains a major problem in the tropics and is the subject of a current global campaign of elimination through vector control and mass treatment with microfilaricidal drugs. Prevention is the aim, as it has been shown that tissue damage long antedates symptoms.

Clinical features

Edema due to lymphatic obstruction, lymphangitis and lymphadenitis are hallmarks of the disease with swelling of legs and vulva. Eventually, genital lesions resembling those of lymphogranuloma venereum (**60**) develop requiring laboratory differentiation.

Diagnosis

The time honoured method of diagnosis of filariasis, the identification of microfilariae in blood specimens taken at night, is still used in many parts of the world. The diagnostic methods of choice, however, are being rapidly superceded by serology and newer tests like PCR, antigen detection using finger prick blood taken during the day and ultrasound to visualise adult worms

Groin node biopsies show extensive replacement by fibrosis. Occasionally, dead worms are found within dilated lymphatic embedded in fibrous tissue, often accompanied by tissue eosinophilia

Treatment

Diethylcarbamazine is the drug of choice for filariasis.

33. HYDATID DISEASE

Hydatid disease is caused by the adult and larval stages of cestodes (tapeworms) belonging to the genus Echinococcosis, particularly *Echinococcus granulosus* and *multilocularis* The primary host is usually the dog. Human infestation results from ingestion of ova present in canine feces. Hydatid cysts are most commonly found in the liver and are very rare in the vulva where they form painless firm or soft subcutaneous swellings.

Diagnosis

The diagnosis of extragenital hydatid disease is based on ultrasound of hydatid cysts and serology. The serologic tests should begin with a screening test, such as ELISA or hemagglutination, and then should be verified using a western-blot method in order to detect the reaction with 8kDA fraction of the Echinococcus antigen. The final diagnosis is based on the histological examination of a hydatid lesion or detecting the protoscolices of tape worms in cystic fluid.

Vulvar hydatid disease may be first diagnosed on the histopathology of an excised subcutaneous mass, where the cysts are identified by their distinctive eosinophilic laminated membrane and scolices. Serology, as above, can assist with the diagnosis and be used for follow-up.

Treatment

Treatment of cystic hydatid disease consists of surgical therapy, percutaneous drainage, chemotherapy and long term observation. Highly effective vaccines against *Echinococcus granulosis* are used in animals. Evidence suggests that they would also be effective if used directly in humans. These vaccines are not yet available for human usage.

34. TRICHOMONIASIS

Infection with the flagellated protozoon *Trichomonas vaginalis* in women produces inflammation of the cervix, vagina, urethra and paraurethral glands. The organism is quickly killed by drying so transmission should always be considered sexual. This also causes difficulty with diagnosis because of its poor survival with transport. The infection is confined to the lower genital tract but the possibility of coexistence with other sexually transmitted infections must always be borne in mind. Trichomoniasis has become less common in the last few decades probably because of the widespread use of metronidazole to which the infection is highly susceptible. However, the disease seems to have a habit of turning up unexpectedly in often embarrassing circumstances, for example, as a result of the occasional extramarital encounter.

Clinical features

Vaginal discharge is the most common presentation. It appears firstly a week or two after the sexual encounter responsible. The discharge may be profuse, irritating and associated with dysuria. Examination reveals a cervicovaginitis characterised by punctate erosions or hemorrhages giving rise to the appearance of "strawberry cervix". The vaginitis bears a close resemblance to that of desquamative inflammatory vaginitis (**79**), with which it must not be confused.

Most but not all women harboring *T. vaginalis* have these symptoms and signs. However, it is uncommon for men to be aware that they are infected with trichomonads. If symptomatic, urethral discharge is the likely complaint in the male. Trichomoniasis does not cause systemic illness.

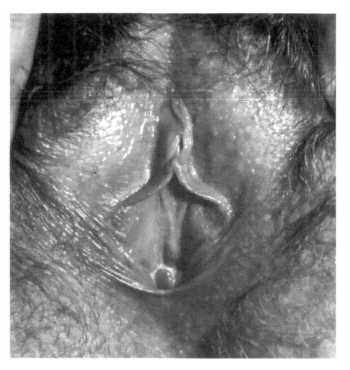

Figure 9.8. Trichomoniasis showing the purulent discharge and lack of vulvitis.

Diagnosis

PCR is the most sensitive method, particularly for samples that are less than optimal. Examination of a saline wet mount slide is a quick and relatively reliable investigation. The organism can be readily cultured but, as already stated, transport to the laboratory can be the problem.

To make a wet mount, separate the labia and introduce a cytology brush the length of the vagina then mix it with one drop of normal saline on a slide, apply a cover slip and examine immediately under 100x magnification with the condenser diaphragm shut down. Numerous polymorphonuclear leucocytes (PMN) will be seen and substitution of the normal bacillary flora by cocci. The trichomonads can usually be readily found in a large proportion of the fields and are identified by their characteristic movement. They are about 7 to 10 microns, larger than a PMN but smaller than a squamous epithelial cell. Unlike a parabasal cell, with which they may be confused, they have a small ovoid nucleus to one side of the cell. They have an anterior, hair-like flagella (hence the name of the genus) and an undulating membrane. These move constantly, imparting the once seen, never forgotten, jerky movement.

Trichomoniasis may be firstly diagnosed on a cervical cytology smear as the infection produces fairly characteristic changes in the epithelial cells. The trichomonads themselves stain poorly with Papanicolaou stain. Histology is not appropriate for diagnosis as the inflammatory reaction is non-specific and organisms are not normally visible.

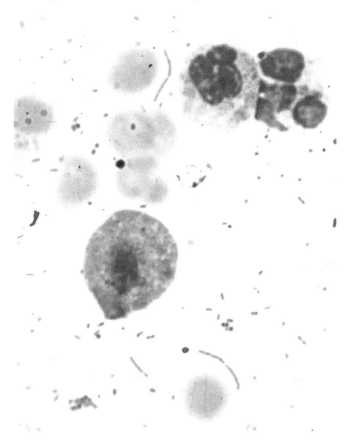

Figure 9.9. *Trichomonas vaginalis* stained with Wright stain. Note its size in relation to the red blood cells adjacent and the flagellum at 6 o'clock.

Treatment

Treatment is generally simple because of the susceptibility of the organism to metronidazole or tinidazole. Recommended dosage is 200mg three times daily for 7 days for metronidazole or 2g of tinidazole as a single dose. Sexual partner(s) should receive simultaneous treatment and this may create difficulties. Sometimes the above dosage appears ineffective and needs to be doubled. Metronidazole rectal suppositories (500mg or 1g) used vaginally may be useful in resistant cases. Thus, follow-up of these patients is recommended.

35. AMEBIASIS

Amebiasis is a rare cause of genital ulceration. It is caused by the protozoon, *Entamoeba histolytica*. Its most serious effects, sometimes lethal, are intestinal. It may need to be considered in the differential diagnosis of vulvovaginal ulceration which may resemble malignancy (ameboma) and be associated with fistula formation. However, amebae may also colonise a malignancy due to loss of host defences. The disease has been described in children.

Diagnosis

Traditionally, amebiasis is diagnosed by microscopy of scrapings or histology. Now, however, a combination of serologic and antigen detection tests or PCR offers the best approach to diagnosis.

Histologic examination of amebic ulcers show extensive necrosis in the base, which may underline the adjacent intact epidermis, and a non-specific inflammatory infiltrate. Vulvar lesions may show extensive pseudoepitheliomatous hyperplasia with only small punctate areas of ulceration. Amebae are found in the slough of the ulcer and are highlighted by the PAS stain. They are the same size as and have a superficial resemblance to histiocytes, but differ by the presence of a single eccentric small round nucleus, about the size of a red blood cell, with a prominent central karyosome. Phagocytosed red blood cells in the cytoplasm are another diagnostic feature. They may be multiple and slightly redder than amebic nuclei.

Treatment

E. histolytica is sensitive to metronidazole. The recommended adult dosage is 800mg 3 times daily for 10 days.

36. LEISHMANIASIS

Leishmaniasis is essentially a zoonosis resulting from the bite of the sandfly which has become infected with protozoa of the genus *Leishmania* acquired from canines and rodents. Different species of *Leishmania* produce different clinical syndromes. The species responsible for visceral leishmaniasis (kala azar) are different from the species responsible for cutaneous leishmaniasis

with which this manual is concerned. The disease is rare in most developed countries but relatively common in many parts of the Mediterranean, Asia, Africa, the Middle East and Central and South America.

Clinical features

Most lesions of cutaneous leishmaniasis are extragenital depending on where the sandfly bites. The typical lesion starts as a minute, pruritic papule which infiltrates the surrounding dermis in a nodular, congested manner. A crust forms and its removal (by scratching) leaves an ulcer which gradually extends. Leishmaniasis may need consideration in the differential diagnosis of vulvar ulceration, particular in the above global regions or in women who have visited these regions.

The cell mediated immune response of the host, influences the manifestations of this infection. Thus, localised cutaneous leishmaniasis and spontaneous resolution are associated with a high level of immune response whereas a poor response is associated with diffuse cutaneous leishmaniasis with numerous nodular lesions, plaques and ulcers. Leishmaniasis may complicate HIV infection.

Diagnosis

Traditionally, the diagnosis is usually made by identifying the organism in tissue or smear. It may also be cultured by a complex procedure available in reference laboratories. These methods are being superseded by more sophisticated detectors such as PCR, ELISA, latex agglutination and immunochromographic strip testing.

In acute lesions, biopsy reveals a massive infiltrate of lymphocytes, foamy histiocytes containing parasites, epithelioid histiocytes, giant cells, plasma cells and eosinophils. The parasites are round to oval basophilic structures measuring 2-4 microns. They have an eccentrically located kinetoplast. The lack of a capsule is helpful in distinguishing them from *Histoplasma capsulatum*. Although the organisms can be seen on routine hematoxylin and eosin staining, they are better seen with Giemsa, preferably on a split-skin smear. Organisms tend to localise at the periphery of the macrophages, the so-called marquee sign.

With increasing chronicity, there is acanthosis, pseudoepitheliomatous hyperplasia and reduction in the number of parasitised macrophages. In AIDS cases, there may be masses of parasitised macrophages with scant plasma cells. An immunoperoxidase antibody is available.

Treatment
Localised nodules may be treated with cryotherapy using liquid nitrogen. Medication which has been used with variable benefit includes pentavalent antimony, amphotericin B, pentamidine isethionate, ketoconazole and rifampicin. The pentavalent antimonial drugs have been the most effective. However, resistance is growing and research into new drugs is being undertaken. No vaccine is available.

Fungal

37. CANDIDA ALBICANS VULVOVAGINITIS
C. albicans is responsible for the commonest female genital disease, vulvovaginal candidiasis. It is a dimorphic yeast. Its two forms are pseudohyphae (filaments) and blastoconidia (spores). An increasing number of non-albicans yeasts (38) are appearing in cultures from vaginal swabs and it is essential to differentiate these yeasts from *C albicans* because they are non-pathogenic or of uncertain pathogenicity whereas *C. albicans* is significantly pathogenic in most women from whom it is cultured. One should avoid non-specific terms such as 'yeast infections' and insist that cultures growing the Candida genus are speciated.

Most women will experience at least one episode of clinical vulvovaginal candidiasis in their lifetime and, considering this high frequency of the disorder, it is unfortunate that much misinformation on candidiasis exists. However, the last few years have seen a greater understanding of its pathogenicity, which must be recognised in order to correctly manage this often highly distressing disease.

The yeast is widespread in nature and most likely reaches the vagina via oral ingestion and perineal contamination. It should not be regarded as a sexually transmitted disease. Estrogen stimulated vaginal epithelial maturation provides glycogen, which has been shown to be a preferred substrate for the yeast. The irritating yeast metabolites (which include alcohol) exit the vagina and produce contact dermatitis of the sensitive vulvar epithelium, thereby producing most of the clinical features of the disorder. In most cases, the organism is detected in the vagina and not where the symptoms are experienced externally. Nevertheless, occasionally, long-standing cases are seen where the yeast is found persisting in the stratum corneum of the vulvar skin after elimination from the vagina.

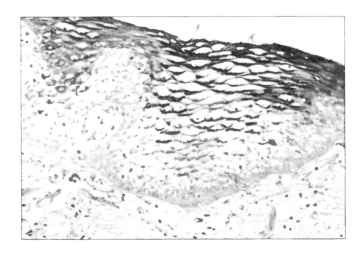

Figure 9.10. Estrogenised vaginal epithelium stained with PAS to show the glycogen granules in the intermediate and superficial cells.

Clinical features
Like many very common clinical disorders, candidiasis can present unusual features and frequently complicates other vulvar epithelial disorders. This condition usually occurs only in females with estrogen levels of the proliferative phase of the menstrual cycle or higher. That is, the newborn, females between puberty and the menopause and postmenopausal women using estrogen replacement. There are, however, important exceptions: Diabetes mellitus predisposes females of all ages to *C. albicans* vulvovaginitis, presumably because of increased blood and urinary glucose (providing a substrate attractive to all yeasts) and diminished resistance to infection. This yeast may readily colonise those infected with human immunodeficiency virus or patients using immunosuppressive agents, sometimes to a life-threatening degree. A most important predisposing factor is antibiotic usage. These drugs are yeast

growth promoters and many women with troublesome candidiasis can pinpoint the onset of their complaint to one or more courses of antibiotics.

Vulvar pruritus is the leading symptom. Some women become aware of change in their vaginal secretions and describe a thick, cheesy discharge with a characteristic odour. The discharge is seldom purulent. Dyspareunia may become intense. The male partner may experience genital irritation from the yeast metabolites giving rise to the misconception of sexual transmission. Premenstrual exacerbation of the symptoms is a feature of this infection because of the increase in vaginal glycogen following the ovulatory peak in estrogen.

Untreated or inappropriately treated vulvovaginal candidiasis can produce serious long-term consequences. These concern genital skin pathology and genital function. Lichen simplex chronicus (**72**) with or without fissuring, excoriation and secondary infection result from the continual scratching and rubbing and is a common example of the former. Sexual function is inevitably impaired if the condition persists long enough because, as with other uncomfortable genital disorders, the ability to become aroused fails and many women will develop secondary vaginismus. Repeated attempts at intercourse under these circumstances results in self-perpetuating dyspareunia and may be one of the commonest causes of the so-called 'vestibulitis syndrome'.

Clinical signs can vary from none (placing a heavy reliance on microbiology) to the severest inflammatory changes, even (rarely) with blisters and ulceration. Typically, however, there is mild to moderate erythema surrounding the introitus. The vaginal epithelium may appear normal or inflamed and exhibit the telltale 'thrush spots'. These consist of vaginal squamous cells matted together by the fungal filaments. They may be a millimetre or two only or constitute a cheese-like membrane coating much of the vaginal wall.

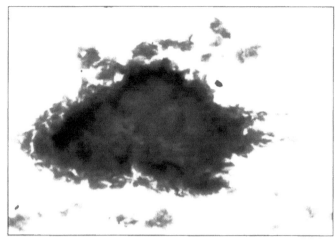

Figure 9.11. A "thrush spot" showing vaginal squamous cells matted together by the fungal mycelium with a few pseudohyphae pulled out as the smear has been made. 100X magnification.

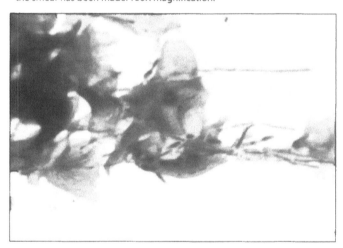

Figure 9.12. Same "thrush spot" as in Fig. 9.11 under 640X magnification showing the relationship between pseudohyphae and vaginal epithelial cells.

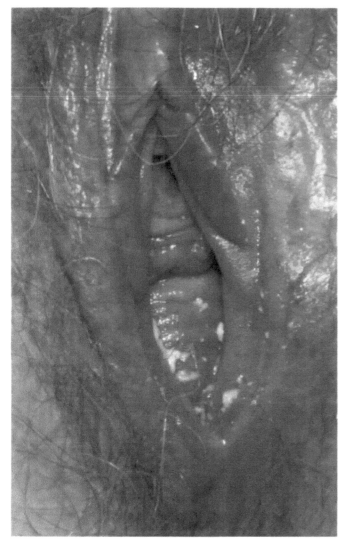

Figure 9.13. Candidiasis.

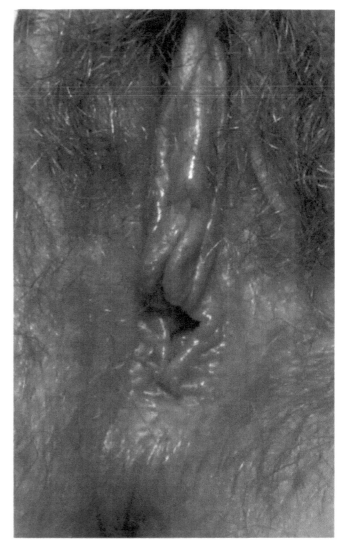

Figure 9.14. Candidiasis presenting as contact dermatitis.

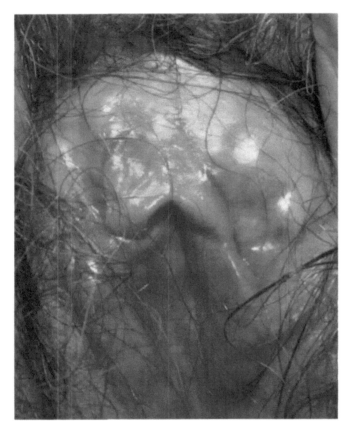

Figure 9.15. Candidiasis presenting with painful fissures.

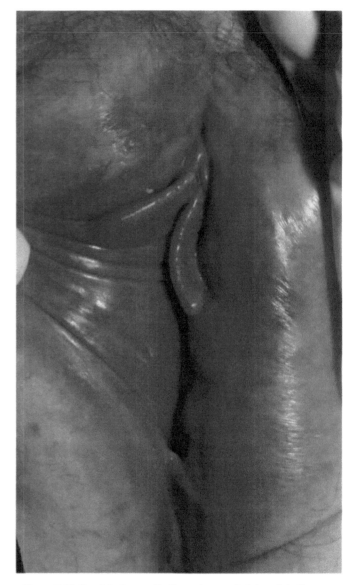

Figure 9.16. Candidiasis complicating vulvar psoriasis in a diabetic.

Diagnosis

A swab is passed the length of the vagina with the labia separated and sent for culture. Unless the woman has used a candidacide within the preceding week (and it is important to enquire), this is the most reliable means of diagnosis. Microscopy (Chapter 1) is about 80% reliable.

Histology has a sensitivity of about 50% compared to culture. Vulvovaginal candidiasis comes into the differential diagnosis of any erythematous rash that shows polymorphs in the stratum corneum and acanthosis on biopsy, particularly psoriasis, impetigenised eczema or excoriated lichen simplex chronicus. The diagnostic pseudohyphae and yeast-forms are not seen on H & E section but require a PAS for visualisation, a mandatory stain on inflammatory vulvar biopsies. Histopathology diagnoses a "fungal infection" and does not readily distinguish between Candida and dermatophytosis.

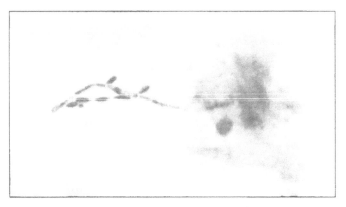

Figure 9.17. C. albicans showing pseudohyphae (the filaments) and budding blastoconidiae.

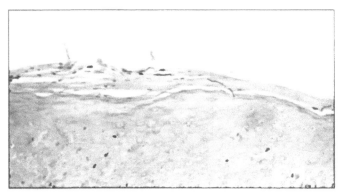

Figure 9.18. Biopsy of vulva from a longstanding case of C albicans infection. It has been stained with PAS and pseudohyphae can be seen in the stratum corneum.

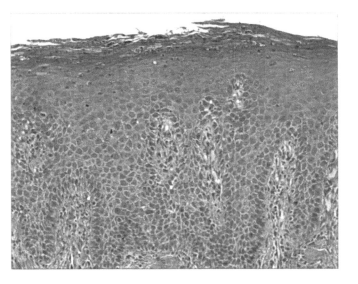

Figure 9.19. Candidiasis: intracorneal pustules and regular acanthosis. These changes may be perfectly mimicked by psoriasis.

Treatment

Many preparations are effective in the treatment of candidiasis. A vaginal imidazole (such as miconazole, clotrimazole or econazole usually as a vaginal cream), inserted nightly for one week, is recommended as the standard treatment for *C. albicans* vulvovaginitis.

Treatment of recurrent candidiasis

There is no generally agreed definition of recurrent candidiasis. However, the infection may be deemed recurrent if there is a proven recurrence less than six months after a similar episode has been successfully treated. Unless further measures are undertaken, experience suggests that recurrences, at an unacceptable frequency, are likely.

Laboratory confirmation of each suspected infection is an integral part of the management. The woman should be advised to have a vaginal swab taken whenever she suspects a recurrence.

There are several strategies for the prevention of recurrent infection. One week of vaginal imidazole is still the treatment of choice when clinical (proven) infection occurs.

Alteration of the vaginal environment

This may be accomplished by a change of contraception to depot medroxyprogesterone acetate (which provides estrogen-free ovulation suppression). For women taking hormone replacement therapy, a lower dose of estrogen can be used.

Long-term vaginal therapy

The nightly insertion of 100,000 units of nystatin in a vaginal cream, tablet or pessary (including during menstruation) can virtually be guaranteed to keep a woman free of candidiasis without producing any significant discharge or irritation during the day. This therapy should continue for six months in the more troublesome cases. It is the treatment of choice for pregnant women who have had more than one proven infection during the pregnancy. Under these circumstances, this prophylaxis should continue until delivery.

Long-term oral therapy

Ketoconazole, fluconazole and itraconazole are effective oral anticandidal drugs. They do not reliably attain concentration in vaginal secretions which is sufficient for them to be recommended as the sole treatment for clinical infection but they are definitely effective for prophylaxis. There is evidence that fluconazole is the most effective and least toxic. The usual dosage of fluconazole for prophylaxis is 100 mg orally twice weekly.

Ketoconazole 200 mg orally daily is over 80% effective in preventing recurrence, but reports of hepatotoxicity and occasionally other adverse effects reduce its attractiveness. Sometimes recurrences will occur unless the dosage is raised to 200 mg twice daily. Six months continuous treatment is recommended.

Treat each recurrence thoroughly

Many women, given ready access to microbiological diagnosis and safe in the knowledge that they can get rapid treatment for each recurrence, will settle on just that - medication with each proven recurrence. In the event of multiple recurrences a recommended regimen is 7 to 14 days continuous use (including during menstruation) of vaginal imidazole cream and a simultaneous course of ketoconazole 200 mg twice daily for five days. In many cases this regimen will reduce the frequency of recurrences.

38. NON-ALBICANS YEAST INFECTION

Although *Candida albicans* is by far the commonest yeast detected by culture of vaginal swabs, particularly in symptomatic women, yeasts of other species of the genus Candida are being detected with increasing frequency. The commonest of these is *Candida* (previously known as *Torulopsis) glabrata.* Other commonly detected species include *C. krusei, C. parapsilosis and C. guilliermondii.*

There is no doubt regarding the potential pathogenicity of *C. albicans* when found in the vagina but the same cannot be said of the non-albicans species. There are two clinically important aspects of non-albicans yeasts. Firstly, they seldom give rise to vulvovaginitis.

Secondly, they are relatively resistant to the azoles and polyenes so effective in the treatment of *C. albicans* vulvovaginitis. It is this latter aspect which probably explains the increasing rate of detection of non-albicans yeasts. That is, they are being selected out with the over-the-counter availability and widespread usage of the azoles and polyenes.

Clinical features

When a non-albicans yeast alone is detected during the investigation of vulvovaginitis, it is advisable to seek another cause and not assume that this yeast is responsible. For example, it is common to see patients with genital contact dermatitis from over use of imidazoles who grow a non-albicans yeast but whose dermatitis resolves with cessation of all medication in spite of persistence of this yeast. However, occasionally women are seen with pruritus, vulvar erythema and possibly discharge. Profuse numbers of non-albicans blastoconidia may be seen on smears made from their vaginal swabs. It is probably reasonable to attempt eradication of the yeast under these circumstances, if no other cause for the presentation can be identified.

Diagnosis

From the above, it can be seen that it is essential to speciate all yeasts grown on vaginal swabs and not to accept a report of "Candida species identified". The germ tube test is done in microbiological laboratories to distinguish albicans from non-albicans species.

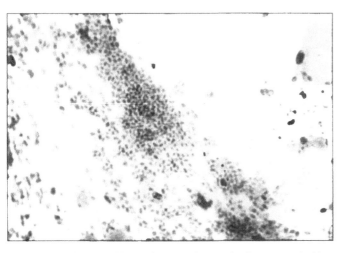

Figure 9.20. Candida glabrata. This vaginal smear has been stained with Wright stain and the purple staining spores can be seen mixed mainly with cervical mucus.

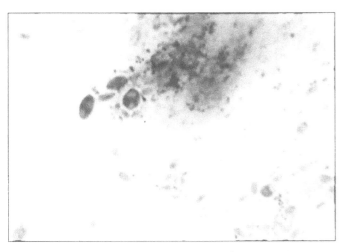

Figure 9.21. Candida glabrata spores 640X magnification (Wright stain).

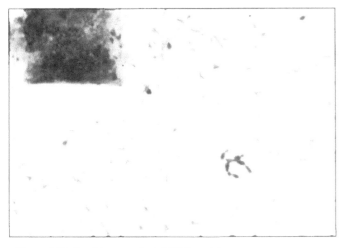

Figure 9.22. Candida parapsilosis (Wright stain).

Treatment

Boric acid is effective against all yeasts including non-albicans species. It can be used as a douche or in gelatin capsules of 500 mg inserted high in the vagina 3 times daily. Gentian violet is also effective but messier. As previously stated, imidazoles and polyenes tend to be ineffective for these yeasts.

39. TINEA CRURIS

Tinea cruris is caused by infection with a dermatophyte, a fungus which normally only parasitises keratin (contrast *Candida* species which affect most commonly the non-keratinised epithelium of the vagina). This disease is also known as ringworm of the groin or dhobie (an Indian laundry worker) itch. The commonest dermatophytes responsible are *Trichophyton rubrum, T. mentagrophytes and Epidermophyton floccosum* which are also common causes of tinea of the feet.

Clinical features

More common in warmer climates (heat and moisture), the patient presents with vulvar itch. She may be known to suffer from tinea pedis or have shared towels or clothing with someone so afflicted.

Examination reveals a well demarcated, erythematous lesion extending from the labia beyond the genitocrural folds out to medial aspect of the thighs. There may be peripheral scaling, vesiculation, nodule or pustule formation and central clearing may be apparent. The vagina is not affected. The clinical appearance may be altered by the empirical use of topical corticosteroids producing the so-called "tinea incognito". With any inflammatory rash not responding to corticosteroids, there should be a high index of suspicion of primary or secondary fungal infection.

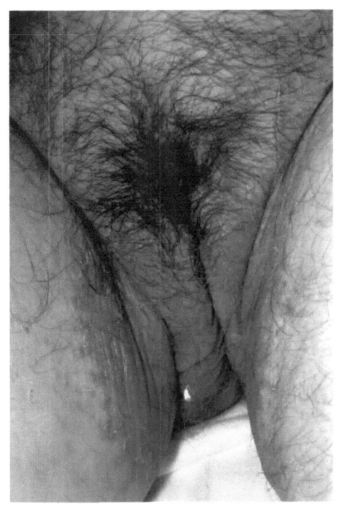

Figure 9.23. Tinea cruris. Note the fine scale on the edge of the lesion on the right thigh.

Diagnosis

Microscopy of scrapings in KOH or culture should provide the diagnosis. The organism is readily cultured.

There is a wide range of histological change. Alterations of the stratum corneum are the key sign, where there may be combinations of neutrophils, compact hyperkeratosis and parakeratosis. The epidermis usually shows mild spongiosis and acanthosis. The dermis shows a mild superficial lymphocytic infiltrate, occasionally with eosinophils and neutrophils. There may be a folliculitis. Like candidiasis, the histopathological features of dermatophytoses may closely resemble psoriasis and excoriated eczematous disease. PAS stain is essential to visualise the organisms.

Treatment

Topical treatment with imidazoles or terbinafine may help but oral medication is necessary for cure, particularly with *T. rubrum*. The following regimens may be used: griseofulvin 500 to 1000mg daily for 4 to 6 weeks, terbinafine 250mg daily for 4 to 6 weeks or itraconazole 100 to 200mg daily for one week of the month for two months.

40. PITYRIASIS VERSICOLOR (TINEA VERSICOLOR)

This relatively mild fungal infection of the stratum corneum is caused by a complex of lipophilic yeasts, often found on healthy skin, now referred to as *Malassezia furfur*. Vulvar involvement is usually only seen in women who manifest the disorder elsewhere, usually upper trunk.

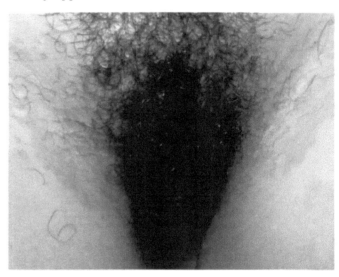

Figure 9.24. Pityriasis versicolor.

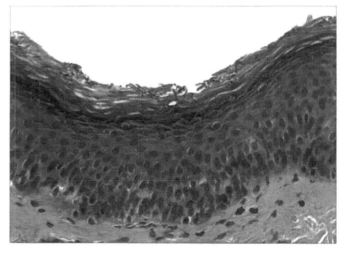

Figure 9.25. Pityriasis versicolor: the routine H & E slide shows the typical "spaghetti and meatballs" organisms in the stratum corneum. By comparison, candidiasis requires a PAS stain to show the organisms.

Clinical features

Pityriasis versicolor may be an incidental finding (particularly on the vulva) in an asymptomatic woman or produce minimal pruritus only. The macules are not very prominent, well demarcated, slightly scaly and slightly erythematous. In dark skinned patients, and occasionally in the light skinned, the macules may be paler than the surrounding skin.

Diagnosis

The morphology of *M. furfur* in scrapings is diagnostic, rendering culture unnecessary. The yeast mycelium consists of short, fragmented filaments with spherical, thick walled conidia, the so-called 'spaghetti and meat balls' appearance.

Treatment

Topical or oral azoles, such as ketoconazole, are effective. Relapse is common.

41 WHITE PIEDRA

White piedra (piedra - Spanish: stone) is a symbiotic infection of the hair shaft by the fungus *Trichosporon beigelli* and certain bacteria. It is more common in tropical climates and is associated with poor hygiene. The lesions may be confused with the nits of pediculosis pubis.

Clinical features

Genital hairs take on a grey or white appearance with tiny, white, adherent nodules on the hair shaft.

Diagnosis

T .biegelli produce characteristic colonies on Sabouraud agar. Microscopic examination of a KOH mount of the hairs may provide the diagnosis.

Treatment

The genital hair is removed by shaving and the area is treated with ketoconazole shampoo or clotrimazole cream. The condition may prove persistent.

Bacteria

PYOGENIC VULVAR INFECTIONS

The vulva, like skin elsewhere, is subject to infection with pyogenic bacteria, usually *Staphylococcus aureus, Streptococci*, coliforms, occasionally others and mixtures of these. The results are essentially the same as extragenital skin infections with these organisms.

Clinical features

42. IMPETIGO refers to superficial infection of the epidermis by the Group A streptococcus and/or *Staphylococcus pyogenes*. It is characterised by superficial lesions with vesicles going on to form crusts. It is uncommon on the vulva. **43. FOLLICULITIS**, where the infection with associated erythema, small pustule formation and discomfort occurs at the level of the ostium of the hair follicle or group of follicles, is common. It is seen on the pubis, labia majora, buttocks and after waxing the 'bikini line'. Deeper infections, often of a solitary hair follicle with *Staphylococcus aureus* or coliforms can go on to **44. ABSCESS** formation (furuncle or boil). In this case, there will be an acutely painful swelling, usually of a labium majus or pubis, with erythema, tenderness and possibly inguinal lymphadenitis. **CARBUNCLE** is the term applied when folliculitis spreads to adjacent tissues resulting in a suppurative lesion with multiple heads. It is more likely to occur in diabetics and the immunocompromised. **45. CELLULITIS** is a diffuse, spreading infection of the loose dermal tissues usually from infection with *Streptococcus pyogenes*. It may result from secondary infection of another dermatosis or excoriation. There is diffuse erythema and swelling and possibly fever and malaise. In the immunocompromised or infirm, cellulitis can be very serious. Erysipelas is a distinctive type of cellulitis with an elevated border which spreads rapidly. Vesiculation may develop at the lower border. Predisposing factors include lymphoedema and diabetes.

Superficial streptococcal infection of anogenital skin accounts for a significant minority of complaints in this area by prepubertal girls. The skin may be bright red and fissured, particularly perianally when it may cause pain on defecation and fecal retention. Purulent vaginal discharge and dysuria may occur. Group A streptococcus will be grown from surface swabs.

The most serious consequence of these pyogenic infections is **46. NECROTISING FASCIITIS** where tissue necrosis (gangrene) occurs. This often lethal complication is generally confined to the elderly with other factors such as diabetes and surgical trauma.

Another manifestation of pyogenic bacterial infection in this area is staphylococcal **47. TOXIC SHOCK SYNDROME**, a life-threatening condition due to a toxin produced by certain strains of *Staphylococcus aureus*. It was first described in healthy menstruating women who use tampons but may also complicate wound infections. Patients present with sudden onset fever, hypotension, mucositis, vomiting, diarrhoea and a rash that resembles a viral exanthem or erythema multiforme.

The above organisms may secondarily infect the cysts that occur in this area such as those of Skene's duct (adjacent to the urethral meatus) or, most importantly, Bartholin's duct (see below).

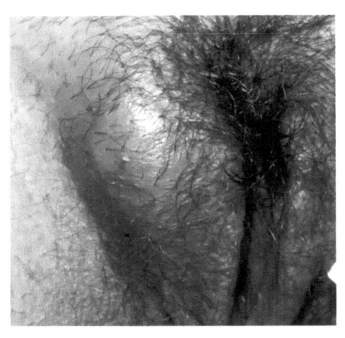

Figure 9.27. Abscess of right labium majus.

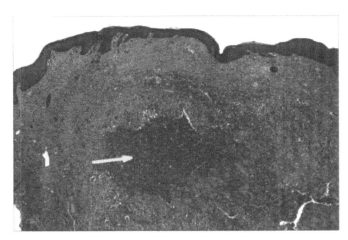

Figure 9.28. Folliculitis: the labium majus shows a nodular inflammatory infiltrate in the dermis with dilatation and polymorphs in the infundibulum of a follicle.

Diagnosis

The diagnosis will usually be made clinically with or without culture of the responsible pathogen.

Histologically, the bullous form of impetigo, which is the common form to be biopsied, shows an intraepidermal pustule containing polymorphs, fibrin, degenerating keratinocytes including acantholytic cells and bacteria. In cellulitis, there is marked dermal edema with numerous polymorphs but no abscesses. In necrotising fasciitis, there is necrosis involving the epidermis, dermis and upper subcutis associated with sheets of polymorphs. Inflammation of the walls of vessels, sometimes with occlusive thrombi, may be seen.

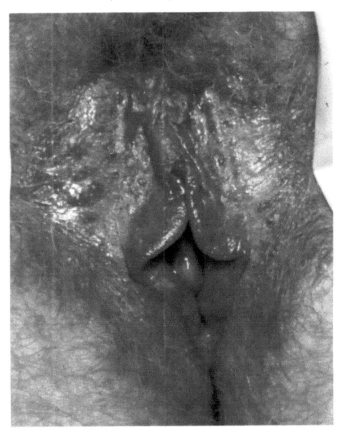

Figure 9.26. Folliculitis.

Treatment

Ideally the treatment of these pyogenic infections should always be based on the identification and sensitivity of the organism or organisms responsible. In practice, this may not be possible or necessary, especially with the minor or superficial infections. These are usually amenable to topical treatment with antibiotic ointments such as those containing mupirocin, neomycin, bacitracin or sodium fusidate or a potent antiseptic such as povidone iodine applied directly to the lesion. Care must be taken with the latter as most potent antiseptics are particularly irritating to genital skin.

The treatment of impetigo is topical mupirocin or neomycin after removal of crusts. More severe cases may require appropriate systemic antibiotic therapy. The deeper and more extensive infections usually require systemic antibiotic therapy, again, preferably after identification of the organism. Cellulitis is most commonly streptococcal in origin and can therefore be expected to be responsive to penicillin.

Superficial streptococcal infection in prepubertal girls will require oral penicillin or erythromycin, preferably for two weeks.

Abscesses must be drained by incision or needle aspiration. Any necrotic tissue must be removed and surgical drainage instituted.

48. INFECTION OF BARTHOLIN'S GLAND

Bartholin's glands are normally impalpable, mucus secreting glands situated at the vaginal introitus at the posterior end of each labium minus. They may became inflamed either as the result of infection by a specific organism with a predilection for the gland, such as the gonococcus (49) or, more commonly, by non-specific infection of a cyst of the gland. These cysts result from obstruction of the duct, usually at or near its opening. This obstruction may result from congenital atresia or narrowing or from infection with the gonococcus but in most cases the cause of the obstruction is unknown. The cysts are usually several centimetres in diameter and are not painful unless infected. Once infected, they enlarge and became acutely painful, constituting the commonest vulvar surgical emergency. Rarely, the gland becomes chronically inflamed for other reasons and the etiology is uncertain.

Clinical features

The woman, almost always in the reproductive years, may or may not have been aware of an antecedent lump (cyst). She presents with an acutely painful swelling on one side of the vulva. Although the woman may ultimately develop infections of both Bartholin's gland, the acute presentation tends to be unilateral.

Examination reveals a tender, red, spherical swelling at the posterior end of the labium minus which may be partly or wholly stretched over it. Depending on the development of the abscess and the infecting organism, there may be ipsilateral inguinal lymphadenitis and/or surrounding cellulitis.

The much less common chronic Bartholinitis presents a quite different picture: Dyspareunia is the likely complaint and the chronically inflamed gland can be felt between finger and thumb as a tender lump, one to two centimetres in diameter at the posterior end of the labium minus, possibly on both sides.

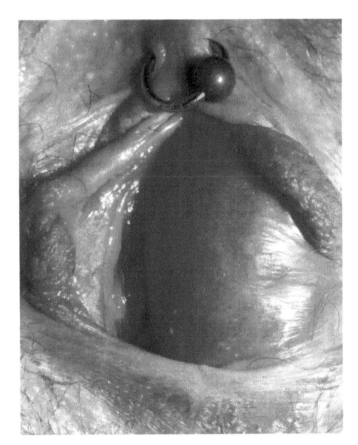

Figure 9.29. Infected cyst of left Bartholin's gland. The stud in the clitoral hood was an incidental finding.

Diagnosis

The contents of an inflamed Bartholin's gland may be sterile, grow mixed organisms, usually vaginal in origin, or occasionally a specific organism such as *Neisseria gonorrhoeae*. It is important to send a swab of the contents for culture even though antibiotics should seldom need to be used in the treatment of these abscesses.

Cysts are lined by one or more of mucinous, transitional or squamous mucosa. Bartholin's gland tissue may be seen adjacent to the cyst. The pathology of a Bartholin's duct abscess is non-specific.

Treatment

The ideal treatment for an infected Bartholin's cyst is the operation of marsupialization performed on the day of presentation. In this procedure, an ellipse of introital skin and underlying cyst wall/pyogenic membrane, about 1/3 the diameter of the cyst itself, is excised, preferably under general anesthesia. The cyst wall is then united to the skin of the cut edge by several, fine, interrupted, absorbable sutures. This procedure should provide a permanent cure (on that side, at least). Compromise procedures such as simple incision or needle aspiration and antibiotics are commonly associated with recurrence. Furthermore, if the cyst is emptied, marsupialization will not be possible until recurrence occurs.

The chronically inflamed Bartholin's gland can be excised. However, because of the vascularity of the area and lack of a plane of dissection, this is not a procedure to be undertaken lightly.

49. GONORRHEA

Neisseria gonorrhoeae, the gonococcus, is a gram-negative diplococcus with typical morphology and is responsible for one of the most important sexually transmitted diseases, gonorrhoea. It infects non-cornified epithelium. In the female, the columnar epithelium of the cervix, the epithelium of the urethra, Bartholin's and periurethral glands are the primary sites of involvement. Ascent of the infection can result in pyosalpinx and infertility.

Clinical features

Approximately 10 or more days after exposure, the woman will experience increased vaginal discharge with or without intermenstrual bleeding and menorrhagia. In a minority, the infection ascends and salpingitis with abdominal pain and fever will be present.

On examination, cervicitis will be apparent and it may be possible to express pus from the urethra or a Bartholin gland. Vulvar ulceration occasionally occurs. Adnexal tenderness and induration may be present on bimanual examination.

Gonorrhoea in children is nearly always due to sexual abuse. Children tend to get an acute gonococcal vulvitis, which is rare in adults

Diagnosis

The finding of Gram negative, intracellular, kidney shaped diplococci on smears made from the swabs from symptomatic patients is fairly certain and is confirmed by culture on selective media and identification by phenotypic methods. Swabs for culture must be taken from urethra, cervix, anus and pharynx. The most sensitive test for gonorrhea, and particularly useful for asymptomatic patients, is PCR/LCR (ligand chain reaction) of swabs from the urethra or cervix or from urine. The usual approach is to use urine (first void) after not passing urine for two hours.

Treatment

Penicillin with or without probenecid has been the classic treatment but antibiotic resistance has become a major problem. Modern regimens may also be influenced by co-infection, particularly with *Chlamydia trachomatis* and include tetracycline, ampicillin, cephalosporins and spectinomycin. Antibiotic selection may require guidance from the results of sensitivity testing in vitro.

50. ACTINOMYCOSIS

Actinomycosis is a sporadically occurring endogenous polymicrobial inflammation in which fermentative actinomycetes of the genera Actinomyces, particularly *Actinomyces israelii,* Propionibacterium and

Bifidobacterium act as the principal pathogens. While any tissue may be affected, the two most important clinical diseases are cervicofacial and gynecological. Gynecological disease is principally IUD-related endometritis and only rarely is the vulva involved.

Clinical features

This infection is encountered most commonly in gynecology in the patient with a long standing intrauterine contraceptive device. The device can be responsible for endometritis from which *A. israelii* is isolated. This may present with vaginal discharge. Genital skin involvement is rare and will present as a discharging abscess, possibly with sinus or fistula formation and surrounding induration. Pus from these lesions characteristically contains 'sulphur granules', which are lobulated masses of intertwining filaments. Regional lymph nodes may be affected.

Diagnosis

Actinomycosis is notoriously difficult to diagnose in a timely and reliable fashion. The diagnosis depends on finding actinomycetic granules histologically and these may be very scarce and require the examination of many sections. Actinomycosis appears as abscesses surrounded by an acute and chronic inflammation and fibrosis. Within the abscesses, the diagnostic actinomycetic granules appear as balls of radiating bacterial filaments.

Culture is not recommended as the results are too difficult to interpret, due to the ubiquitous nature of the organism, which may be normal residential flora.

Treatment

Actinomyces is sensitive to the antibiotics used in the treatment of Gram positive infections. Penicillin is the most useful but high dosage and prolonged treatment is usually necessary. Surgical excision and drainage may also be necessary.

51. ERYTHRASMA

Erythrasma is a mild, possibly asymptomatic but chronic skin infection caused by a group of related coryneform bacteria usually called *Corynebacterium minutissimum*. The lesions produce coproporphyrin and fluoresce pink under Wood's light.

Clinical features

The infection is seen most commonly in the toe clefts but may be found in the groins, genitofemoral regions and natal cleft as well as axillae and other sites. Lesions are superficial, sharply marginated, red or brown and become finely creased and/or scaly.

Diagnosis

Corynebacterium minutissimum may be cultured from scrapings.

Erythrasma is one of the invisible dermatoses and the biopsy appears normal. The small cocco-bacilli can be seen in the stratum corneum on PAS, Gram or silver stains.

Treatment

Topical clotrimazole or miconazole are effective against *C. minutissimum*. Oral erythromycin may be used for extensive lesions.

52. TRICHOMYCOSIS

Trichomycosis is a rare condition resulting from colonisation of genital hair by *Corynebacteria spp.* The affected hairs appear grey and stiff with minute concretions which may be yellow, black or red. Sweat discoloration and malodor may occur. The condition responds to topical antibacterials.

53. DIPHTHERIA

Cutaneous diphtheria may need to be considered in the differential diagnosis of genital ulceration in populations with a low rate of immunisation. The lesions are the result of primary or secondary infection with *Corynebacterium diphtheriae* which is usually associated with throat infections.

Clinical features

The ulcer may be found in the genitocrural flexure. It tends to be superficial, oval or irregularly linear with an overhanging edge and a floor consisting of a grey, adherent membrane. Regional lymph nodes may be enlarged.

Diagnosis

Diagnosis is by culture of a specimen collected by swab.

Treatment

Diphtheria antitoxin and penicillin or erythromycin constitute the treatment of diphtheria.

54. CHANCROID (SOFT CHANCRE)

Haemophilus Ducreyi is the gram-negative, anaerobic bacillus responsible for chancroid, a sexually transmitted infection characterised by genital ulceration and suppurating inguinal lymphadenitis. The disease derives its name from the softness of its ulcer or chancre in contrast to the ulcer of syphilis, the hard chancre.

Clinical features

A week or so after exposure, symptoms that may herald the onset of this condition are pain on voiding and/or defecation, vaginal discharge, dyspareunia or rectal bleeding. The chancre begins as a tender papule which breaks down to become an ulcer. Vesicles do not occur in this condition. More than one ulcer may form and they may become confluent. The edges of the ulcer are soft, ragged and undermined and tend to be remarkably free of pain in the female thereby permitting untreated sex workers to continue spreading the disease. The lesions occur around the introitus and may spread into the vagina. Many patients develop a bubo. This refers to the suppurating inguinal lymph gland, usually unilateral, which is a feature of chancroid. If the bubo ruptures, inguinal ulceration can occur.

Diagnosis

Smears of pus may show Gram negative rods forming parallel chains, the "school of fish" appearance. Smear diagnosis is confirmed by culture from ulcer scrapings or pus from buboes on selective agar. *H. ducreyi* is also diagnosed by PCR.

Chancroid ulcers appear non-specific in routine histology. There is tissue necrosis, fibrin, red blood cells and polymorphs, mixed inflamed granulation tissue and a peripheral infiltrate of lymphocytes and plasma cells. Microabscesses may be present. Adjacent epidermis may show hyperplasia. The organisms may be seen in Giemsa or silver stains as short chains in the ulcer base.

Treatment

H. ducreyi is variably susceptible to many antibiotics, particularly the more recently developed cephalosporins. Ceftriaxone can be curative in a single intramuscular dose of 250mg. Aspiration of a bubo may be required.

55. DONOVANOSIS

The disease, donovanosis, and its causative organism, *Calymmatobacterium granulomatis,* have both had confusing name changes in the past. These include most recently granuloma inguinale, granuloma venereum and *Klebsiella or Donovania granulomatis*. Donovanosis is an infection usually, but not always, sexually transmitted, resulting in genital ulceration with occasional extragenital lesions. It is more common in tropical climates.

Clinical features

One to several weeks after probably repeated exposure, single or multiple papules appear. These break down to form clean, granulomatous lesions which may be painless and gradually spread. The labia are primarily involved but vaginal and cervical extension occasionally results in abnormal vaginal bleeding. Inguinal lymphadenitis is not a feature of the infection but spread of the ulceration itself to the groin may occur.

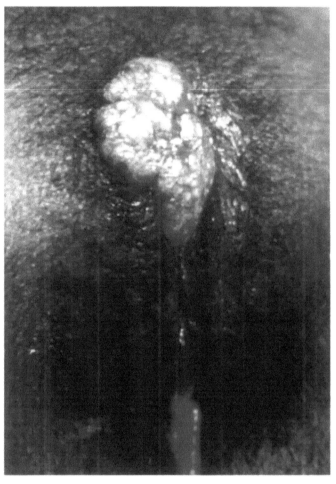

Figure 9.30. Donovanosis. Photo courtesy of Dr. Stuart Aitken.

Diagnosis

Diagnostic tests have improved recently with *Calymmatobacterium granulomatis* now able to be cultured and a polymerase chain reaction (PCR) available. Donovanosis, however, is still readily diagnosed clinically. It is confirmed on Giemsa-stained smears or tissue sections. These show large macrophages containing red-stained, intracytoplasmic encapsulated ovoid structures, 1-2 microns long, with prominent polar granules (Donovan bodies).

Biopsy shows central ulceration and adjacent pseudoepitheliomatous hyperplasia. Plasma cells and pale-staining macrophages (in which the parasites may be seen on Giemsa -stained sections) predominate at the base of the lesion. Scattered neutrophil microabscesses are seen. Pseudoepitheliomatous hyperplasia may be confused with squamous cell carcinoma, which, however, may also occur in long-standing donovanosis

Treatment

Many antibiotic regimens are used with varying success. Azithromycin is currently recommended (1g orally once weekly for 4 weeks or 500mg orally daily for 7 days).

56. MALAKOPLAKIA

Malakoplakia, from the Greek, "malakos" meaning soft and "plakos" meaning plaque, is an uncommon inflammatory disease presenting as soft yellow to pink plaques and nodules. The pathogenesis is an impaired immunological response of monocyte phagocytosis to a variety of mundane and unusual bacterial infections. The most common isolate is *E coli*. Virtually any site in the body may be implicated, but most cases involve the genitourinary system, including the urethra. Skin involvement is rare, but when it occurs, the perianal region is most commonly described. The vagina is another site where malakoplakia has been reported. A number of cases have responded to prolonged courses of antibiotics, which may be combined with local excision.

Pathology

Histological examination shows masses of foamy histiocytes (von Hansemann cells), many of which contain intracytoplasmic calcified spherules, termed Michaelis-Gutman bodies.

57. TUBERCULOSIS

Mycobacterium tuberculosis is responsible for tuberculosis, a highly complex disease capable of affecting any part of the body. It is associated with poverty and a low standard of public health and is a not uncommon infection in patients infected with the human immunodeficiency virus.

The vulva and vagina are least commonly affected by genital tuberculosis (fallopian tube most commonly) and when this region does manifest the disease, the extragenital manifestations are likely to be of greater importance to the patient. As with cutaneous tuberculosis elsewhere, the clinical features are extremely variable. The disease may need to be included in the differential diagnosis of vulvar nodules, ulcers with ragged edges, fungating masses and suppurating lymph nodes, from early childhood onwards.

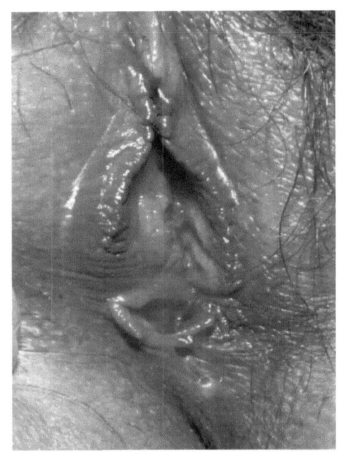

Figure 9.31. Vulvar ulcer in patient with active pulmonary tuberculosis.

Diagnosis

The diagnosis may be made histologically. Culture is more productive and is the standard method. The highest yield is with polymerase chain reaction but contamination can be a problem.

Histologically, the dermis shows tuberculoid granulomas characterised by surrounding lymphocytes, a tendency to confluence and caseation. Langhans' giant cells are characteristic but may not be common. The epidemis may be hyperplastic and transepidermal elimination of granulomas may be observed. Tuberculous bacilli may be found with difficulty in tissue sections or pus on Ziehl-Neelsen staining

Treatment

Treatment of tuberculosis is with systemic antituberculotic therapy with drugs including isoniozid, rifampicin, pyrazinamide and ethambutal, usually in combination. The emergence of strains resistant to these drugs is an increasing problem worldwide.

58. SYPHILIS

Syphilis is a sexually transmitted infection remarkable for the extraordinary diversity of its clinical manifestations. It has been called the great imitator. Its particular importance to the subject of this manual is in the differential diagnosis of genital ulceration. However, wherever there is skin, syphilis needs to be borne in mind when disorders of this organ present with unusual features.

Treponema pallidum is the minute spirochete responsible for syphilis. Its small size requires dark field microscopy or electron microscopy for its demonstration. Untreated, the infection eventually involves most tissues of the body producing different effects over the years. Thus, it is customary to refer to early (primary and secondary) syphilis within the first few months and late or tertiary syphilis occurring one or more years later. As the spirochete is capable of crossing the placenta, there is also a congenital form of the disease.

Clinical features

Approximately 3 weeks after contracting the infection, a dull macule appears in the introital region, becomes raised and then ulcerated. The ulcer, or chancre, is rounded and has a firm edge and a well defined indurated base. Lymph nodes become palpable but, like the chancre, are not particularly tender unless secondarily infected.

Three to 6 weeks later, secondary syphilis develops often as a systemic illness with extragenital skin lesions. Genital manifestations include condylomata lata which are large, raised areas occurring on the vulva and other moist, warm areas. They differ from viral warts by having a flat surface. So-called "mucous patches" may also be found on the vulva. These are very superficial ulcers.

The gumma is the hallmark of late syphilis. This is a granulomatous inflammatory nodule associated with tissue destruction and fibrosis. The extragenital manifestations of tertiary syphilis are likely to be of greater importance to the patient than any gummatous involvement of the genitals.

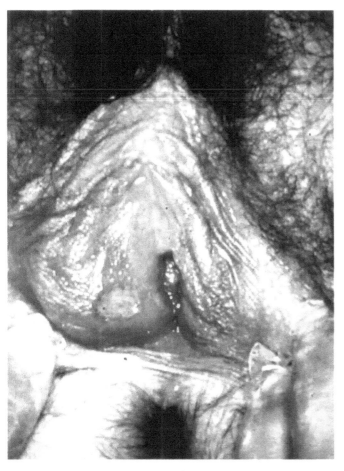

Figure 9.32. Chancre. Photo courtesy of Dr. Ian Denham.

Diagnosis

While microscopy and fluorescence of a smear or tissue from a chancre may identify the spirochaete, the sensitivity is low. The basis of diagnosis of syphilis is serology. Screening is by combinations of the Venereal Disease Research Laboratory (VDRL), rapid plasma reagin (RPR) tests and the *Treponema pallidum* hemagglutination assay (TPHA). Some HIV patients have atypical serologic tests. Confirmation is by IgG fluorescent treponemal antibody absorption test (IgG FTA Abs) or 19- S-IgM FTA Abs.

The histological features of syphilis are as protean as the clinical and depend, to some extent, on the stage. In general, there are acanthosis, a lichenoid tissue reaction, a superficial and deep inflammatory infiltrate (mainly lymphocytic but including plasma cells and histiocytes) and sometimes granulomas. Blood vessels show narrowing due to endothelial cell swelling and proliferation. When faced with any of these manifestations, the pathologist should readily think of syphilis and suggest serology, particularly as interpretation of spirochetal stains in tissue is usually very difficult. Syphilis may be confused with other diseases. In particular, pseudoepitheliomatous hyperplasia in syphilis may mimic squamous cell carcinoma, the lymphoid infiltrate may be nodular and mimic lymphoma, and the granulomatous reaction may mimic granuloma annulare or sarcoidosis.

Treatment and Follow- up

Penicillin remains the antibiotic of choice for syphilis. Follow up testing by VDRL or S-IgM FTA Abs at 3,6,12 months and annually for 4 years after treatment is recommended.

59. CHLAMYDIA TRACHOMATIS OCULOGENITAL INFECTION

C. trachomatis, an obligate intracellular bacterium, is a common cause of sexually transmitted disease, particularly pelvic inflammatory disease, which may be silent, and cause blindness (the end stage of trachoma). It differs from all other bacteria because of its peculiar life cycle which mostly takes place within the host cell thereby making identification difficult. The organism has 3 biotypes, one of which is responsible for lymphogranuloma venereum (60). Infection in females tends to be less symptomatic than in males further impairing understanding of the disease. Clinically, it tends to resemble gonorrhoea because of its predilection for the columnar and transitional epithelia of the urogenital tract. Infection from the maternal genital tract during delivery often causes chlamydial disease of the eye and respiratory tract in neonates

Clinical features

Cervicitis results in a mucopurulent discharge, the commonest symptom. Any urethritis is relatively mild but may cause dysuria. Again like the gonococcus, it is a cause of Bartholinitis.

Diagnosis

Diagnosis is by polymerase chain reaction (PCR) or ligase chain reaction (LCR) performed on cervical swabs taken with special collection swabs or on first voided urine, 2 hours after not passing urine.

Treatment

Tetracycline, ampicillin and doxycycline are all highly effective against *C. trachomatis* oculogenital infection.

Prevention through screening has become a priority and is facilitated by PCR examination of tampons and urine.

60. LYMPHOGRANULOMA VENEREUM (LGV)

This sexually transmitted disease is caused by a biotype (serovars L1, L2, L3) of the *Chlamydia trachomatis* responsible for the oculogenital infection (59). Unlike the oculogenital strains, these biotypes are able to infect lymphoid tissue. It has caused confusion historically because of clinical similarity to syphilis (LGV has early and late manifestations) and chancroid. Other names for it include lymphogranuloma inguinale and tropical bubo. LGV has a world-wide distribution but is most common in West Africa, India, South-East Asia, South America and the Caribbean. It is rare in industrialised countries.

Clinical features

The earliest manifestation is a papule on the posterior vaginal wall, fourchette or elsewhere on the vulva or posterior lip of the cervix. The papule breaks down to form an eroded area, shallow ulcer or herpetiform lesion. Women develop, less frequently than men, the inguinal lymphadenopathy characteristic of the infection. This is a lymphadenitis that can suppurate, break down and form ulcers and sinuses.

A particularly nasty late form of LGV is known as esthiomene (Greek: eating away). Genital lymphangitis and edema result in the vulvar subcutaneous tissue undergoing induration, enlargement and ulceration. This can affect the area, clitoris to anus.

Pathology

The primary ulcer is not commonly biopsied or recognised as LGV. It appears as a non-specific chronic ulcer with frequent plasma cells and some endothelial cell swelling. Thus, it may resemble syphilis. The secondary stage lesion consists of granulomas similar to those seen in cat-scratch disease. These have stellate areas of central necrosis containing polymorphs and cell debris surrounded by palisaded epithelioid histiocytes. Fibrosis becomes prominent in older lesions.

Diagnosis

Serology using the LGV complement fixation test is most commonly used to establish diagnosis. Titres greater or equal to 1:64 are consistent with the diagnosis of LGV. The microimmunofluorescent test is considered more sensitive but is less available. A micro-IF titre greater or equal to 1:512 is considered positive. The organism can also be grown in tissue culture on material collected from ulcers, buboes or rectal swabs.

Treatment

LGV is sensitive to many antibiotics including tetracycline, chloramphenicol, erythromycin, minocycline and rifampicin.

61. BACTERIAL VAGINOSIS

Bacterial vaginosis (BV) is unique amongst the disorders in this manual because it produces symptoms, clinical signs and diagnostic changes but does not produce any disorder of vulvar or vaginal tissues. BV represents a disturbance of the vaginal microbial ecosystem and is one of the commonest causes of patients complaining of vaginal discharge.

For reasons which are poorly understood, the normal vaginal flora, in the reproductive years predominantly lactobacilli, is replaced by largely anaerobic, gram variable coccobacilli consistent with *Gardnerella vaginalis*, Bacteroides species and others including peptostreptococci and Mobiluncus species.

BV is a relatively harmless disorder but of recent years, reports have been appearing suggestive of a link between BV in pregnancy, premature labor and chorioamnionitis. The disorder has been cited as a possible risk factor in pelvic inflammatory disease. Much more research is needed on these more sinister possibilities.

Whether or not BV should be considered as a sexually transmitted infection also remains uncertain. It has been found in virgins and its high recurrence rate is unaffected by treatment of the sexual partner. On the other hand, it is more common in those with multiple sexual partners and the organisms have been cultured from the urethras of the partners of most, but not all, of the women with BV.

Clinical features

Malodorous discharge is the leading symptom of BV. It is the odor, possibly more than the volume of the discharge, which the woman finds most annoying. There is no associated irritation or dyspareunia unless the patient causes irritation by excessive hygiene and/or use of deodorants in an effort to rid herself of the odor. Many women seem unconcerned about having obvious BV presumably because they and/or their partners accept the above symptoms as normal.

The signs of BV are quite characteristic but should still always be confirmed as described below. The discharge is white, unlike the yellow coloration imparted by pus and may contain small bubbles (produced by the anaerobic bacteria). The lack of any associated inflammatory changes (unless the patient has caused any) distinguishes BV from discharge due to vaginitis or cervicitis. Occasionally, BV does coexist with other vaginal infections and this will alter the clinical features depending on the other infecting agent.

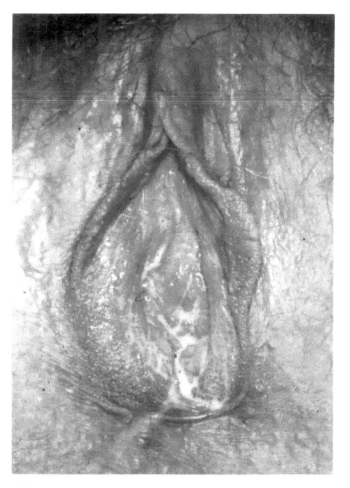

Figure 9.33. Bacterial vaginosis showing the characteristic non-purulent discharge and lack of vulvitis. Photo courtesy of the late Herman Gardner MD of Gardnerella fame.

Diagnosis

Confirmation of BV is best made by microscopic examination of the discharge. Culture of the discharge is important for differential diagnosis but not essential to diagnose BV.

Diagnosis can be made on a stained smear or a wet mount preferably examined with phase contrast. The characteristics are replacement of the usual flora with a profusion of minute coccobacilli imparting a 'dirty, smudged' appearance under low magnification. The coccobacilli adhere to some of the epithelial cells in large numbers and give the cell border an irregular outline, the so-called "clue cell". Moderate to profuse numbers of clue cells are required to make the diagnosis of bacterial vagnisosis. Culture is not recommended for bacterial vaginosis alone but, if it has been performed for another condition, then BV may be suspected by the range of isolates listed above. Polymorphonuclear leukocytes (PMNs) are absent or found only in association with cervical mucus (contrast vaginitis, when PMNs predominate).

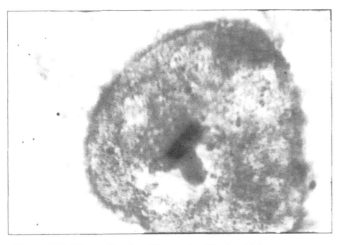

Figure 9.34. "Clue cell" under oil immersion (Wright stain).

Treatment

In view of the relatively harmless nature of BV, explanation of the nature of the disorder may be all that the patient requires, particularly when advised the symptoms wax and wane over time and are likely to get no worse than those experienced at presentation.

Should she still request abolition of the symptoms, clindamycin vaginal cream inserted high into the vagina for 7 consecutive nights is the most effective currently available treatment. Oral or vaginal metronidazole has been used but not with the consistent success of vaginal clindamycin. As already stated, no benefit has been shown from treating the sexual partner.

Recurrence is common a few months after treatment, another reason for not rushing into medication.

A change of contraception to depot medroxyprogesterone acetate will generally render the woman unaware of BV by reducing the volume of vaginal secretions (by means of estrogen-free ovulation suppression). This is often a preferable alternative to repeated courses of clindamycin.

Viruses

62. HERPESVIRUS INFECTION

Genital herpes is caused by the herpes simplex virus (HSV), a member of the Herpesviridae family which includes varicella zoster virus, cytomegalovirus and Epstein-Barr virus. It is one of the commonest sexually transmitted diseases. There is good evidence that its incidence has doubled in the last couple of decades, whereas the incidence of many sexually transmitted infections has fallen. One to two million new cases are managed annually in the USA and 1 in 5 of the population are seropositive to HSV type 2.

Genital herpes is most commonly caused by HSV type 2 whereas orofacial herpes ('cold sores') is usually caused by HSV type 1. In the minority of cases of genital herpes caused by HSV1, the disease tends to be less severe and have a substantially (6 to 10 times) lower incidence of recurrence.

The most serious complication of genital herpes is transmission to the neonate with the production of potentially lethal neonatal herpes. Fortunately, this occurs relatively uncommonly. HSV has been identified as a cofactor in the acquisition, transmission and progression of human immunodeficiency virus disease. These aspects aside, genital herpes seldom causes particularly disabling disease and does not have the permanent sequelae of, say, gonorrhoea and syphilis. Nevertheless, its psychosocial effects are profound and behove the clinician to manage the patient with great care and to particularly avoid incorrect diagnosis.

Herpes virus exists in two forms, one active and replicative and the other latent and dormant. The latent form follows the primary infection and the viral particles persist in this form in the sensory ganglia usually supplying the site of the clinical lesions. As a result, the virus persists throughout the host's lifetime and currently available drugs and host immunity are incapable of eradicating these viral particles.

Asymptomatic viral shedding has been identified as responsible for most of the transmission of the disease to the sexual partner and to the neonate.

Clinical features

Female genital herpes is an episodic illness characterised by the production of vesicles which break down to form shallow ulcers. In addition to the vulva, sites affected include anus, buttocks and cervix. Extragenital HSV2 infection can produce lesions in the oropharyngeal region and even on the fingers. It is customary to speak of primary and recurrent episodes of genital herpes. However, there is now evidence that many so-called primary attacks are merely the first episode of which the woman is aware and the infection has been acquired long before this particular clinical manifestation.

The classical sequence of events is as follows. Approximately one week after acquiring the infection, itching, erythema and pain are experienced in the vulvar region but extending from the mons pubis to the buttocks and occasionally thighs. Some women experience prodromal fever, headache, malaise and muscle pain. Small, painful vesicles appear in the area of discomfort and break down fairly quickly to form shallow ulcers usually less than a centimetre in diameter. Similar lesions form on the cervix and are responsible for vaginal discharge but vaginal lesions are uncommon. The urethra may be involved, with severe dysuria occasionally resulting in acute retention of urine requiring catheterisation. The lesions disappear without scarring in 2 to 3 weeks. Inguinal lymphadenitis is common, irrespective of secondary infection.

At least one more episode is common 6 or more weeks later. The secondary attack is usually much less severe, with fewer and smaller vesicles and ulcers. Some women go on to have recurrences at intervals of one or more months, sometimes at the same stage of the menstrual cycle. Fortunately, true recurrent herpes is the exception rather than the rule but fear of it is widespread in women at risk. Untreated, recurrences of genital herpes lessen with time, making the condition a younger person's disorder.

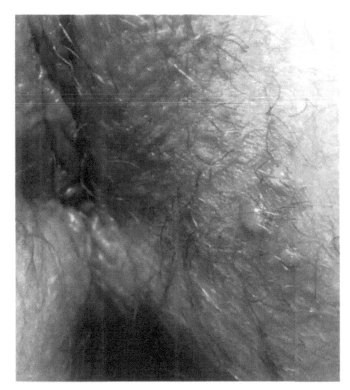

Figure 9.35. Herpes simplex blisters.

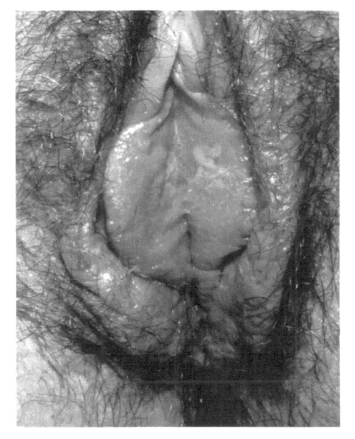

Figure 9.36. Herpes simplex ulcers. Medial aspect left labium minus and posterior right labium majus.

Diagnosis

Rapid diagnosis can be obtained by microscopic examination of a smear made from a freshly opened vesicle after staining with Giemsa, Wright or with immunofluorescence (Tzanck test). The cytopathic effects of the virus should be readily apparent. The virus can also be readily cultured. PCR-based technology has become the method of choice in some laboratories and looks like becoming the "gold standard" for diagnosis but the techniques are too expensive for routine use. Furthermore, due to the extreme sensitivity of PCR, the presence of herpes virus DNA on PCR does not necessarily imply pathogenicity.

Histology shows an intraepidermal vesicle that contains polymorphs, fibrin and squamous cells. Squamous cells show ballooning degeneration, acantholysis, multinucleation and intranuclear inclusions. The dermal changes are an infiltrate of polymorphs and lymphocytes with activated lymphocytes present. Occasionally, herpes may appear confined to a follicle. When herpes is associated with HIV infection, it may appear verrucous with little inflammation, or deeply ulcerated with pseudoepitheliomatous hyperplasia, a combination that can look very much like squamous cell carcinoma of the vulva, clinically and histologically.

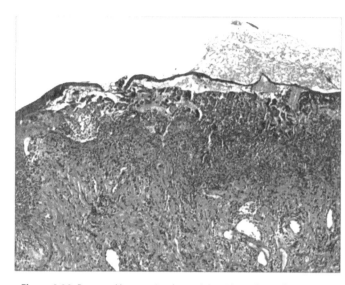

Figure 9.38. Ruptured herpes simplex vesicle with marked inflammation.

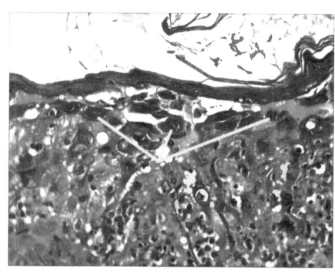

Figure 9.39. Cytopathic effects of herpes simplex: multinucleation, early acantholysis and gray to purple intranuclear inclusions.

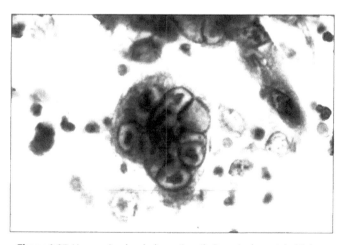

Figure 9.37. Herpes simplex dyskaryotic cells. Papanicolaou stain, high magnification.

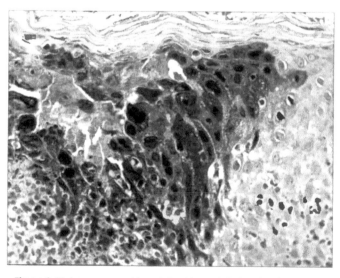

Figure 9.40. Immunoperoxidase stained herpetic lesion showing a marked reaction in the nuclei and cytoplasm of squamous cells.

Treatment

Genital herpes is essentially self-limiting, so with each episode one needs to decide whether or not to treat at all, apart from palliative measures such as analgesics. The anti-viral agents aciclovir, valaciclovir and famciclovir are not curative but will prevent recurrences and, if introduced quickly at sufficient dosage, will lessen the severity and duration of an individual episode. Their greatest use lies in the prevention of recurrences in the woman who is having more than, say, 6 episodes yearly. In this case a prophylactic dosage should be used for one or more years.

No topical preparation (including topical antiviral agents) has been shown to be superior to placebo in the treatment of herpes.

HSV infection in pregnancy

A major source of anxiety regarding genital herpes is the widespread knowledge in the community that the neonate may be infected with the virus by the mother - with a potentially lethal outcome. In fact, neonatal herpes is an uncommon disorder with an incidence variously given as between 1 in 2,500 to 1 in 33,000 births. Furthermore, when it occurs, in the majority of the cases, the source of the infection cannot be shown to be the mother.

The neonate is at greatest risk when a primary episode of herpes with HSV 2 occurs at the time of birth. Conversely, the least risk is with recurrent herpes due to HSV1. Thus, management will be guided where possible by the results of serology and viral swabs.

The usual recommendations for treatment where primary herpes occurs in pregnancy are as follows: No treatment is recommended in the first trimester but consideration should be given to the use of one of the above anti-virals later in the pregnancy. At or near delivery, cesarean section is recommended in addition to giving an anti-viral to mother and baby. Swabs should be taken from the baby immediately after delivery.

With recurrent herpes, the benefits of an anti-viral and cesarean remain uncertain. However, most obstetricians would probably perform cesarean if the woman had clinical herpes at or near term, irrespective of whether it was primary or recurrent.

63. HERPES ZOSTER

Herpes zoster virus (human herpesvirus 3, also known as varicella zoster virus - VZV) is the cause of varicella (chicken pox), when widespread or shingles, when confined to a nerve segment. It is nowhere near the problem on the vulva as that caused by herpes simplex virus. Nevertheless, vulvar herpes zoster (as shingles) has been reported.

Shingles arises from reactivation of the virus in the posterior root ganglia, where it has survived following earlier varicella. Neuritis results and pain is the likely presentation. This will be associated with unilateral, grouped blisters on an erythematous base. The lesions may become generalised in the immunosuppressed patient. Post-herpetic neuralgia is common, particularly in the elderly.

Diagnosis

It is important to distinguish herpes zoster from herpes simplex because of prognosis and the sexual transmissibility of herpes simplex. This is done by serology or viral culture as the histological features of herpes simplex and zoster are identical.

64. CYTOMEGALOVIRUS (CMV) INFECTION

CMV is one of the commonest infecting agents of our species. It is a rare cause of genital ulceration, usually only in the immunosuppressed.

Diagnosis

The diagnosis is usually made on biopsy of genital ulceration in an immunocompromised patient. CMV may be confirmed using serology and/or PCR.

Histologically, CMV infection shows a variable chronic inflammatory infiltrate in which diagnostic inclusions may be seen, particularly in endothelial cells. Intranuclear inclusions are large rounded amphiphilic bodies and the less common cytoplasmic inclusions are multiple, coarse basophilic granules. Immunoperoxidase staining is available and characteristically shows more positive cells than can be readily found on routine staining.

Treatment

Treatment is seldom required but some success has been reported with antiviral agents used when the disease threatens life or sight (retinitis).

65. EPSTEIN BARR VIRUS (EBV)

EBV may rarely cause a severe vulvovaginitis as a primary manifestation of infectious mononucleosis of teenagers and young adults. Diagnosis is serologic.

66. HUMAN PAPILLOMA VIRUS (HPV)

HPV is one of the most important infecting agents in gynecology. It is believed to have infected the genital tracts of over one half of the world's sexually active population making it the commonest sexually transmitted infection. Over 36 HPV types are trophic for anogenital epithelium where the virus exists in a mostly latent (subclinical) form. Its most serious manifestations are cervical neoplasia, less commonly vulvar neoplasia and laryngeal papillomatosis in the offspring of mothers manifesting HPV infection. Fortunately, laryngeal papillomatosis is relatively uncommon (1000 or more new cases annually in the USA). This section will be largely devoted to the commonest clinical manifestation of anogenital HPV infection, warts or condylomata acuminata (singular: condyloma acuminatum).

Human papillomaviruses contain a circular, double-stranded DNA genome about 7900 pairs long. There are over 85 distinct but related genotypes so far molecularly cloned and sequenced with some 65 more provisionally identified by polymerase chain reaction (PCR) amplification. PCR analysis of tissue samples can now be followed by type specific probing sometimes identifying more than one type in the same sample. The different HPV types are trophic for different epithelia with different pathogenic effects, all initially benign. Thus, HPV types -6 and -11 are associated with condylomata acuminata and laryngeal papillomatosis, whereas potentially oncogenic types include -16, 18, 31, 33, 35, 39, 45, 52, 58 and 70. The latter are associated with VIN (130) and VAIN (196) and will be discussed in section 8.

The transition from latent to clinical infection may be associated with immune system and/or tissue change such as physical or biological trauma, stress, pregnancy or immunodeficiency from any cause including iatrogenic and HIV infection. No cure or vaccine for HPV currently exists although much research is taking place with this aim. Thus, treatment is directed solely at elimination of the manifestations of the infection.

In the 1980's, HPV was thought to be responsible for some vulvovaginal lesions other than condylomata, VIN and VAIN. These microscopic lesions were included in the causes of genital discomfort and the misnomer "HPV vulvitis" was often used. Further research has refuted this concept. This is fortunate, because much harm was done to women with these pain syndromes, with attempts to eliminate the virus with tissue destructive modalities such as laser.

Clinical features

The incubation period of this infection is relatively long. Thus, the time from the sexual episode during which the infection was acquired to the appearance of visible warts extends from 3 weeks to months or possibly years. It is the sensation of a lump or growth which attracts the patient's attention rather than itch or pain. Advanced cases may complain of quite severe discomfort and discharge.

Examination reveals the characteristic warty papules which usually appear around the introitus posteriorly but spread to the labia minora, clitoral region, perineum and anus. In a minority, these condylomata acuminata extend into the vagina and may be found on the cervix. The lesions may further spread and coalesce to form cauliflower-like masses. Rapid growth is common in pregnancy. Each lesion has a spiky (acuminate) surface which is more obvious with magnification.

Women often present with a few early lesions which may be difficult to differentiate from the skin tags (squamous papillomata) so common in this region. The difference between these lesions may be obvious if examined with magnification after the application of 5% acetic acid, which turns warts white but has little or no effect on skin tags. Vestibular papillomatosis (3), a variation of normal, may also cause confusion and can be differentiated by the above means.

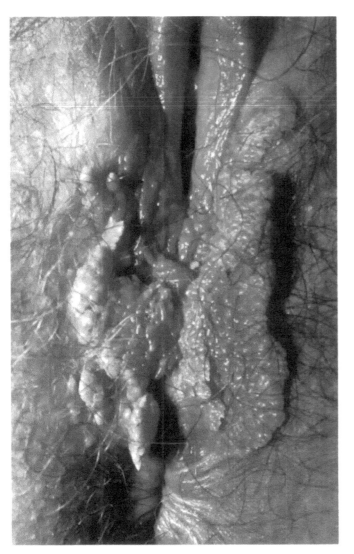

Figure 9.41. Condylomata acuminata.

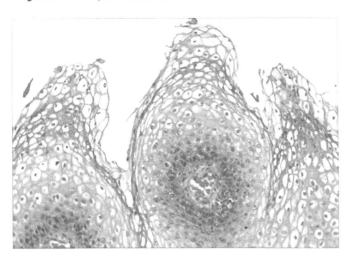

Figure 9.42. Urethral condyloma acuminatum with acuminated (sharp-pointed) projections of squamous epithelium showing koilocytosis.

Diagnosis

The diagnosis is usually made clinically or on biopsy. If necessary, paraffin embedded tissue can be subjected to PCR where the detection of HPV DNA is close to 100%. There is a commercially available nucleic acid test that detects oncogenic virus on a specially collected cervical swab. Other infections, such as candidiasis or trichomoniasis, are often found in conjunction with genital warts. Thus, a vaginal swab should be taken from all new cases.

Condylomata acuminata rather than flat warts are the typical form seen on the vulva. The main histological changes are marked acanthosis, basal cell hyperplasia, hyperkeratosis and papillomatosis. Cytological changes consist of vacuolisation of squamous cells of the upper prickle cell layer and coarse keratohyaline granules of the granular cell layer. The cytological changes are much less prominent than those of many other types of wart and may not be seen in clinically obvious condylomas. Under such circumstances, the pathologist needs to qualify the report to indicate that the diagnosis is not definite. The histological differential diagnosis is seborrheic keratosis.

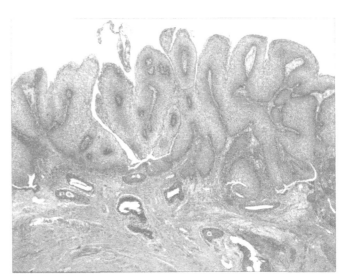

Figure 9.43. Urethral condyloma formed by papillomatosis covered by thickened squamous epithelium.

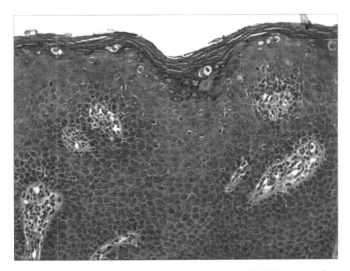

Figure 9.44. Vulvar condyloma: cytopathic evidence of HPV infection of perinuclear haloes and nuclear irregularity distinguishes a condyloma from a seborrheic-keratosis, but is not always seen.

Treatment

Any concomitant infection must be treated or recurrence of the warts is more likely.

Chemical applications are the first line of treatment in most cases. Podophyllin 25% in tinct. benz. co. and trichloracetic acid are suitable chemicals with a high success rate. Each is corrosive and must be used with great care or ulceration can result. Podophyllotoxin, the active principle of the above podophyllin preparation is now available in 0.5% solution and is relatively safe for the patient to apply to herself with the aid of a mirror (2 applications daily for 4 days a week for up to 4 weeks). Ideally, chemical applications (apart from podophyllotoxin) should be carried out by the medical attendant on a weekly basis until the lesions have disappeared. The chemical should be applied only to the lesions themselves with petroleum jelly smeared on the surrounding skin for its protection.

Podophyllin is cytotoxic and can be absorbed into the circulation. Its use is contraindicated in pregnancy and should be restricted where lesions are large and/or confluent.

A recent therapeutic development showing considerable promise is the immunomodifier imiquimod. Imiquimod is not antiviral, it induces interferon when applied to genital warts with subsequent tumor necrosis. It is available in 5% cream form and is applied to the warts nightly, 3 times weekly for 4 to 16 weeks depending on response. It will clear the warts completely in most, but not all women, with a very low recurrence rate. Its cost currently prevents wide usage.

Alternatives to chemical application are diathermy destruction or laser vaporisation. These require local or general anesthesia and possibly carry a higher risk of ulceration with no significantly less risk of recurrence than that seen with chemical application.

A vaccine against type 16 HPV has been produced and is being trialled

Giant condyloma

Giant condyloma is a rare manifestation of HPV infection of the vulva resulting in a large, fungating, verrucous, brown, trabeculated tumor that resembles a non-metastasising carcinoma. It is also known as giant condyloma of Buschke-Loewenstein .

In spite of its formidable appearance, it is relatively benign and grows without distant spread in a "pushing pattern". It may appear at the leading edge of a vaginal prolapse.

Treatment is by wide local excision. Chemical applications and physical means of destruction should not be attempted.

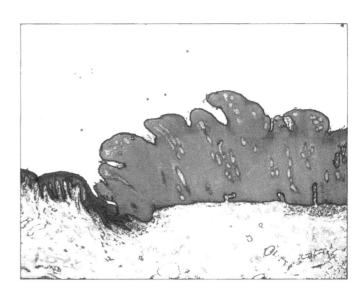

Figure 9.45. Giant vulva condyloma. This condyloma covered a large part of the vulva. Such lesions need to be distinguished from verrucous carcinomas, which are typically non-HPV related.

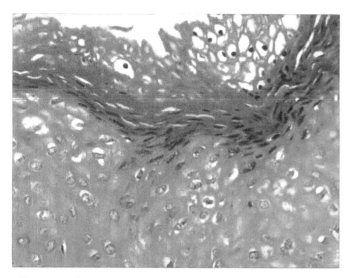

Figure 9.46. Giant vulvar condyloma. Koilocytosis in seen in the surface layers.

67. MOLLUSCUM CONTAGIOSUM

Molluscum contagiosum virus (MCV) is a member of the Poxviridae family and has worldwide distribution. It is responsible for a contagious skin disorder manifested by a variable number of characteristic skin nodules that can occur anywhere on the body, most commonly on the neck, trunk, groin and thighs in children. Lesions spread widely on areas of atopic dermatitis under treatment with corticosteroids and in the late stages of AIDS when they are likely to be refractory to treatment. However, sexual transmission may be the explanation when the lesions are found only in the anogenital area.

Clinical features

The incubation period is between two weeks and six months. Each lesion is a pale, shiny, hemispherical papule usually with a central pore which gradually grows up to 5 to 10 millimetres in diameter. Where genital lesions occur in children, the mode of transmission is uncertain. In young adults, the molluscs predominantly affect the genitalia and the disease is usually sexually transmitted.

Diagnosis

Diagnosis is usually clinical, as the lesions are distinctive. Otherwise, diagnosis may be made on the histology of a lesion or microscopy of material curetted or expressed from the centre of a lesion

Histology shows distinctive pear-shaped, lobules of squamous cells attached to the epidermis and protruding into the dermis. Some appear centred on follicles. Infected cells show cytoplasmic inclusions which change as cells mature. Initially, the inclusions are eosinophilic but towards the surface, they enlarge and become basophilic. They progressively compress the nucleus and when, towards the epidermal surface, the nucleus is lost, the inclusion appears to take over the whole cell. The appearances are distinctive and there is no differential diagnosis, although lesions may be small and require levels to demonstrate.

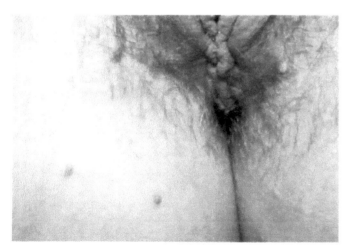

Figure 9.47. Molluscum contagiosum.

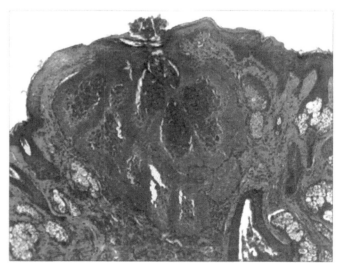

Figure 9.48. Molluscum contagiosum: a cluster of lobules of squamous cells resembling a bunch of grapes descending into the dermis.

Treatment

The lesions can be treated with cryotherapy, expression of the contents of the papule by squeezing its base with forceps or application of povidone iodine. Alternatively, curettage may be used. This also provides material for histology if confirmation of the diagnosis is required.

68. HUMAN IMMUNODEFICIENCY VIRUS (HIV) INFECTION

The acquired immunodeficiency syndrome (AIDS) refers to the clinical manifestations of infection with HIV. First isolated in 1983, HIV is a retrovirus, an RNA virus that replicates via a DNA intermediary. In developed countries, AIDS was originally associated with male homosexuals and intravenous drug users but the incidence of this disease in females is rapidly rising world wide. Factors recognised as responsible for this rise are poverty, prostitution, heterosexual contact (particularly with bisexual men) and intravenous drug users - plus the coexistence of other sexually transmitted diseases interfering with epithelial integrity such as herpes simplex and syphilis. The risks of HIV transmission is also increased in the presence of such STDs because they have been shown to upregulate CCR5, which is a specific vaginal endothelial receptor and coreceptor for HIV transmission. Homozygous genetic defects in the CCR5 gene is the reason some sexual exposures to infection do not result in AIDS. Research is in progress to find a topical agent which blocks the CCR5 receptor.

In patients infected with both HIV and syphilis, the syphilis serology may be negative due to the immunosuppression. This is an example of the difficulties likely to be encountered in the management of two infections which share the ability to manifest themselves in any organ over a prolonged period.

Clinical features

The interval between acquiring HIV infection and the development of clinical disease varies from 14 days to seven years or longer. Extragenital manifestations of AIDS are likely to alert the clinician to the diagnosis. There is no difference in the incidence of opportunistic infections between males and females with the disease.

Sexually transmitted infections are of particular relevance to the vulva with regard to HIV infection. The viral illnesses molluscum contagiosum, herpes and warts show more numerous, larger and atypical lesions. A severe form of ulcerative herpes virus infection with pseudoepitheliomatous hyperplasia affecting the vulva may closely resemble carcinoma, clinically and pathologically.

Ulcerative genital lesions, for example syphilis, are associated with an increased sexual transmission of HIV and, in the presence of HIV, chronic diseases such as syphilis may follow an atypical and shortened course. Scabies, candidiasis and dermatophytosis may be more severe.

Human papillomavirusus (HPV) infection. types 16 and 18 with oncogenic potential are associated with HIV. Thus, HIV infection is associated with an increased incidence of HPV-related premalignant and malignant squamous lesions of the cervix, vagina, vulva, perineum, perianal region and anus. High-grade squamous intraepithelial lesions are part of the CDC classification of HIV and invasive cervical cancer is an AIDS-defining condition. VIN has been reported 29 times more frequently in HIV-infected women than controls. A case of squamous cell carcinoma of the vulva in a 12 year old with vertical transmission of HIV has been recorded. Other important AIDS-related neoplasms that do not specifically target the vulva are Kaposi's sarcoma, uncommon in females and non-Hodgkin's lymphomas.

HIV infected patients suffer an increased incidence of a wide range of dermatoses. There is no predilection for the vulva, although it may be involved as part of a generalised rash. Pruritic papular eruption is the commonest cutaneous manifestation of HIV. Other common diseases are psoriasis, particularly in flexures and drug reactions. Drug reactions are strikingly frequent and often severe.

Diagnosis

The diagnosis of HIV is by serology (EIA) with HIV western blot to confirm. False negative results may occur in the window period (4-6 weeks post infection).

Treatment

AIDS is treated with protease inhibitors and retroviral agents. The highly active antiretroviral therapy (HAART) has more side effects in women with a higher incidence of lipodystrophy. Mortality and opportunistic infections have been substantially reduced. However, treatment may lead to more clinical manifestations of some infections. This is due to improved immune function in immunodeficient patients which restores pathogen-specific immune responses and inflammation in tissues affected by pathogens.

Syphilis has been found to be unusually resistant to treatment in patients infected with HIV.

REFERENCES

Abercrombie PD, Korn AP Vulvar intraepithelial neoplasia in women with HIV AIDS Patient Care STDS 1998; 12: 251-4

Basoglu M, Gul O, Yildirgan I, Balik AA, Ozbey I, Oren D. Fournier's gangrene: a review of fifteen cases. Am Surg 1997; 63: 1019-21

Blair JD, Livinsgtone DG, Vongsnichakul R Tampon-related toxic-shock syndrome. Histopathjologic and clinical findings in a fatal case. Am J Clin Pathol 1982; 78: 372-6

Bleker OP, Smalbraak DJ, Schutte MF. Bartholin's abscess: the role of Chlamydia trachomatis. Genitourin Med 1990; 66: 24-5

Bowden FJ, Tabrizi SN, Garland SM, Fairly CK. Sexually transmitted infections: new diagnostic approaches and treatments. Medical J of Australia 2002; 176: 551-7.

Brady S, Wilson JD. Closing the feedback loop: an audit of the use of imiquimod for the treatment of genital warts. J E A D V 2004; 18:314-7.

Brook I Anaerobic bacteria in suppurative genitourinary infections. J Urol 1989; 141: 889-93

Burstein GR, Workowski KA Sexually transmitted diseases treatment guidelines. Curr Opin Pediatr 2003; 15: 391-7

Carey JC, Klebanoff MA Bacterial vaginosis and other asymptomatic vaginal infections in pregnancy. Curr Womens Health Rep 2001; 1: 14-9

Cheng, Sola X et al. Genital ulcers caused by Epstein-Barr virus. J Am Acad Dermatol 2004; 51:5:824-6.

Cho SY, Kang SY Significance of scotch-tape anal swab technique in diagnosis of Enterobius vermicularis infection. Kisaengchunghak Chapchi 1975; 13: 102-14

Coonrod DV Chlamydial infections Curr Womens Health Rep 2002; 2: 266-75

Czelusta A, Yen Moore AY. Sexually transmitted diseases in HIV infected patients. J Am Acad Dermatol 2000; 43: 409-432

Dayna G, Diven J. An overview of poxviruses. J Am Acad Dermatol 2001; 1-14.

Dennerstein G, Ellis DH. Oestrogen glycogen and vaginal candidiasis. Aust N Z J Obstet Gynaecol 2001; 41(3):326-8.

Dennerstein G, Scurry J, Garland S, Brenan J, Fortune D, Sfameni S, O'Keefe R, Tabrizi S. Human papillomavirus vulvitis: a new disease or an unfortunate mistake? Br J Obstet Gynaecol 1994; 101:992-8.

Dennerstein G. The treatment of Candida vaginitis and vulvitis Aust. Prescriber 2001; 24: 62-4

Dias P, Hillard P, Rauh J Skene's gland abscess with suburethral diverticulum in an adolescent. J Adolesc Health care 1987; 8: 372-5

Diven PG An overview of poxviruses J Am Acad Dermatol 2001; 1-14

Edlow JA. Erythema migrans Med Clin North Am 2002; 86: 239-60

Fagan WA, Collins PC, Pulitzer DR. Verrucous herpes virus infection in human immunodeficiency virus. Arch Pathol Lab Med 1996; 120: 956-8

Friedmann W, Schafer A, Kretschmer R CMV of the vulva and vagina. Geburtshilfe Frauenheilkd 1990; 50: 729-30

Helling-Giese G, Sjaastad A, Poggensee G, Kjetland EF, Richter J, Chitsulo L. et al Female genital schistosomiasis (FGS): relationship between gynaecological and histological findings. Acta Trop 1996; 62: 257-67

Hoerauf A. Control of filarial infections: not the beginning of the end, but more research is needed. Curr Opin Infect Dis 2003; 16: 403-10

Holmes KK, Mardh P, Sparling PF, Lemon SM, Stamm WE, Piot P, Wasserheit JN. Sexually Transmitted Diseases 3rd edition 1999. International. McGraw-Hill

International Herpes Management Forum (useful website with additional information on Varicella zoster virus, Epstein-Barr virus and Cytomegalovirus): www.ihmf.org/

Jamkhedkar PP, Hira SK, Shroff HJ, Lanjewar DN Clinico-epidermiologic features of granuloma inguinale in the era of acquired immune deficiency syndrome. Sex Transm Dis 1998; 25: 196-200

Ko C, Elston D. Pediculosis. J Am Acad Dermatol 2004; 50:1-12.

Koutsky LA et al. A controlled trial of a human papillomavirus type 16 vaccine. New Engl J Med 2002; 347:1645-51

Kreuter A, Schugt I, Hartmann M, Rasokat H, Altmeyer P, Brockmeyer NH Dermatological diseases and signs of HIV infection. Eur J Med Res 2002; 21: 57-62

Laven JS, Vleugels MP, Dofferhoff AS, Bloembergen P. Schistosomiasis haematobium as a cause of vulvar hypertrophy. Eur J Gynecol Reprod Biol 1998; 79: 213-6

Mabey D, Peeling RW Lymphogranuloma venereum Sex Transmit Infect 2002; 78: 90-2

Majewski J, Jablonska S. New treatments for cutaneous human papillomavirus infection. J E A D V 2004; 18:262-4.

Mardh PA Bacterial vaginosis: a threat to reproductive health? Historical perspectives, current knowledge, controversies and research demands Eur J Contracept Reprod Health Care 2000; 5: 208-19

Mc Crary J et al. Varicella-zoster virus. J Am Acad Dermatol 1999; 41:1-14.

Mehregan DR, Mehregan AH, Mehregan DA Cutaneous malacoplakia: a report of two cases with the use of anti-BCG for the detection of organisms. J Am Acad Dermatol 2000; 43: 351-354

Melby PC Recent developments in leishmaniasis. Curr Opin Infect Dis 2002; 15: 485-90

Patel SR, Wiese W, Patel SC, Ohl C, Byrd JC, Estrada CA. Systematic review of diagnostic tests for vaginal trichomoniasis. Infect Dis Obstet Gynecol 2000; 8: 248-57

Peters WA 3rd Bartholonitis after vulvovaginal surgery Am J Obstet Gynecol 1998; 178: 1143-4

Priestly CJF, Jones BM, Dhar J, Goodwin L. What is normal vaginal flora? Genitourin Med 1997;73:23-28.

Ramdial PK Transepithelial elimination of late cutaneous vulvar schistosomiasis Int J Gynecol Pathol 2001; 20: 166-72

Rompalo AM Can syphilis be eradicated from the world. Curr Opin Infect Dis 2001; 14: 41-4

Sanders CJ, Mulder MM. Periurethral gland abscess: aetiology and treatment. Sex Transmit Infect 1998; 74: 276-8

Sardan K, Koranne RV, Sharma RC, Mahajan S. Tuberculosis of the vulva masquerading as a sexually transmitted disease. J Deramtol 2001; 28: 505-7

Sarkar R, Kaur C, Thami GP, Kanwar AJ. Genital elephantiasis. Int J STD AIDS 2002; 13: 427-9

Schwebke JR Update of trichomoniasis Sex Transmit Infect 2002; 78: 378-9

Sobel JD, Wiesenfeld HC, Martens M, Danna P, Hooton TM, Rompalo A, Sperling M, Livengood C, Horowitz B, Von Thron J, Edwards L, Panzer H, Chu TC. Maintenance Fluconazole Therapy for Recurrent Vulvovaginal Candidiasis. N Engl J Med 2004; 351:9:876-883.

Steen LJ, Carbonara PA, Schwartz RA. Arthropods in dermatology. J Am Acad Dermatol 2004; 50:819-42.

Tanyuksel M, Petri WA Jr. Laboratory diagnosis of amebiasis. Clin Microbiol Rev 2003; 16: 713-29

Taylor-Robinson D, McCaffrey M, Pitkin J, Lamont RF Bacterial vaginosis in climacteric and post-menopausal women Int J STD AIDS 2002; 13: 449-52

Veliath AJ, Bansal R, Sankuran V, Rajaram P, Parkash S. Genital amebiasis Int J Gynaecol Obstet 1987; 25: 249-56

Walker DG, Walker GJ Forgotten but not gone: the continuing scourge of congenital syphilis. Lancet Infect Dis 2002; 2: 432-6

Walthar M, Muller R. Diagnosis of human filariases (except onchocerciasis) Adv Parasitol 2003; 53: 149-93

Williams TS, Callen JP, Owen LG. Vulvar disorders in the prepubertal female. Pediatr Ann 1986; 15: 588-9

Zhang W, Li J, McManus DP. Concepts in immunology and diagnosis of hydatid disease. Clin Microbiol Rev 2003; 16: 18-36

Chapter 10

4. NON-INFECTIOUS DERMATOSES

A. Spongiotic dermatitis

Dermatitis (synonymous with eczema) is the prototype of inflammation in the skin and is characterised by dilatation of post-capillary venules in the papillary dermis and edema (spongiosis) of the epidermis. In the acute phase, edema will be manifested by blisters and pain but in the subacute and chronic phase, scale and itch will reflect the edema and inflammation. There are two main groups: exogenous or contact dermatitis and endogenous dermatitis. The latter group refers to atopic dermatitis or dermatitis where the origin appears to be psychogenic or uncertain.

Biopsy, when these conditions are present, is frequently helpful but cannot be relied upon to distinguish one from another. Thus, their pathology will be described jointly.

CONTACT DERMATITIS

Contact dermatitis may be the second commonest (after candidiasis) cause of vulvar discomfort. Like candidiasis, it frequently complicates other dermatoses, usually as a result of inappropriate treatment. A thorough understanding of this condition is essential for the management of the majority of vulvar complaints, especially when they are long standing. Contact dermatitis is subdivided into primary irritant and allergic, depending on its pathogenesis.

69. Primary irritant dermatitis is spongiotic dermatitis produced by local irritants without an immune basis but with a wide range of susceptibility. Vulvar skin has been shown to react more intensely to irritants than forearm skin. The condition is characterised by damage to the lipid containing epidermal barrier and the inflammatory response depends on the strength of the irritant. Frequent, over-zealous washing with excessive use of soaps is a commonly implicated factor. Other irritants can include urine, sweat and local applications such as imidazoles. Vulvovaginal candidiasis is a biologic contact dermatitis of the primary irritant type.

An important form of irritant contact dermatitis is diaper dermatitis or nappy rash. It is seen in infants and incontinent adults. High pH ammoniacal urine activates protease and lipase in feces, adding potent chemical trauma to skin which is macerated and exposed to the friction of the napkin. Secondary infection with Candida and other microorganisms and other irritants such as soap, antiseptics and deodorants aggravate the problem. There may be underlying atopic dermatitis or psoriasis.

70. Allergic contact dermatitis is less frequent but is a true delayed hypersensitivity reaction. The allergen penetrates the epidermal barrier and is presented by Langerhans Cells to T cells to form a clone of sensitized lymphocytes. This sensitization persists indefinitely and rechallenge results in spongiotic dermatitis which is usually mild with pruritus, erythema and scale. In severe cases there may be swelling, blistering and oozing. The causative allergen may be obscure and patch testing, which is a test of delayed hypersensitivity, may be necessary to elucidate the cause.

Sensitivity to medicaments is the most important cause of allergic contact dermatitis and this may explain a therapeutic failure. The ubiquitous paper bag filled with creams and potions used by the patient is well known to dermatologists and this includes over-the-counter as well as prescribed remedies.

Local anesthetic creams, particularly those containing benzocaine, and neomycin are common sensitizers. The stabilizer ethylenediamine and preservatives in cream bases, such as parabens, chlorcresol and benzyl alcohol, may all cause allergic reactions.

Sensitivity to corticosteroids is well documented although rare. Topical imidazoles may cause local irritation but are uncommon sensitizers. Latex sensitivity may be the cause of a contact reaction to condoms.

Perfume sensitivity is common and women are exposed to a plethora of fragrances in soaps, shampoos, body washes and detergents. Local genital exposure to perfumed sanitary napkins and fragranced toilet paper may be important.

From several series of patch tests carried out on patients with vulvar dermatitis it appears that allergic contact dermatitis is an uncommon primary cause of vulvar symptoms but is usually a secondary sensitization of inflamed skin.

Clinical features

Itch is the leading symptom. The patient may be able to relate the onset of the disorder to the application of some form of medication or the use of a hygiene product. Good history taking is important. In more severe cases, swelling, blistering and even ulceration and bleeding may occur. Fissuring of spongiotic skin may be painful (rather than pruritic) due to exposure of the nerve endings in the dermis.

Examination may reveal surprisingly little relative to the magnitude of the complaint. However, there will usually be diffuse erythema with or without swelling and fissuring. Fissuring tends to occur in the interlabial sulci, the folds adjacent to the clitoris and the perineum. Linear excoriations or erosions and eventually lichenification result from scratching and rubbing. Lichenification is manifest by epidermal thickening, exaggerated skin markings ("magnifying glass skin") and usually whitening due to maceration of the exaggerated horny layer.

In diaper dermatitis, erythema and other inflammatory changes are maximal where the skin has been in contact with the diaper, sparing the folds of the groin.

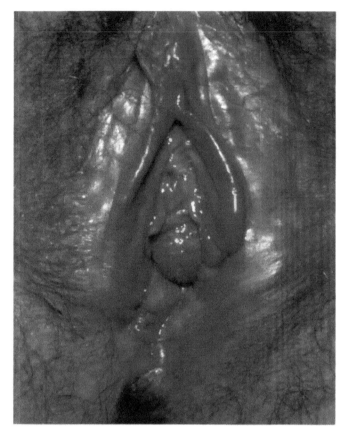

Figure 10.1. Contact dermatitis.

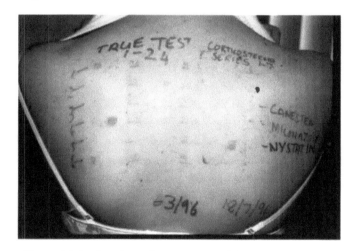

Figure 10.2. Patch testing in the investigation of allergic contact dermatitis. The patches have been removed from the back of the patient's chest after 48 hours showing 3 positive reactions on the left hand side and one on the right.

Diagnosis

Exclusion of infection by vaginal swabbing is essential, particularly as candidiasis may be clinically indistinguishable from or coexist with contact dermatitis.

There is a small but definite place for patch testing when allergic contact dermatitis is suspected and management is proving difficult. It is a test of delayed hypersensitivity where the agents being tested are left in contact with the skin of the back for 48 hours. The application of the patches and interpretation of the results is best managed by a specialized service.

Biopsy will often be helpful in the management of these patients, when the diagnosis is in doubt or when the response to treatment is not as expected (see pathology section below).

Treatment

The measures outlined in Chapter 2 may all be required but avoidance of the chemical or chemicals responsible for the contact dermatitis is paramount. The latter may prove surprisingly difficult particularly when compulsive behaviour is involved, for example with hygiene. Topical steroids will hasten resolution but should not be relied upon as the cure.

For diaper dermatitis, super-absorbent, disposable diapers should be used, soap and other irritants avoided. Bath oil can be added to the water used for bathing and emollients such as equal parts of liquid and white soft paraffin may be applied with benefit. Hydrocortisone 1% cream with an imidazole if indicated may be applied and the diaper should be left off as long as possible.

71. ATOPIC DERMATITIS

Atopy refers to a genetic predisposition toward the development of hypersensitivity reactions against environmental antigens. The atopic syndrome is dermatitis, asthma and allergic rhinitis. While atopic dermatitis usually starts in infancy and is self-limiting, it may continue into adult life or even start in adult life. It is a complex immune reaction mediated by the TH2 subgroup of T helper cells. Resulting cytokines interact with B cells often resulting in raised serum levels of IgE. Exogenous factors may be superimposed.

Clinical features

Atopic dermatitis is a not uncommon cause of vulvar pruritus before and after puberty. The clues to diagnosis are the history of infantile eczema, asthma and/or

hay fever and the extragenital skin involvement. The hair bearing skin of the vulva is affected in a similar manner to the characteristic sites, namely skin flexures, particularly cubital and popliteal fossae and nipples.

The lesions may be quite well demarcated. There may be mild erythema, swelling, scale and commonly linear excoriations and lichenification.

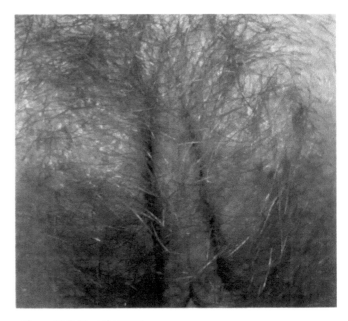

Figure 10.3. Discoid eczema.

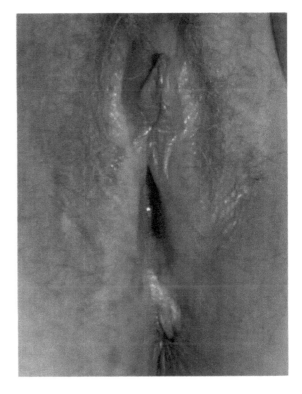

Figure 10.4. Atopic dermatitis.

Treatment

The principles of treatment of atopic dermatitis are outlined in Chapter 2. There is a heavy reliance on topical steroids. The new immunosuppressives tacrolimus and pimicrolimus are also now being used in the treatment of this disorder.

Pathology

Spongiotic dermatitis is the commonest cause of rashes in general dermatology. Likewise on the vulva, spongiotic dermatitis heads the list of biopsy diagnoses in most published vulvar biopsy audits. These all show parakeratosis, spongiosis, lymphocyte exocytosis, psoriasiform hyperplasia and a superficial perivascular lymphohistiocytic dermal infiltrate, which may or may not contain eosinophils (Figs. 10.5 and 10.6). Histology cannot be relied upon to distinguish one from another.

Spongiosis is the histological phenomenon of intercellular edema of squamous cells and is manifest by increased clear spaces between squamous cells with consequent highlighting of the desmosomes. Spongiosis, as distinct from cell shrinkage processing artefact, is always accompanied by increased lymphocytes within the squamous epithelium (lymphocyte exocytosis). Spongiosis may be seen in many dermatoses but is commonest in spongiotic dermatitis

With time and continued irritation, spongiotic dermatitis comes to resemble lichen simplex chronicus. Histologically, the changes of *chronic* spongiotic dermatitis are psoriasifiorm hyperplasia and dermal fibrosis and the diagnostic features of spongiotic dermatitis of parakeratosis, spongiosis and inflammatory cells may no longer be identified. Excoriation (from scratching) is characterised by parakeratotic scale crust, spongiosis and lymphocyte exocytosis in the upper epidermis, changes which resemble fungal infection and psoriasis.

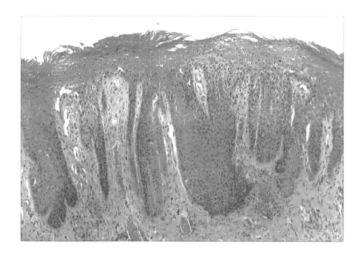

Figure 10.5. Vulva. Spongiotic dermatitis due to atopic dermatitis with evidence of irritation: parakeratosis and regular acanthosis, dermal fibrosis.

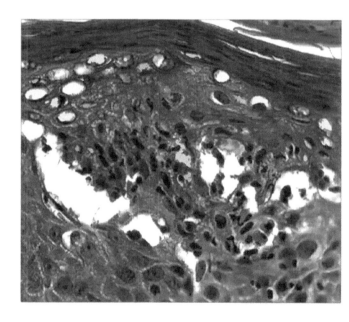

Figure 10.6. Vulva. Acute contact dermatitis with a collection of eosinophils in the prickle cell layer.

B. Psoriasiform dermatitis

Psoriasiform dermatitis is defined as a non-infectious dermatosis where the tissue reaction is characterised by acanthosis with regular elongation of rete ridges. The two main vulvar psoriasiform dermatoses are lichen simplex chronicus and psoriasis

72. LICHEN SIMPLEX CHRONICUS

Lichenification is the term used in clinical dermatology to describe thickening of the skin in response to rubbing or scratching. Lichen simplex chronicus (LSC) is one of the commonest of the skin disorders and refers to lichenified skin where no other pathology is diagnosed. The woman may have started the process in response to a pruritic disorder, such as atopic dermatitis or candidiasis (in remission when she presents) or she may have started traumatizing the area because of a behavioral anomaly. Irrespective of the cause, an itch-scratch cycle is established and the condition will self-perpetuate.

Vulvar LSC is common and has caused gynecologists much confusion and concern. Until the last decade or so, the term leukoplakia was used to describe the condition where the thickened skin took on a white appearance due to maceration in the moist environment of the vulva. Although purely a descriptive term, leukoplakia was considered a diagnosis and confused with premalignant disorders. Historically, numerous inappropriate vulvectomies were performed for "leukoplakia" and the term should no longer be used.

Clinical features

Itch, often of long duration (even decades), is the presenting symptom. It tends to be worse at night when the patient is in bed and this is the time when much of the scratching takes place. Exacerbation with stress and sleep disorders is common and should be asked about. Because LSC tends to be external to the introitus, it may or may not interfere with sexual function. The woman will have tried numerous treatments, prescribed, over-the-counter and home remedies and it is important to enquire about these. Trauma to the area by means more subtle than scratching may be used such as the use of rough towels or even brushes. For this reason, a hygiene history can be helpful. The woman with vulvar LSC frequently suspects that the condition is infection related.

Examination will reveal a variable degree of thickening of the skin mainly of the labia majora, pubis, perineum or perianal region. Hair may be absent or distorted as a result of the chronic trauma. Exaggeration of skin markings is a useful sign. If moist, the thickened keratin layer will become white. Fissuring and/or excoriation may be apparent.

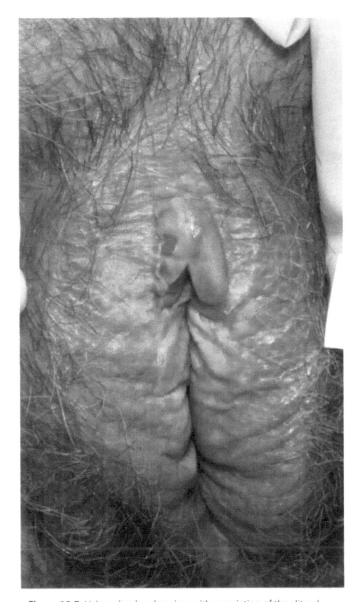

Figure 10.7. Lichen simplex chronicus with excoriation of the clitoral hood.

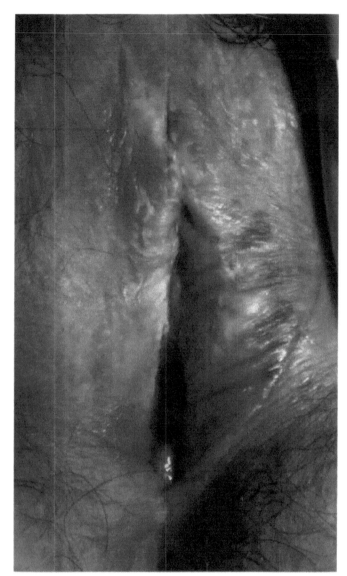

Figure 10.8. Lichen simplex chronicus with fissuring of the interlabial sulcus to the right of the clitoris.

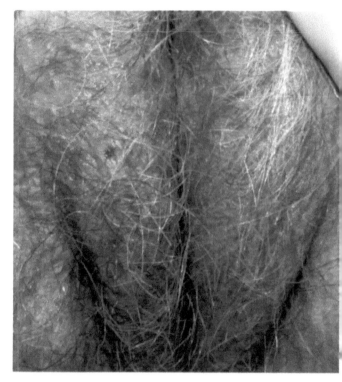

Figure 10.9. Lichen simplex chronicus mainly of right labium majus with excoriation.

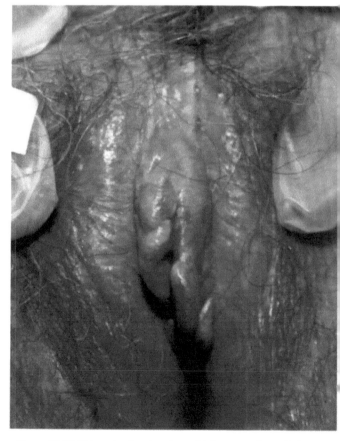

Figure 10.10. Lichen simplex chronicus with fissures and excoriations that have partly healed.

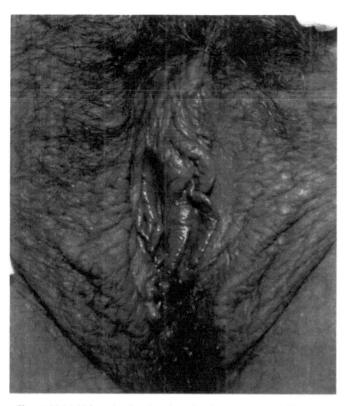

Figure 10.11. Lichen simplex chronicus showing exaggerated skin markings and sparse hair as a result of rubbing.

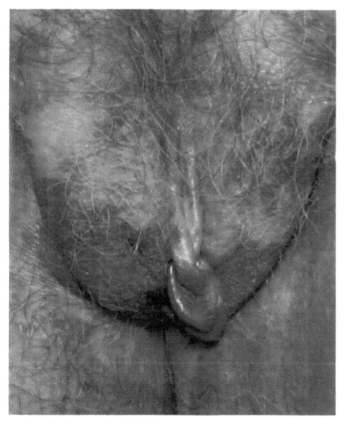

igure 10.12. Lichen simplex chronicus with vitiligo.

Pathology

While there are characteristic clinicopathological features of LSC, the diagnosis also rests on exclusion of other causes of chronic itch. It is essential to look for candidiasis in these patients and a vaginal swab must be sent for culture. Be warned, however, that a non-albicans yeast will be grown not infrequently because *C. albicans* will have usually been selected out by the anticandidals these patients will have tried and to which non-albicans yeasts are usually resistant. Non-albicans yeasts rarely cause pruritus resulting in LSC.

A serum ferritin estimation may be useful as iron deficiency has been implicated as a contributing factor in some cases of LSC.

Because clinical diagnosis may be straightforward, it is not unreasonable to commence treatment without histological confirmation. However, should the patient not respond as expected in, say 2 to 3 weeks, then biopsy is indicated

The histological changes of lichen simplex chronicus are hyperkeratosis, hypergranulosis, acanthosis with regularly elongated rete ridges, dermal fibrosis, in particular, vertical streaks of coarse collagen in the papillary dermis and a mild superficial perivascular lymphohistiocytic infiltrate.

There is only a moderate correlation between clinical and histological diagnoses of LSC. We have found that when skin with a clinical diagnosis of LSC is biopsied, in about 20% of cases, another dermatosis, particularly spongiotic dermatitis, may be identifiable histologically. Conversely, when clinicians have diagnosed another chronic dermatosis on the vulva, in about 20% of cases the pathologist sees only the changes of lichen simplex chronicus.

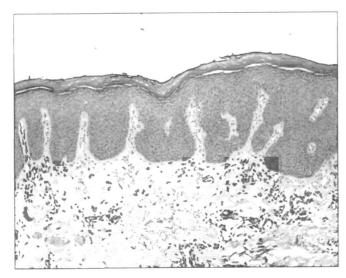

Figure 10.13. Vulva. Lichen simplex chronicus. Hyperkeratosis, regular acanthosis, dermal fibrosis and mild dermal superficial perivascular lymphocytic infiltrate.

Treatment

It is necessary to break the itch-scratch cycle by topical steroid usage and behavioral modification (similar to contact dermatitis). LSC is likely to require mid-strength or potent steroids (see Table 1 in Chapter 2). Formal counseling may be beneficial for the patient with LSC, particularly in the clinic setting and the reader is referred to the psychologist's chapter in this manual. The patient must understand that topical steroids alone will rarely cure LSC. Sedation, particularly nocturnal, may be necessary in the more severe cases in order to stop the patient scratching. Occasionally admission to hospital to carry out the above treatment in a controlled environment is required and is remarkably beneficial when all else seems to fail.

73. INTERTRIGO

Intertrigo (Latin: rubbing between) is a common complication of obesity. It is a dermatological response to frictional trauma. Thus, it is commonly seen in the genitocrural folds of obese women where skin surfaces are constantly in contact resulting in friction, sweating and secondary infection with *Staphylococcus aureus* and *Candida albicans*.

Clinical features

The patient may seem unaware of what appears to the examiner a significant rash or complain of itching, discomfort or moisture in the area.

The lesion is a well demarcated, erythematous, macular rash with the cardinal sign of accurate matching of the lesions when the rubbing surfaces are brought together.

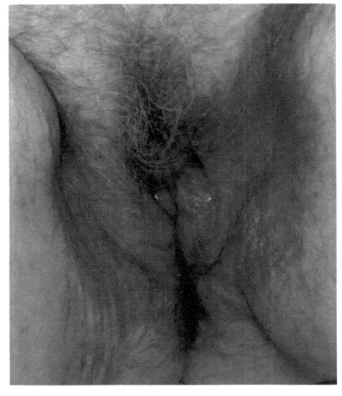

Figure 10.14. Intertrigo.

Diagnosis

In more difficult cases, swabs and skin scrapings should be sent for culture and glucose tolerance assessed. Biopsy may be necessary because of easy confusion with other flexural eruptions including psoriasis, contact dermatitis and tinea cruris. Histologically, intertrigo is indistinguishable from lichen simplex chronicus.

Treatment

Separation of the involved surfaces should be attempted although this may be difficult without significant weight loss. If the woman is diabetic, good control of the diabetes is important. Elimination of bacterial and candidal infections are essential. Topical corticosteroids and saline soaks are other useful measures. The multifactorial etiology of intertrigo may justify the use of 'shot gun therapy' such as triamcinolone acetonide/neomycin sulphate/gramicidin/nystatin cream.

74. PSORIASIS (including seborrheic dermatitis)

Psoriasis is a genetic condition which affects about 2% of the population. It is an autoimmune disease mediated by the TH1 subgroup of helper T cells. Increased expression of TH1 cytokines in psoriasis causes the inflammatory response and rapid cell turnover. It is the latter which gives rise to the characteristic silvery scale of the disorder typically seen on the knees, elbows and scalp. Triggering factors may be respiratory infections, stress and drugs including beta blockers and lithium.

Onset may be at any age but peak incidence occurs from 15 to 25 and 45 to 55 years. Diaper rash in babies sometimes resembles psoriasis ('psoriasiform diaper rash'). This may be an early manifestation of psoriasis. Psoriasis occasionally presents for the first time on the vulva and can cause diagnostic confusion when this happens.

75. Seborrheic dermatitis is an ill defined condition which clinically and histologically is identical to psoriasis involving the scalp and skin flexures. The pathogenesis of seborrheic dermatitis has always been obscure, although it has been claimed that *Malassezia* (previously known as *Pityrosporum*) yeasts are the cause. That being the case, it could provide an explanation for the reported increased incidence with early Human Immunodeficiency Virus (HIV) infection. Psoriasis has an increased incidence with HIV infection and *Malassezia* yeasts may increase because of a favorable milieu for their growth.

Seborrheic dermatitis, as seen on the face and in other non-genital sites, shows histological features which are seen on the epidermal lips of follicular ostia and overlap dermatitis and psoriasis.

While seborrheic dermatitis has been listed as one of the commonest vulvar dermatoses in some of the older gynecological textbooks, it has dropped out of favor. We did not feel the need to make a diagnosis of seborrheic dermatitis in 1200 consecutive new patients seen at the Dermogynaecology Clinic at the Mercy Hospital for Women, Melbourne, but diagnosed vulvar psoriasis in 20 women (and considerably more with spongiotic dermatitis) in the same cohort.

Clinical features

The clue to the diagnosis of vulvar psoriasis is the presence of the characteristic extragenital lesions and a search should be made for these when this diagnosis is suspected. These lesions may not be widespread and the patient may not have been previously aware that she was a psoriasis sufferer and may have, for example, assumed a scaly psoriatic scalp lesion was dandruff.

Pruritus is the usual symptom. It may vary from mild to quite severe. Women may not be aware that they have vulvar psoriasis until they develop infection with *Candida albicans*.

Vulvar psoriasis may cover most of the vulvar skin with characteristic involvement of the natal cleft with fissuring where the process is well developed. The lesion is well demarcated (unlike dermatitis) and erythematous but, unlike extragenital psoriasis, scale is absent. The labia minora, clitoris, vestibule and vagina are spared. The prognosis is variable but relapse is generally the rule.

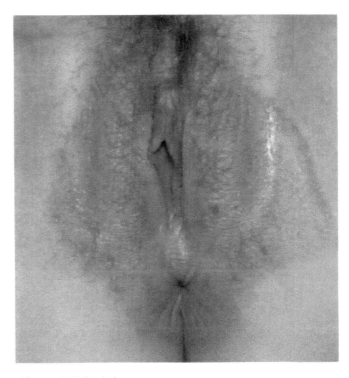

Figure 10.15. Psoriasis.

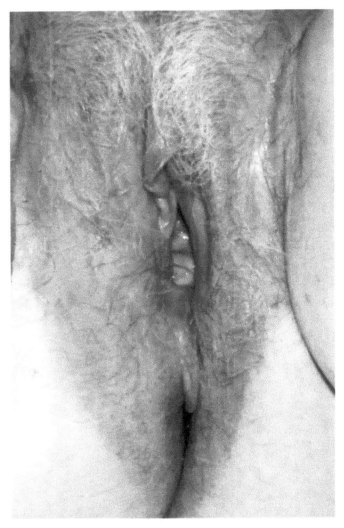

Figure 10.16. Psoriasis.

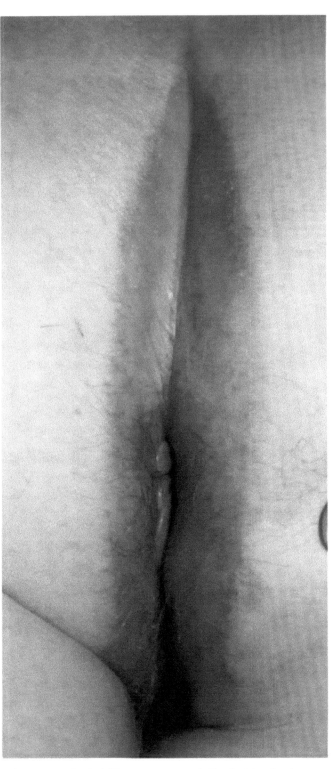

Figure 10.17. Psoriasis. The same patient as in Fig 10.16 showing the characteristic extension into the natal cleft.

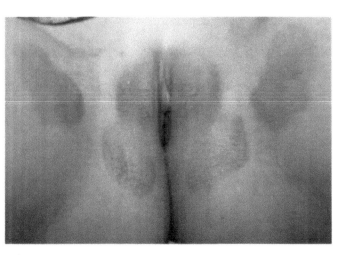

Figure 10.18. Psoriasis in a prepubertal girl.

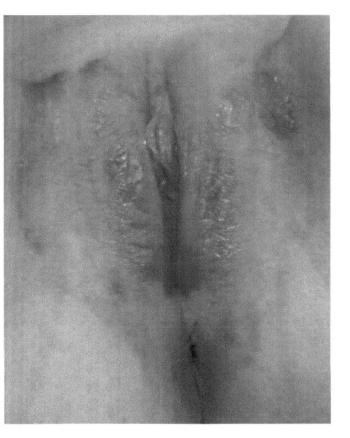

Figure 10.19. Childhood psoriasis. Note labial and perineal lichenification.

Pathology

C.albicans infection may be responsible for the patient's awareness of the psoriasis, so a vaginal swab is essential.

The histological changes of psoriasis are polymorphs at the summits of parakeratotic mounds, subcorneal collections of polymorphs associated with spongiosis, acanthosis with regular elongation of rete ridges, frequent mitoses and suprapapillary thinning. The dermal changes are edematous papillae with dilated vessels and occasional polymorphs and a superficial perivascular lymphohistiocytic infiltrate. Early lesions have less parakeratosis and polymorphs and mainly show mild irregular acanthosis, reactive changes in squamous cell nuclei and increased mitoses. Chronic lesions tend to lose some of their diagnostic features and come to resemble lichen simplex chronicus. It should be remembered that these changes may be seen in fungal infection, the principle differential diagnosis.

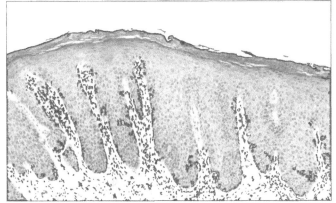

Figure 10.20. Vulvar psoriasis. The features are parakeratosis, regular acanthosis, papillary dermal edema and perivascular lymphocytic infiltrate.

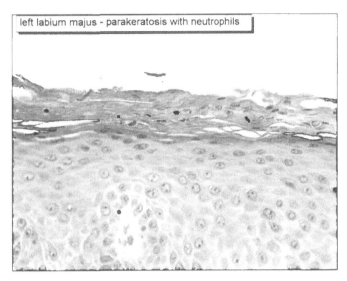

left labium majus - parakeratosis with neutrophils

Figure 10.21. Vulvar psoriasis with parakeratosis containing a mound of neutrophils.

Treatment

Topical corticosteroid therapy is effective for vulvar psoriasis and the other treatments for extragenital psoriasis should not be necessary. Patient education on the care of compromised genital skin is important and secondary infection should be sought and treated appropriately.

76. REITER'S SYNDROME (CIRCINATE VULVITIS)

Reiter's syndrome consists of the combination of arthritis, urethritis and conjunctivitis. It is associated with *Chlamydia trachomatis* or some other infections. There have been occasional case reports of this syndrome also manifesting vulvar ulceration, pustules, erosions, erythema and verrucous lesions affecting most of the vulva out to and including the genitofemoral folds. In a couple of reports, the erosions were grouped in a circinate distribution resembling the more common circinate balanitis of the male, hence the name 'circinate vulvitis'.

Pathology

On biopsy, the vulvar lesions have demonstrated hyperkeratosis, acanthosis, microabscesses deep in the epidermis and a dermal inflammatory infiltrate with focal multinucleated giant cells. Direct immunofluorescence is negative.

C. Lichenoid Dermatitis

Lichen is a firm, mossy plant that grows on the surfaces of rocks and tree trunks. The fanciful resemblance of lichen to the firm flat-topped violaceous papules of a common dermatosis provides its name, lichen planus. Lichen planus is the prototype of a family of conditions termed the 'lichenoid dermatoses' that share two key histological features: vacuolar degeneration of the basal layer of the epidermis and a band-like infiltrate of chronic inflammatory cells in the dermis, usually hugging the epidermis. Their common pathogenesis involves a lymphocyte-mediated attack on the basal keratinocyte. Graft versus host disease (GVH) provides an understandable model for the lichenoid dermatoses. In GVH, viable T lymphocytes from the bone marrow of a donor attack various cells of the recipient in patients who have had a bone marrow transplant. The autoimmune nature of many of the lichenoid dermatoses is reflected in an increased familial incidence and an association with each other and with autoimmune internal organ diseases. The lichenoid dermatoses that affect the vulva include the most important chronic vulvar dermatosis, lichen sclerosus.

77. LICHEN SCLEROSUS

Lichen sclerosus is a chronic dermatosis that may be seen at virtually any age except the perinatal period, in either sex and on virtually any site on the body except the palms and soles. It is commonest in females (sex ratio 4-6:1), the early post-menopausal years (mean 55 years) and on the vulva (95%).

Vulvar lichen sclerosus (LS) has been increasingly well recognised as a distinct entity as a result of the greater use of biopsy and because the histopathology of LS is usually straightforward and characteristic. Previous confusing terminology has also impaired its recognition. The following terms have been used in the past to describe the condition and have no place today: lichen sclerosus et atrophicus, kraurosis vulvae, leukoplakia, dystrophy, guttate scleroderma, guttate morphea and white spot disease.

The vulva is the commonest site of occurrence of LS but the average gynecologist would only see a small number of new cases in a lifetime. It is, however, one of the commonest diseases seen in clinics specialising in vulvar disorders.

The cause of LS is unknown but it does have features suggesting an autoimmune basis. Circulating autoantibodies to extracellular matrix protein 1 ("Nature's biological glue") have been demonstrated in the majority of patients. The levels of these antibodies are particularly high in late disease. The condition will recur in the same place after excision. No infective agent has ever been implicated in its cause.

Clinical features

Most women present in middle age or older, although a minority of cases are prepubertal girls. Vulvar itch is the commonest presenting symptom. Dyspareunia may occur as the condition advances. The patient or her medical attendant may be alarmed by the appearance of the condition.

The vulva surrounding the introitus, perineum and often around the anus (figure of 8 distribution) assumes a white appearance, which may be even and symmetrical, or patchy. The outer labia majora, pubis and vagina are spared. Ecchymoses form readily. Telangiectasia, vesicles and bullae are less common. The process usually thickens the skin but tissue paper-like thinning also occurs. A most important sign is alteration of the vulvar architecture. There may be a variable degree of resorption of the labia minora and phimosis of the clitoral hood. Introital stenosis may occur resulting in fissuring of the fourchette and/or the vestibule anteriorly when intercourse is attempted. The epidermis is readily scratched or rubbed off, particularly over ecchymoses, resulting in erosion or ulceration. In a small percentage of cases, relatively asymptomatic extragenital lesions of similar appearance are found on the upper trunk or occasionally elsewhere.

Most (but not all) childhood LS regresses at puberty but the condition tends to be very chronic in the older woman. Childhood LS may be mistaken for sexual abuse with disastrous consequences if the possibility is mentioned to the parents. Biopsy under general anesthetic is preferable to such a mistake.

LS very occasionally coexists with genital lichen planus producing substantially greater anatomical distortion.

LS has been considered potentially premalignant because it is not infrequently found adjacent to vulvar squamous cell carcinoma and long term follow-up studies have shown carcinoma developing in 1-4%. Our experience has been that it is extremely rare to see invasive cancer complicate adequately managed LS. Nevertheless, any suspicious change, particularly ulceration not responding readily to treatment, must be examined for malignancy by biopsy and/or cytology of scrapings taken with a scalpel blade.

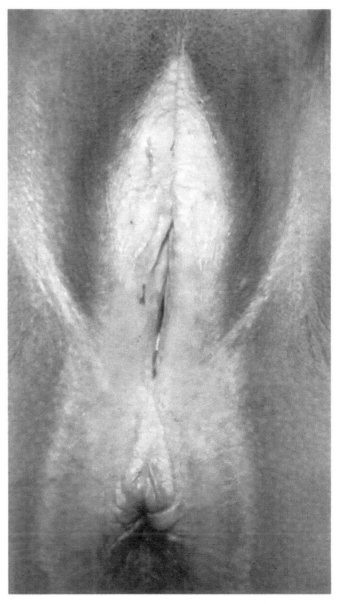

Figure 10.22. Lichen sclerosus showing the characteristic figure of 8 distribution.

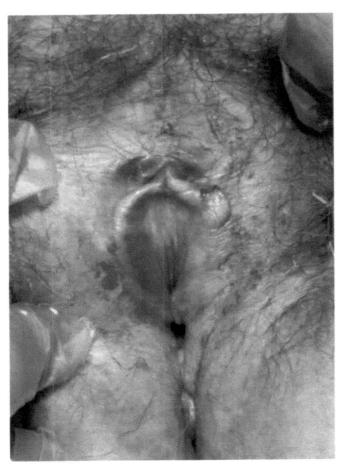

Figure 10.23. Lichen sclerosus showing ecchymoses especially lateral to the partly absorbed labia minora.

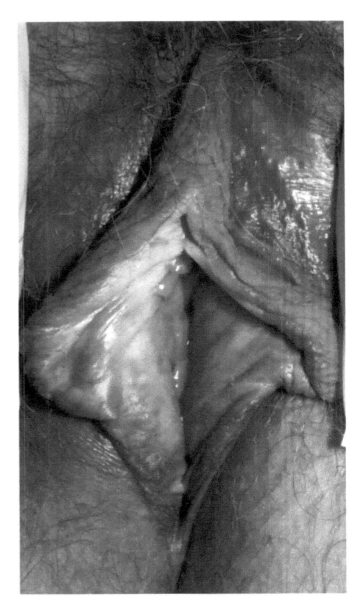

Figure 10.24. Asymmetric lichen sclerosus.

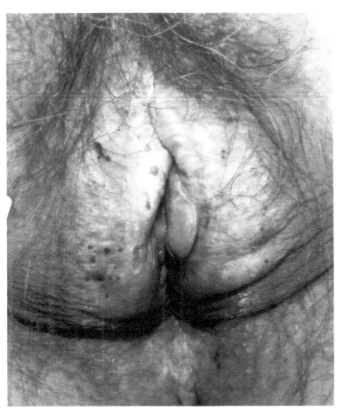

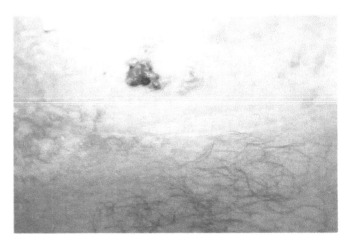

Figure 10.27. Extragenital lichen sclerosus on lower abdomen.

Figure 10.25. Lichen sclerosus with patchy, marked lichenification and small ecchymoses.

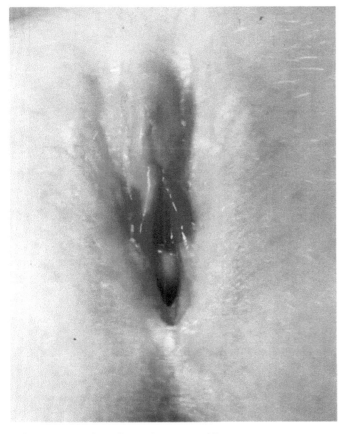

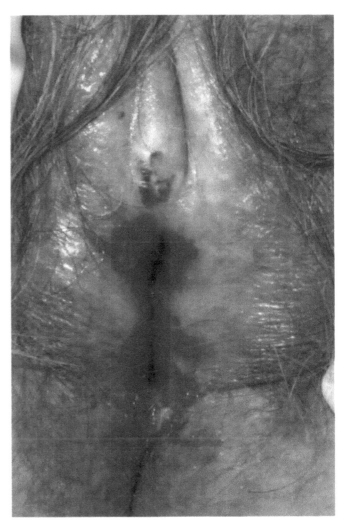

Figure 10.26. Lichen sclerosus in an 8 year old.

Figure 10.28. Lichen sclerosus with atypia on biopsy (VIN).

Pathology

LS is usually diagnostic on biopsy. The features are a band of homogenised collagen in the upper dermis, basal layer vacuolar degeneration and a lymphocyte-rich inflammatory infiltrate beneath the homogenised collagen. In 90% of vulvar LS, the epidermis shows acanthosis (hyperplasia), not atrophy as found in extragenital lichen sclerosus and as suggested by the old name "lichen sclerosus et atrophicus". The dermal changes of LS appear to evolve through stages of edema, hyaline change and fibrosis.

In long-standing disease, the diagnostic feature of hyalinisation of the dermis is lost to fibrosis and the changes gradually merge with lichen simplex chronicus. Even in these late stages, however, there may still be focal changes of a lichenoid tissue reaction. Eventually, the appearances are difficult to distinguish from long-standing lichen planus and lichen simplex chronicus The non-specific histology of late lichen sclerosus may contrast with clinically obvious, severe lichen sclerosus.

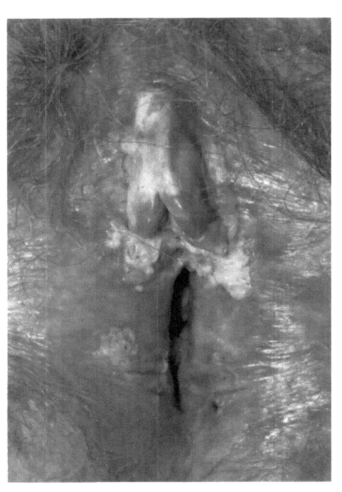

Figure 10.29. Lichen sclerosus with early invasive carcinoma.

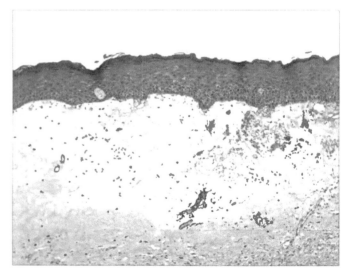

Figure 10.30. Lichen sclerosus early lesion in a 10 year old girl. Acanthosis, early basal layer vacuolar change and a broad zone of cell poor edema.

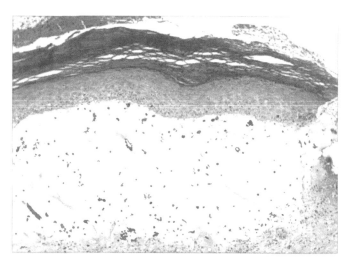

Figure 10.31. Lichen sclerosus early lesion in a woman of reproductive age. Acanthosis, early basal layer vacuolar change and a broad zone of cell poor edema in the upper dermis

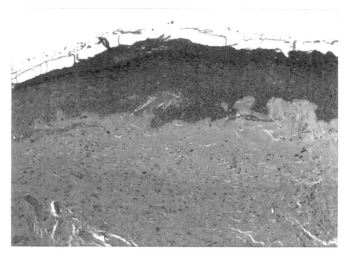

Figure 10.32. Lichen sclerosus, established lesion. Hyperkeratosis, acanthosis, basal layer degeneration and dermal hyalinisation and fibrosis

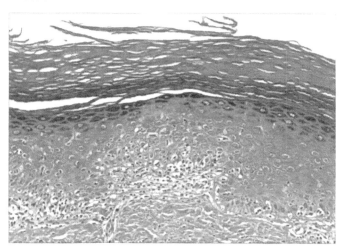

Figure 10.33. Lichen sclerosus old lesion. Hyperkeratosis, acanthosis, basal layer degeneration, dermal fibrosis and inflammation. There is no edematous-hyaline layer

Treatment

Topical steroid therapy should render the woman free of symptoms and halt the progression of any anatomical distortion. Mild steroids tend to be ineffective so treatment should commence with a potent or super-potent steroid and a mid-strength steroid used for maintenance. The woman needs to understand that the skin is compromised. Chemical and physical trauma are to be minimised but, if this is done and with the use of steroid therapy, LS should not significantly impair her quality of life, including sexual relations.

Most cases will respond to the steroid in a cream vehicle but occasionally other forms of administration will be preferable. These include aerosols intended for the respiratory tract, especially when the lesions are moist, or intralesional injection in the most difficult cases. Always remember that the commonest cause of LS not responding to steroids is *C. albicans* infection, so some of these women will need to have a vaginal swab taken from time to time.

Treatments used in the past, for which there is probably no place, are vulvectomy, laser surgery and topical testosterone and estrogen. Should treatment be requested for introital stenosis precluding intercourse, transposition on a pedicle of healthy skin from the labium majus is preferable to simple vulvoplasty.

LS is unaffected by pregnancy and is not a contraindication to a vaginal delivery. Because of the association with cancer, albeit slight, these patients should be kept under 6 to 12 monthly review even when symptoms are controlled.

78. LICHEN PLANUS

Lichen planus (LP) is an uncommon vulvovaginal disorder but one of the most serious because it produces epithelial erosion (partial loss of epithelial thickness in contrast to ulceration where there is full thickness loss). Its cause is unknown. Occasionally it is a manifestation of a drug reaction. An association with hepatitis B and C viruses has been recently noted. In the USA up to 5% of LP patients, particularly those with severe erosive disease, are hepatitis C positive. It can affect the mouth in a similar manner to the vulva and vagina. When both regions are similarly involved and when unusual sites such as esophagus are also involved, the term vulvovaginogingival syndrome is sometimes used.

Clinical features

Most women with LP present between the ages of 30 to 60 years. Soreness and dyspareunia are the usual symptoms, often of sufficient severity to preclude intercourse. Vulvar dysuria, discharge and even bleeding on contact may occur. Extragenital lesions will be present in a minority of cases. Oral lesions can occur with LP giving rise to discomfort, particularly with eating.

Gynecological examination reveals patchy erosion, usually of the medial aspect of the labia minora extending to a variable degree into the vagina. The eroded areas are red, moist and have a well defined edge. They may vary in size from pin point up to several centimetres in diameter. An occasional pathognomonic sign, more common in association with the oral lesions, is associated white lines of hyperkeratosis called Wickham's striae. In severe cases, adhesion formation between the eroded vaginal walls can result in partial obliteration of the vaginal lumen.

Oral lesions should be specifically sought. They resemble the genital lesions and occur on the buccal mucosa and gums. Occasionally the characteristic violaceous papules of LP will be found on the skin elsewhere.

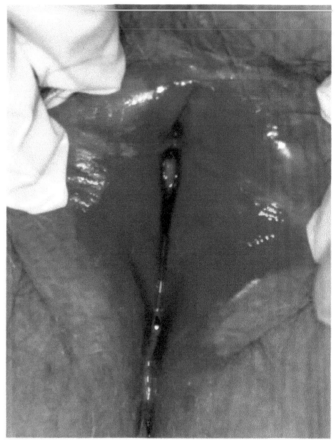

Figure 10.34. Lichen planus.

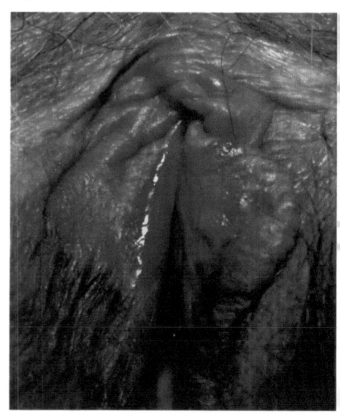

Figure 10.35. Lichen planus mainly affecting the right labium minus.

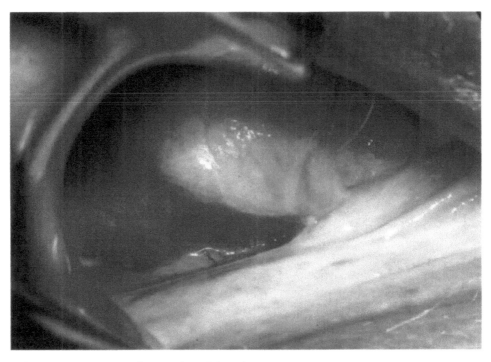

Figure 10.36. Patchy vaginal erosion due to lichen planus.

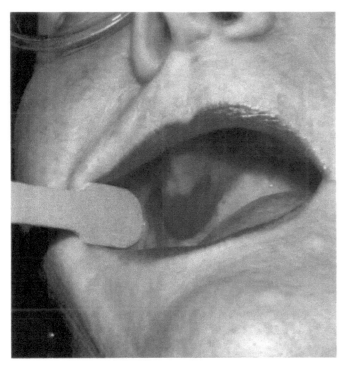

Figure 10.37. Oral lichen planus.

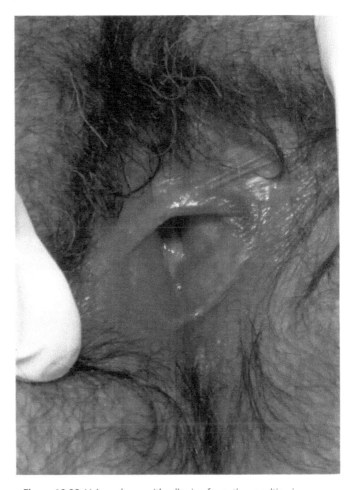

Figure 10.38. Lichen planus with adhesion formation resulting in introital stenosis.

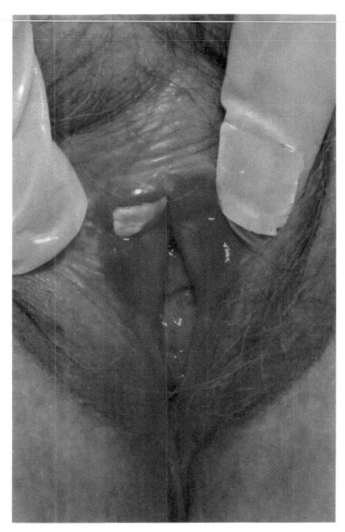

Figure 10.39. Lichen planus with a patch of lichenification.

histological features in chronic cases. The erosive form of lichen planus shows thinning of the squamous epithelium with a lack of maturation of squamous cells and a band-like infiltrate of lymphocytes with variable numbers of plasma cells. Basal layer vacuolar degeneration is usually not seen.

The diagnosis of lichen planus can be difficult. Biopsy may be able to offer no more than non-specific "lichenoid tissue reaction", "erosive vulvitis" or "erosive vaginitis". Gynecologists may be unfamiliar with its protean clinical manifestations and dermatologists may not be experienced in examining the vagina. Extragenital lesions should be looked for and, although uncommon, are easier to diagnose than vulvar disease. A particularly useful aid to diagnosis and means of assessing response to treatment is vaginal cytology and the reader is referred to the section on office pathology in chapter 3.

Because genital LP may resemble atrophic vaginitis or be worsened by estrogen deficiency, a serum estradiol may be a useful investigation in the older woman.

Pathology

The key histological features of LP are basal layer vacuolar degeneration with apoptotic keratinocytes (Civatte bodies) and a dermal, band-like, lymphocyte-rich inflammatory infiltrate. These changes are most easily recognised in keratinised skin. In long standing cutaneous disease, the diagnostic features are lost and the appearances come to resemble lichen simplex chronicus, although focal lichenoid inflammation may remain. The presence of pigment incontinence (melanin-containing macrophages) in the upper dermis is an indication of past basal layer damage. These changes merely indicate a long-standing, lichenoid tissue reaction and are not diagnostic of LP. Lichen sclerosus, with which LP may be associated, causes identical

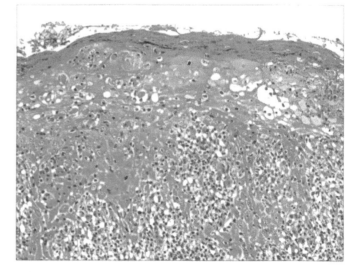

Figure 10.40. Non-erosive lichen planus of the vulva with acanthosis, basal layer degeneration and a closely applied dermal chronic inflammatory cell infiltrate.

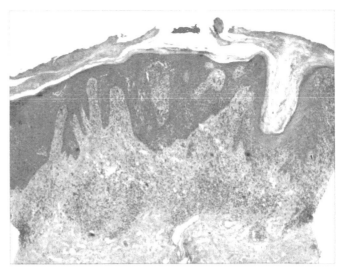

Figure 10.42. Lichen planus, hypertrophic variant (leg). Hyperkeratosis, follicular plugging, marked acanthosis with long irregular ridges, dermal fibrosis and inflammatory infiltrate.

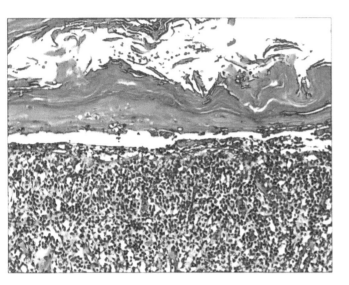

Figure 10.41. The bullous variant of lichen planus showing dermo-epidermal splitting due to basal layer vacuolar degeneration, apoptotic keratinocytes and lymphocytic infiltrate.

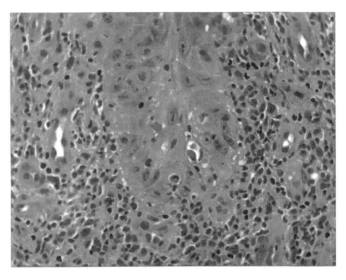

Figure 10.43. Lichen planus, hypertrophic type (leg). The tip of a rete ridge shows basal layer degeneration and adjacent lymphocytic infiltrate.

Hypertrophic LP is a rare form of LP that has been reported also occurring on the vulva in association with HIV infection. It appears as warty growths that not only may resemble carcinoma clinically and histologically but also appear to show a propensity to transform into carcinoma. On the vulva, hypertrophic LP may become infected, painful and macerated. Histologically, hypertrophic LP looks like pseudoepitheliomatous hyperplasia with a lichenoid tissue reaction. The hyperplastic squamous epithelium often appears as an infundibulocystic proliferation with some resemblance to pseudoepitheliomatous hyperplasia. The lichenoid tissue reaction may be focal and confined to the deepest portions of the squamous proliferation. The diagnosis of hypertrophic LP may be supported by finding LP on the extragenital skin (where it may also be hypertrophic), oral mucosa and nails.

Treatment

Intravaginal cortisone is the most useful form of medication. Finding a satisfactory vehicle for the steroid suitable for vaginal use may be difficult. The single most useful form of treatment for vaginal LP that this author has ever used is triple sulphonamide vaginal cream (no longer available in Australia) into which 1% hydrocortisone has been incorporated and inserted nightly with a vaginal applicator. Clindamycin vaginal cream with 1% hydrocortisone can be similarly useful. Betamethasone 0.05 to 0.1% may be necessary for the more severe case. 10% hydrocortisone acetate rectal foam used with a vaginal applicator can be very effective but initially may have to be used 3 times daily. The direct application of a potent steroid to the lesions is worth trying but difficulty getting the preparation to adhere to the lesions is the problem. Injection of triamcinolone acetonide (possibly best diluted with normal saline or lignocaine) beneath the eroded epithelium may be successful when all other treatments have failed.

An unfortunate, small minority of women with severe genital LP will appear to be unresponsive to vaginal steroid therapy. Other treatments tried with variable success include systemic steroids and hydroxychloroquine, topical cyclosporin, tacrolimus and pimicrolimus. Significant absorption may occur when the latter are used vaginally.

79. DESQUAMATIVE INFLAMMATORY VAGINITIS.

Desquamative inflammatory vaginitis (DIV) is an uncommon but important form of erosive vaginitis. It may be a variant of genital lichen planus (LP) or immuno-bullous disease. It is important because these women present to gynecologists who will probably not have seen the condition beforehand and will assume that the vaginitis is infective in origin and treat accordingly without success. Like LP, DIV is characterised by epithelial erosion in the absence of a demonstrable pathogen, has similar features suggestive of an immune disturbance as the cause and may be associated with the larger erosions characteristic of LP.

Clinical features

DIV is confined to the vagina and cervix. Discharge is the leading symptom. It may be irritating and associated with dyspareunia and vulvar dysuria.

The vaginitis bears an uncanny resemblance to trichomoniasis with minute erosions appearing as small red spots on the vaginal walls and ectocervix. The discharge is purulent. Unlike the classical LP described above, adhesion formation is generally not seen with DIV.

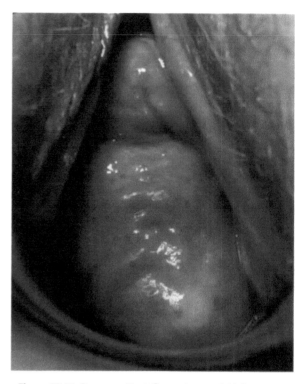

Figure 10.44. Desquamative inflammatory vaginitis in a patient with vaginal prolapse.

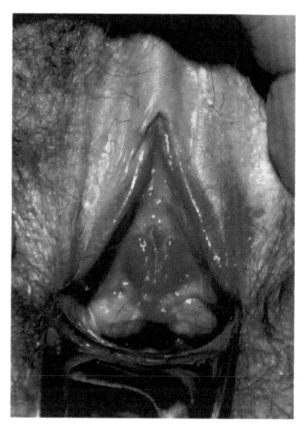

Figure 10.45. Desquamative inflammatory vaginitis.

Pathology

Vaginal and cervical swabs must be examined in all cases but will be negative for all pathogens if DIV is the diagnosis. The cytology of the discharge is characteristic. Polymorphs will be present in profuse numbers and there is a mixture of differentiated squamous cells with parabasal cells from the deeper layers exposed by the erosive process. These findings may resemble atrophic vaginitis, particularly if an estrogen cream has been used. A serum estradiol may aid differentiation in the older woman.

Vaginal biopsies of patients with a clinical diagnosis of DIV show a non-specific erosive vaginitis indistinguishable from that seen in erosive lichen planus.

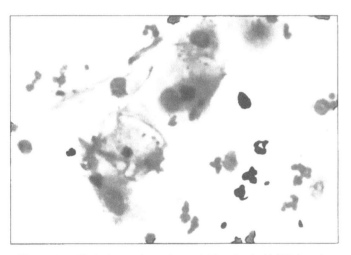

Figure 10.46. Vaginal smear in erosive vaginitis stained with Wright stain.

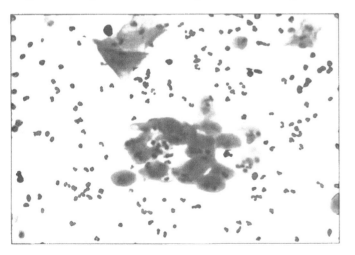

Figure 10.47. Vaginal smear in lichen planus showing regenerative atypia (Papanicoloau stain). Photo courtesy of the Victorian Cytology Service.

Treatment

DIV is more predictably responsive to vaginal steroid than LP. So much so that the disappearance of polymorphs from the vagina after 2 weeks of 10% hydrocortisone rectal foam inserted into the vagina 2 or 3 times daily can almost be considered a therapeutic test. The use of triple sulphonamide or clindamycin vaginal cream without steroid sometimes results in improvement but relapse is common. DIV is a chronic disorder and, once controlled, it is likely that maintenance therapy with intravaginal steroid will be necessary a couple of times a week.

80. VULVITIS CIRCUMSCRIPTA PLASMACELLULARIS (PLASMA CELL VULVITIS OF ZOON)

Vulvitis circumscripta plasmacellularis (VCP) is also known as Zoon's vulvitis because of features it shares with Zoon's balanitis (which was described before VCP). It remains uncertain whether or not it is merely a variant of lichen planus with capillaritis. Clinicians who have managed VCP generally agree that it is a distinct entity because of some characteristic clinical features. Its cause is unknown but it is occasionally seen in association with conditions such as endocrine failure with autoantibodies suggesting on autoimmune basis.

VCP is usually a disorder of middle aged, often postmenopausal women. Rarely, it has been reported at younger ages, including a case report of an 8 year old in whom abuse had been erroneously suspected. The usual symptoms are introital discomfort, soreness and vulvar dysuria, present for months or years.

The characteristic lesions are of one or more well demarcated macules of variable size and shape distributed asymmetrically around the introitus. Their striking feature is their peculiar orange hue due to the hemosiderin content. The macules can be red through orange to brown.

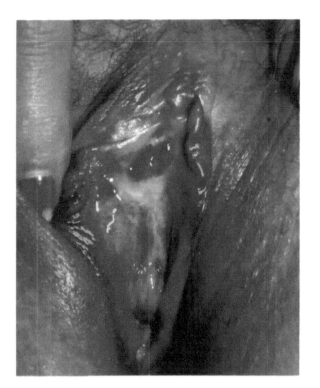

Figure 10.48. Plasma cell vulvitis.

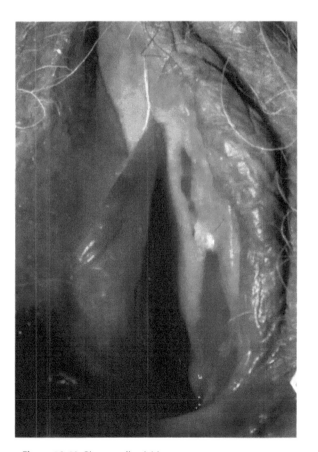

Figure 10.49. Plasma cell vulvitis.

Pathology

A vaginal swab should be negative for pathogens. A careful sexual history may be wise in view of the similarity of the lesions to those of trauma.

Biopsy is the principle investigation and shows many of the features of vulvovaginal lichen planus (see above). In addition there are extravasated red blood cells and hemosiderin containing macrophages (prominent with Perl's stain) in the dermal infiltrate. As the name would suggest, plasma cells are present in large numbers in the dermal infiltrate. This prominence of plasma cells, however, may be non-specific as this may be found in chronic inflammatory cell infiltrates due to any cause in the medial vulva, vagina, anus and mouth.

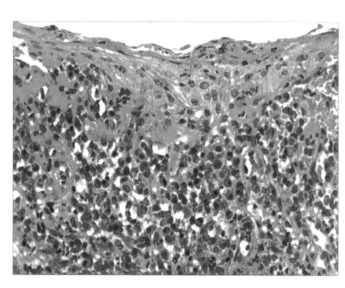

Figure 10.50. VCP of vestibule showing thinning of the epidermis, marked dermal inflammation with numerous plasma cells, hemosiderin, macrophages and extravasated red blood cells.

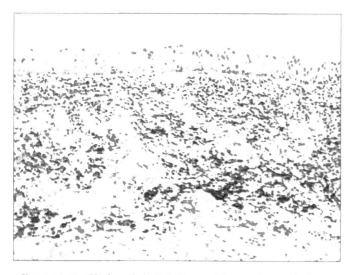

Figure 10.51. VCP of vestibule. Perls' Prussian blue reaction confirming much hemosiderin.

Treatment

If the patient is postmenopausal, estrogen replacement alone can bring about resolution of the lesions. There is variable success with topical steroids. Intralesional injection of triamcinolone may be effective. Interferon alpha injection has been reported as a successful treatment. There would seem to be no place for surgery for VCP.

81. LUPUS ERYTHEMATOSUS

Lupus erythematosus (LE) is an autoimmune disease. There is a spectrum of disease from purely cutaneous LE to a severe systemic disease mediated by immune complex formation. Vulvar lesions are rare and virtually never found on the vulva in isolation.

Clinical features

Cutaneous LE produces well defined erythematous patches which may scar, usually on light exposed areas. It is predominantly a disorder of middle age but can occur at any age. Vulvar lesions may be white plaques or erosions.

Diagnosis

The vulvar lesions of LE are clinically and histologically indistinguishable from erosive lichen planus. By contrast, patients with erosive vulvovaginitis with no other evidence of extragenital disease, when investigated, hardly ever have lupus antibodies in their serum.

Treatment

Antimalarial therapy and/or steroids are used for LE. Intralesional steroid may be necessary for individual patches.

82. GRAFT VERSUS HOST DISEASE

Graft versus host disease (GVHD) is a multisystem disorder which most commonly affects the skin and gut in the setting of an allogenic bone marrow transplant. Patients are mainly leukemic women. Donated T lymphocytes unable to be rejected by the host, proliferate and attack host cells. In the vulvovaginal area, the commonest manifestation is an erosive vulvovaginitis, clinically identical to erosive lichen planus

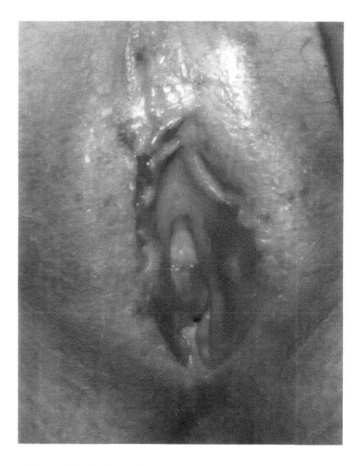

Figure 10.52. Graft versus host disease.

Pathology

The vulvovaginal lesions of GVHD are histologically indistinguishable from those of erosive lichen planus. Infection needs to be excluded.

Treatment
Treatment of genital GVHD is as for lichen planus.

83. FIXED DRUG ERUPTION
Certain drugs may cause a rash in the same site upon re-exposure. The penis is a site of predilection in the male. Only a handful of case reports of this condition affecting the genitocrural area or vagina exist.

Fixed drug eruptions appear as pigmented plaques which flare up to become an erythematous or bullous area upon re-exposure to the offending drug. Drugs that have caused this condition include sulfas, phenolphthalein and non-steroidal anti-inflammatories.

Pathology
The histology is of a lichenoid tissue reaction with necrotic keratinocytes to necrotic epidermis. There is clefting at the dermo-epidermal junction and bullous formation in severe cases. The lesions heal with a brownish tinge, which is seen histologically to be due to pigment incontinence.

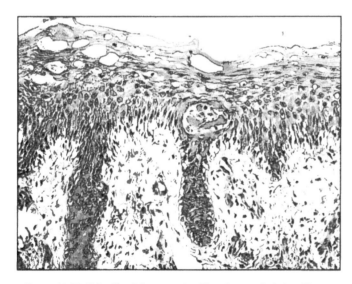

Figure 10.53. Vulva. Fixed drug eruption. There is spongiosis, basal layer vacuolar change and papillary dermal edema.

D. Vesicobullous disorders

The vesicobullous or blistering disorders are uncommon but serious (sometimes life-threatening) skin disorders resulting from a breakdown in the cell attachments within the epidermis or at the interface between the epidermis and the dermis (the basement membrane zone). The defect may be genetic or result from the action of autoantibodies against the adhesion molecules (autoantigens). The latter group are called the immunobullous diseases. The situation of the autoantigens within the epithelium determines the depth at which the breakdown occurs and thus much of the clinical features of the individual disorders. On mucosal surfaces the intraepithelial breakdown will usually present as erosions (partial thickness loss) or ulcers (full thickness loss) rather than blisters.

These disorders will usually be seen and managed by dermatologists and the extragenital manifestations will be of greatest concern to the patient and medical attendant. Those described here may affect the vulva and sometimes the vagina. Occasionally they will present primarily in the genital area and need to be considered in differential diagnosis. Diagnosis will require biopsy and usually immuno-fluorescence best performed on biopsies of perilesional skin. Because of the similarity in pathogenesis of the immunobullous diseases, their treatment will be discussed jointly.

84. PEMPHIGUS AND VARIANTS
The lesions present as scaly, flaccid blisters which may involve the vulva.

Pemphigus vulgaris is the prototype of acantholytic immunobullous disease. IgG antibodies are directed against desmoglein 3, which is important for adhesion of cells particularly on mucosal surfaces, leading to acantholytic blisters which easily break down to leave eroded surfaces.

Blisters arise from uninflamed skin due to acantholysis. They occur within the epidermis just above the basal layer. Initial lesions often occur in the mouth with erosions and ulcers. The vulva may be similarly affected and desquamative vaginitis may develop. Flaccid blisters and erosions may be widespread.

is poor. The condition results from the production of antibodies against desmoglein but also plakin proteins. A polymorphous eruption develops with blisters. Marked mucosal involvement is a feature. Clinically, it resembles erythema multiforme.

Pathology

The characteristic histology is suprabasilar acantholysis with villous projections of the subjacent stroma retaining a single row of basal keratinocytes. Direct immunofluorescence shows an intercellular (desmosomal) pattern with IgG and complement. Circulating antibodies will be demonstrated in indirect immunofluorescence in most cases.

The diagnosis is clinicopathological with support of immunofluorescence. The most helpful pathology comes from untraumatized early lesions. These are hard to find on the vulva and other sites may be preferentially biopsied.

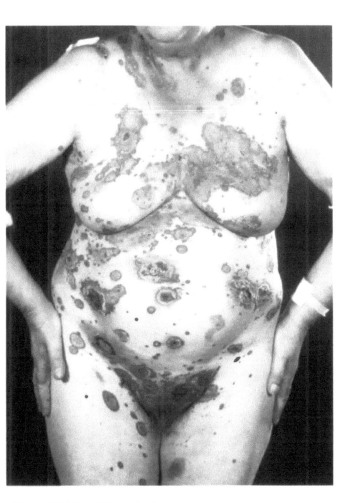

Figure 10.54. Pemphigus vulgaris.

Pemphigus vegetans is a rare form of pemphigus vulgaris featuring thick, hyperkeratotic plaques. It involves the vulva and skin flexures.

The blisters in **pemphigus foliaceus** form relatively superficially in the epidermis beneath the stratum corneum. IgG antibodies are directed against the adhesion molecule desmoglein 1, which is not found in mucosal epithelium. The lesions present as scaly, flaccid blisters which may involve the vulva, particularly mons pubis but not introitus or higher. Scaling may obscure blister formation, causing confusion in diagnosis.

There are several recently described pemphigus variants of which **paraneoplastic pemphigus** is the most important. It is seen in the presence of internal neoplasia, usually one of the lymphomas. The prognosis

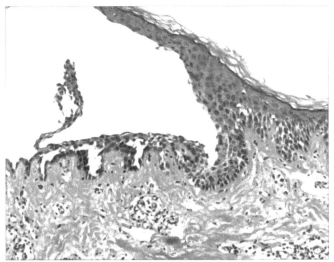

Figure 10.55. Pemphigus (extragenital). Edge of a lesion showing a vesicle and its suprabasilar cleft.

85. BULLOUS PEMPHIGOID

Bullous pemphigoid (BP) is the commonest of the immunobullous diseases. It predominantly affects the elderly but rarely occurs in children. Morbidity may be contributed to by complications of treatment. Antibodies develop against collagen XVII in the basement membrane zone (epitopes of molecular weight

180 and 230 kDa). IgG and C3 are deposited in the basement membrane zone producing subepidermal blisters.

Clinical features

Patients develop tense, itchy blisters on an erythematous or urticarial background, often around the groin. Mucosal involvement is uncommon and seldom severe. Localised, non-scarring pemphigoid with tense bullae confined to the vulva may occur in 7 to 12 year old girls. Such a presentation may be mistaken for child abuse. The disease tends to be self limiting but may last for years.

Pathology

The biopsy is best taken from the edge of a lesion from the upper body rather than the vulva. The key features of bullous pemphigoid are a subepidermal bulla and eosinophils. The eosinophils form a conspicuous component within the bulla and in the dermal infiltrate. The cell poor form of BP contains very few cells within the bulla and prebullous pemphigoid shows only dermal changes. Direct immunofluorescence in BP is an important adjunct to the diagnosis. It shows a linear band of IgG and/or C3 in the basement membrane zone. Circulating antibodies can also usually be detected by indirect immunofluorescence in most patients.

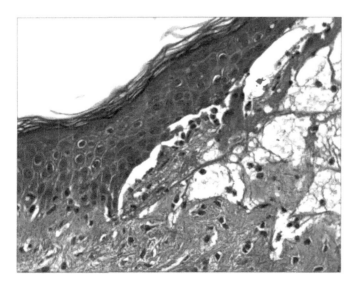

Figure 10.56. Bullous pemphigoid. The biopsy has been taken from the arm. It shows the edge of a subepidermal bulla containing fibrin and eosinophils. An unruptured lesion, such as this, is rarely seen in the vulva.

86. MUCOUS MEMBRANE PEMPHIGOID (CICATRICIAL PEMPHIGOID)

Mucous membrane pemphigoid (previously known as cicatricial pemphigoid) encompasses a heterogenous group of subepithelial blistering disorders of mucous membranes and mucocutaneous junctions, causing scarring. Genitalia are involved in 17% of cases. This unusual form of pemphigoid is the most important type of pemphigoid to affect the vulva and vagina. IgG antibodies are formed to basement membrane zone adhesion molecules, particularly to collagen XVII (BP180) and laminin 5. When laminin 5 is the epitope, there is a significant incidence of systemic neoplasms, particularly of gastro-intestinal tract and endometrium in these patients.

Clinical features

Most patients are over 60 years old. Blisters form and rapidly break down to form erosions, particularly on the mucosal surfaces that are involved in most cases of cicatricial pemphigoid. Mouth, conjunctivae (may cause blindness), nose, pharynx, larynx and genitalia can be affected. Scarring following mucosal erosion is a distinguishing feature of cicatricial pemphigoid. Vulvovaginal cicatricial pemphigoid particularly affects the hairless vulvar skin and vestibular and vagina. Usually, only erosions are seen but there may be blisters at the edge of the lesions. Scarring results in labial fusion and vaginal stenosis.

Pathology

The usual features that are seen are dermal scarring and eosinophils. The diagnostic feature of a subepidermal blister will hardly ever be seen in chronic cases. Rather, the epidermis will be either denuded, or in chronic cases, re-epithelialized. The dermis will always show eosinophils but these will be admixed with other inflammatory cells and, depending on the age of the lesion, the stroma will vary from edematous to fibrous. Fibrosis is seen only in chronic cases. Direct immunofluorescence adds strong support to suggestive histological findings by showing linear IgG and other antibodies at the basement membrane zone.

87. LINEAR IgA BULLOUS DERMATOSIS (LABD)

LABD is a rare immunobullous disease where the autoantibody is IgA which is deposited beneath the epidermis in a linear fashion. The target antigens in LABD (285 and 97kDa) also differ from those of bullous pemphigoid. LABD behaves like bullous pemphigoid, although it shows an increased tendency to affect the genital area.

Clinical features

Children and adults present with itchy, blistering erosions or papules and plaques with blistering around the edges in the genital area, buttocks, thighs, neck and face. Secondary infection following irritation may lead to pustulation in children. Herpetic (grouped) lesions (string of pearls sign) can be a helpful clinical diagnostic feature or can be misdiagnosed as herpes and mistakenly suggest sexual abuse.

Pathology

The key features are a subepidermal blister with either neutrophils or eosinophils predominating. The neutrophils are within the blisters as well as forming papillary dermal microabscesses in adjacent skin, resembling dermatitis herpetiformis. The eosinophilic-rich variant resembles bullous pemphigoid. The diagnostic test is immunofluorescence which shows IgA in the basement membrane zone.

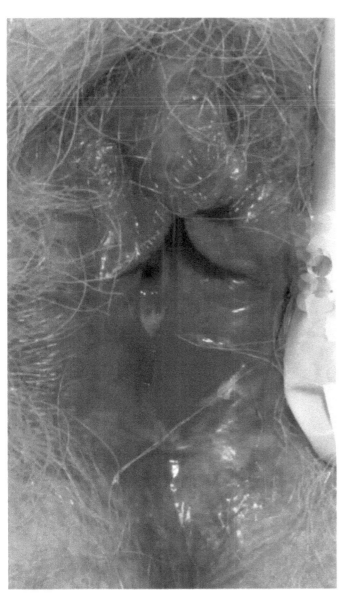

Figure 10.57. Mucous membrane pemphigoid showing freshly ruptured blister.

Herpes gestationis is a form of bullous pemphigoid occurring in pregnancy. Once it has occurred, it will recur with subsequent pregnancies, often with increasing severity. It responds to corticosteroid therapy and has little or no effect on foetal outcome. It needs to be distinguished from the common polymorphous eruption of pregnancy (pruritic urticarial papules and plaques of pregnancy - PUPPP)

ERYTHEMA MULTIFORME

Erythema multiforme (EM) is an immune complex disease frequently due to viral infection, particularly with herpes simplex virus. There are typical target lesions usually on the limbs, without mucosal involvement.

88. BULLOUS ERYTHEMA MULTIFORME (STEVENS-JOHNSON SYNDROME)

This syndrome is a more severe immune complex disease with non-classic erythematous lesions on the trunk and with mucosal involvement with severe erosions of vulva and vagina. Mucosal surfaces alone may be involved. The syndrome is frequently drug related.

89. TOXIC EPIDERMAL NECROLYSIS

This is a potentially lethal blistering disease which may involve over one third of the body surface including mucosal areas. Healing may be associated with scarring. It is drug related and often a manifestation of a drug hypersensitivity syndrome with multi-organ involvement (fever, hepatitis, lymphadenopathy, nephritis, pneumonitis and hematological abnormalities). Drugs implicated include anticonvulsants and allopurinol.

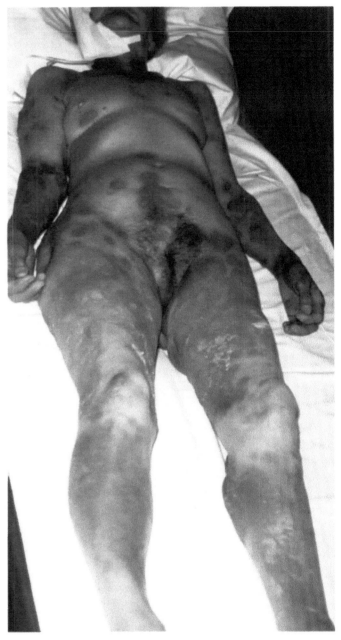

Figure 10.58. Toxic epidermal necrolysis.

Pathology

The most characteristic feature of all forms of EM is the finding of necrotic keratinocytes, which may be scattered to full thickness epidermal necrosis. These are accompanied by intraepithelial lymphocytes, which may overrun the dermo-epidermal junction. The dermis shows variable edema and there is a superficial perivascular dermal lymphocytic infiltrate. Granulocytes may be present, particularly in severe bullous forms. The bullae are formed following a split at the dermo-epidermal junction.

OTHER IMMUNOBULLOUS DISEASES

Immunobullous disorders which are rarer than the above or seldom involve vulva and vagina include dermatitis herpetiformis which is associated with coeliac disease.

Treatment of the immunobullous diseases

Drugs and neoplasia must be excluded as etiological factors. The mainstays of treatment are topical and systemic corticosteroids. Unfortunately, dependency on oral corticosteroids contributes significantly to the morbidity and sometimes mortality of these diseases. Steroid sparing drugs such as azathioprine and mycophenolate mofitil used in conjunction with the steroid may be beneficial. With widespread lesions, fluid balance must be maintained and infection controlled. Tetracyclines may help pemphigoid and dapsone is often used in cicatricial pemphigoid. The use of systemic corticosteroids in toxic epidermal necrolysis is controversial. Intravenous immunoglobulin may be helpful in severe pemphigus and TEN.

90. DARIER'S DISEASE (including papular acantholytic genitocrural acantholysis)

Darier's disease (keratosis follicularis) is a genetic abnormality of keratinization. It is inherited as an autosomal dominant but may arise from mutation on chromosome 12q23-24. There is loss of cell adhesion due to gene mutations in the calcium pump interfering with calcium binding sites on cell adhesion molecules. This leads to acantholysis.

Occasionally acantholytic disease is confined to the flexural crease of the groin with involvement of the vulva, where it presents as flesh coloured papules. This variety is not inherited. The histology is that of an acantholytic dermatosis which resembles both Hailey-Hailey and Darier's disease. The question is whether this phenomenon, known as **(91.) papular acantholytic dermatosis of the groin,** is a separate disease or simply a manifestation of other acantholytic diseases, in particular, Darier's or Hailey-Hailey disease.

Clinical features

Disease onset is usually between the ages of 10 to 30 years but may be any age. Small, crusted papules develop and become confluent on scalp, face, trunk and flexures. The vulva is occasionally involved with white papules but the pubic and inguinal areas may be severely affected. Rarely, the disease may be confined to the vulva. Particularly in hot weather, bacterial infection of the denuded skin is common and presents with weeping and oozing. Herpes simplex virus infection may also complicate the disorder. Flexural and thickened lesions predominate in some patients.

Pathology

The history of an inherited skin disorder and the distribution and appearance of extragenital lesions are important. The finding of palmar keratotic pits and V-shaped splits in the ends of the nails may help distinguish Darier's from Hailey-Hailey disease. The pathology of Darier's disease is identical to that of Grover's disease and these two diseases are distinguished clinically.

The histology is usually characteristic, except in old lesions that may show lichen simplex chronicus. The key features are suprabasilar acantholyis, corps ronds (acantholyic squamous cells with a pyknotic nucleus, perinuclear clear zone and peripheral eosinophilic cytoplasm) and grains (acantholytic parakeratotic cells).

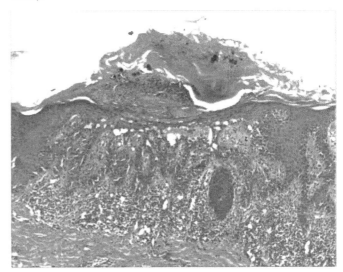

Figure 10.59. Darier's disease.

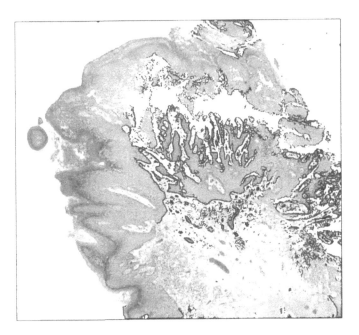

Figure 10.60. Papular genitocrural acantholysis showing hyperkeratosis, acanthosis and suprabasilar and intraepidermal clefting.

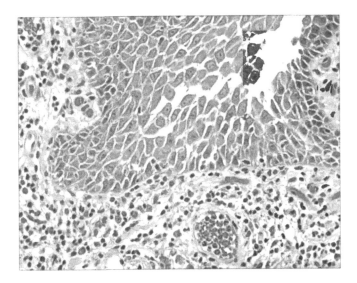

Figure 10.61. Papular genitocrural acantholysis showing multilayered acantholysis resembling Hailey-Hailey disease.

Treatment

Emollients and topical corticosteroids are beneficial. Control of secondary infection may require antibiotics. Oral retinoids will control the manifestations of the disease but its teratogenicity may limit its use in women of childbearing age. Genetic counseling may be indicated.

92. BENIGN FAMILIAL CHRONIC PEMPHIGUS (HAILEY AND HAILEY DISEASE)

This uncommon hereditary (autosomal dominant) disorder of keratinization is not related to true pemphigus. As with Darier's disease, there is loss of cell adhesion by interference with calcium binding sites on cell adhesion molecules resulting in pemphigus-like acantholysis.

Clinical features

The disease begins in young adults, who present with flexural erosions and crusting giving rise to a painful, red rash, sometimes resembling chronic flexural dermatitis, intertrigo or candidiasis. The perineum, perianal area, axillae, submammary folds and neck are the characteristic sites. The vulva is involved, usually as part of contiguous perineal disease. Friction and secondary infection may precipitate the problem. A few patients have developed HPV-related VIN and invasive squamous cell carcinoma.

Pathology

The key pathological feature is acantholysis at all levels of the epidermis giving rise to the characteristic "dilapidated brick wall" appearance.

Treatment

Treatment is essentially the same as Darier's disease but prevention of friction and secondary infection will require attention. Surgery (including CO2 laser) of localised areas may be required.

93. EPIDERMOLYSIS BULLOSA

Other genetic blistering disorders which rarely affect the vulva (and do not affect the vagina) include epidermolysis bullosa (EB). Junctional EB (due to molecular translocation in laminin 5) and dystrophic EB (due to molecular changes in collagen 7) may occur in a severe form involving the diaper area.

E. Granulomatous diseases

Granulomas are circumscribed collections of epithelioid histiocytes due to indigestible antigen, usually lipoprotein. Vulvar non-infectious granulomata are uncommon. When they occur, the cellular infiltrates form plaques which may have an annular (ring shaped) configuration. As these changes involve the dermis, clinical diagnosis is difficult and biopsy is an essential investigation.

94. SARCOIDOSIS

Sarcoidosis is a granulomatous disorder of unknown cause producing epithelioid cell tubercles mainly in the lungs, lymph nodes, liver, spleen, eyes, as well as skin. Some patients with cutaneous sarcoid have no evidence of systemic disease. There is a high incidence in Afro-Americans. Sarcoid of the vulva has only been rarely reported.

Clinical features

The tubercles appear in the skin as yellow to violaceous papules or occasionally plaques, often with surrounding induration. Scarring is unusual. The labia majora and perianal skin may be thus affected.

Pathology

The key feature is the "naked" non-necrotising granuloma. That is, a granuloma without a cuff of lymphocytes and other inflammatory cells.

The minimum diagnostic criteria for cutaneous sarcoid are naked granulomas and exclusion of other causes of granulomas. Clinical evidence of disease elsewhere and raised angiotensin-converting-enzyme strongly support the diagnosis.

Treatment

Intralesional and/or systemic corticosteroids have been used successfully.

95. ANO-GENITAL GRANULOMATOSIS (VULVITIS GRANULMATOSA or MIERSCHER-MELKERSSON-ROSENTHAL SYNDROME)

Granulomatous cheilitis is part of the Miescher-Melkersson-Rosenthal (Melkersson-Rosenthal) syndrome of cheilitis, facial palsy and fissured tongue. Granulomatous vulvitis is the less common analogous condition of the vulva. Granulomatous cheilitis and vulvitis may be seen together. Intestinal Crohn's disease may be associated with identical findings which are then referred to as oral or vulvar Crohn's disease. Sometimes, the intestinal manifestations first appear years later. The question that has not been answered is whether granulomatous cheilitis and vulvitis are forme frustes of Crohn's disease, or whether they are diseases in their own right.

Clinical features

Granulomatous vulvitis is rare. It presents in adult life as persistent inflammation and swelling of the labia majora, perineum and perianal region. The tissues are non-tender and indurated. There may be non-tender enlargement of inguinal lymph nodes and nodularity around the anus.

Pathology

The dermis shows edema, dilated lymphatics and granulomas. The granulomas may be well-formed sarcoidal granulomas, tuberculoid granulomas, or merely collections of one or more giant cells. Dilated lymphatics may contain macrophages in and near them. There are also collections of plasma cells and lymphocytes. Crohn's disease can produce identical findings.

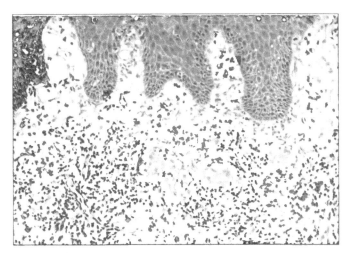

Figure 10.62. Miescher-Melkerssohn-Rosenthal syndrome of the vulva. Granulomas, lymphocytes and edema are seen beneath the epidermis.

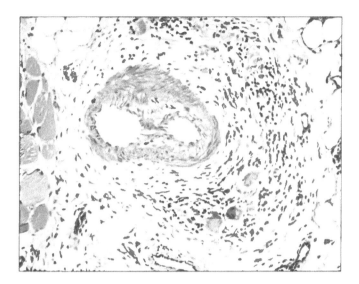

Figure 10.63. Miescher-Melkerssohn-Rosenthal syndrome of the vulva showing dermal granulomas, surrounding lymphocytic infiltrate, dermal edema and dilated small vessels.

Treatment

There is no specific treatment available for anogenital granulomatosis of the vulva although intralesional corticosteroid and resection of lesions have been used.

96. CROHN'S DISEASE

Inflammatory bowel disease best describes a spectrum of often overlapping disorders that have been named Crohn's (granulomatous) colitis, ulcerative colitis and regional enteritis (preferably) or ileitis. It is a cellular immune disease mediated by T cells and their cytokines (for example, TNFα). Vulvar manifestations of Crohn's disease tend to be associated with involvement of the lower colon and rectum (Crohn's colitis). The disorder appears to be increasing in frequency, especially in the young. Cutaneous involvement not in contact with the bowel is referred to as metastatic Crohn's disease.

Clinical features

Most vulvar involvement is seen in women in whom inflammatory bowel disease has already been diagnosed and possibly even treated by bowel resection. Rarely, the genital lesions may be the first manifestation of the disease. The vulva, vagina, perineum and perianal regions may all be affected. Local contiguous involvement from large bowel Crohn's is associated with perianal ulceration, edematous skin tags, sinuses and

fissures. Metastatic Crohn's disease appears as areas of edema and erythema. Painful lumps appear which may break down to form sinuses, ulcers resembling knife cuts or fistulae with skin to vagina and/or anorectal communication. Pain associated with the lesions can be minimal or disabling.

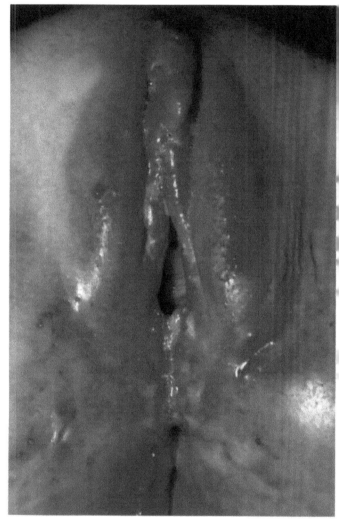

Figure 10.64. Crohn's disease.

Pathology

The key histological features are granulomas, edema and inflammation. Non-ulcerated edematous areas show the same changes as granulomatous vulvitis. These are edema, lymphatic dilatation and chronic granulomatous inflammation. Ulcers, fissures and sinuses show marked non-specific acute and chronic inflammation with suppuration and fibrosis. Granulomas may be difficult to find and, once ulceration has occurred, foreign body granulomas need to be excluded as the cause of any granulomas.

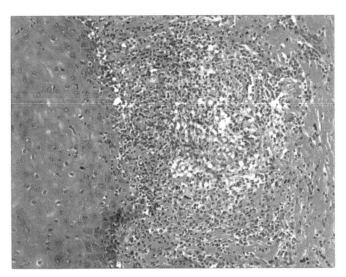

Figure 10.67. Crohn's vulvitis. Just outside the wall of the sinus, there is a granuloma with surrounding lymphocytes.

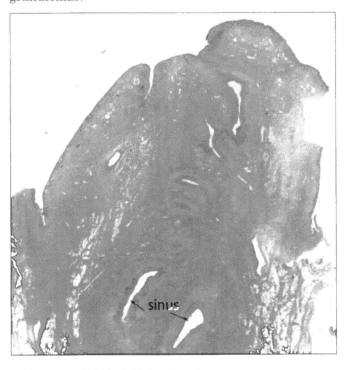

Figure 10.65. Crohn's vulvitis showing a sinus.

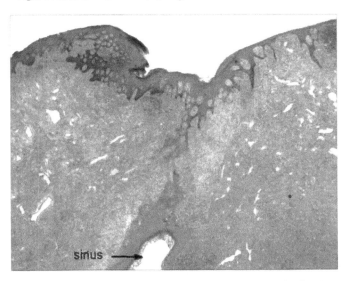

Figure 10.66. Crohn's disease of the labium majus. A sinus in the dermis is bordered by squamous epithelium and surrounded by inflammation.

The diagnosis is clinicopathological. The pathological component relies heavily on the finding of granulomas. When there is no history of Crohn's or no granulomas are found, the diagnosis can be difficult and all the pathologist may be able to offer is to suggest Crohn's disease as a possibility. Chronic lymphatic obstruction due to radiation, surgery or which is congenital is distinguished by the lack of granulomatous inflammation. Hidradenitis suppurativa causes ulcers, sinuses, abscesses and edema which can appear similar to Crohn's disease, clinically and histologically. Any granulomas found, however, will be foreign body granulomas.

Treatment

Fistulae may heal spontaneously or with medical treatment of which sulfa drugs and corticosteroids are the mainstay. Immunosuppressives have been used with success. Surgery is best left as a last resort. Vulvectomy may be necessary for pain relief.

97. FOREIGN BODY GRANULOMA

A granulomatous response may occur if vulvar tissue is the site of entry of foreign bodies such as splinters, vegetation spines, suture material or hair. Infection with cellulitis, abscess formation, delayed healing and sinus formation are more likely under these circumstances.

Foreign body granulomas of skin are seen as erythematous, brown or purple papules, nodules or occasionally, plaques.

Diagnostic imagery with ultrasound or X-ray may be helpful. Excision/biopsy is the likely preferred management.

F. Vasculopathic Disorders

98. URTICARIA (HIVES, WHEALS) AND ANGIOEDEMA

Urticaria is a common skin disease resulting from allergic and non-allergic degranulation of dermal mast cells with liberation of histamine and other vasoactive substances. The condition commonly results from ingestion of certain foods and food additives, usage of drugs or contact with various substances, when the term contact urticaria is applied. In its most severe form, urticaria may develop into anaphylaxis, which may be life threatening. In its chronic form, there may be an underlying vasculitis (urticarial vasculitis) associated with collagen vascular disease or hepatitis C.

Clinical features

Pruritic, erythematous patches progress to wheal formation. The wheal is the characteristic lesion of urticaria. It is pale pink and raised (due to edema) and often surrounded by a flare. Urticaria can occur anywhere on the body. The wheals vary in size and shape and each one is transient, usually subsiding within 24 hours. Angioedema (previously called angioneurotic edema) is a deeper form of urticaria characterised by swelling of subcutaneous and/or submucosal tissues. It may affect eyes, lips and upper respiratory tract as well as genitalia.

It may be possible to identify the offending allergen. Foods such as shellfish and nuts and some food additives are common causes. Penicillin and other antibiotics, aspirin, non-steroidal anti-inflammatory agents and morphine are commonly implicated.

When urticaria persists longer than 6 weeks it is referred to as chronic urticaria. It is twice as common in women. It is a relapsing condition, frustrating both for patient and doctor.

The wheals of contact urticaria occur within minutes following topical exposure to allergens. Potential allergens relevant to vulva and vagina include latex (condoms) and, very rarely, semen. Semen allergy must be distinguished from the more common non-specific irritation by semen which, like sweat, may irritate genital epithelium inflamed for some other reason. Pruritus, swelling and erythema occur within minutes of ejaculation when semen allergy exists and may be prevented by condom usage or withdrawal. The antigens involved are thought to arise from seminal plasma, probably glycoproteins. Acute, life-threatening anaphylactic reactions have been described with both latex and semen.

Papular urticaria is a form of urticaria resulting from insect bites.

Diagnosis

The diagnosis of urticaria is essentially clinical and, because the findings are evanescent, history is crucial. Scratching forearm skin through a drop of the partner's semen will produce a wheal and flare reaction in semen allergy. Latex sensitivity is best demonstrated by the radioallergosorbent test (RAST).

Usually a biopsy will not be performed. If it is, for example for consideration of differential diagnosis, edema will appear as dermal pallor. As pallor is also produced in thin histological sections or pale staining, better histological guides to urticaria are dilated vessels containing granulocytes and a light interstitial infiltrate of eosinophils.

Treatment

Where possible, the offending allergen must be sought and removed. Thus, it is advisable to avoid aspirin, food additives (colourings and preservatives) and some alcoholic beverages or any other suspect food or drug. Antihistamines are most useful. Non-sedating antihistamines (for example, laratadine) are preferable for daytime usage but sedating forms (for example, promethazine) may be preferable for use at night. For more severe, acute urticaria, short term corticosteroids may be necessary. Finally, for severe angioedema and anaphylaxis, adrenaline can be life saving.

99. HENOCH-SCHONLEIN PURPURA

Henoch-Schonlein purpura (HSP) is a form of leucocytoclastic vasculitis occurring mainly in children with lesions on the limbs and buttocks rather than the genitals. It may result from streptococcal infection. It may affect the kidneys with an IgA nephritis.

Clinical features

Rarely, HSP may present as a rash on the vulva of a child. Erythematous macules become papular urticarial and purpuric. The purpuric spots or petechiae are extravasations of red blood cells and cannot be blanched by pressure. The lesions resolve but may recur. Abdominal and joint pains may occur.

Pathology

HSP appears as a leukocytoclastic vasculitis with endothelial swelling and rarely fibrinoid necrosis of superficial dermal small vessels. There is an intravascular and perivascular surrounding polymorph-rich infiltrate. Frequent breakdown of polymorphs appears as nuclear debris (leukocytoclasis).

If biopsy is performed, it must be combined with a sample for immunofluorescence. The finding of a leukocytoclastic vasculitis with IgA immunofluorescence in vessel walls is diagnostic.

Treatment

Treatment is supportive. Penicillin is indicated if streptococcal infection is present. Renal function should be watched. Corticosteroids may be required.

100. PYODERMA GANGRENOSUM

Pyoderma gangrenosum can occur on skin anywhere but rarely affects the vulva where it may need to be considered in the differentiation of vulvar ulceration. It is a neutrophilic dermatosis and, although its cause is not understood, may be a cellular immune reaction. There may be associated inflammatory bowel disease, polyarthritis, neoplasia (usually lymphoma) or myeloproliferative disease.

Clinical features

The earliest lesion is a small hemorrhagic blister or pustule which develops into a painful chronic or rapidly spreading ulcer with a characteristic blue edge. The ulcers heal with a cribriform (net-like) scar. Children particularly may have perigenital or perianal lesions.

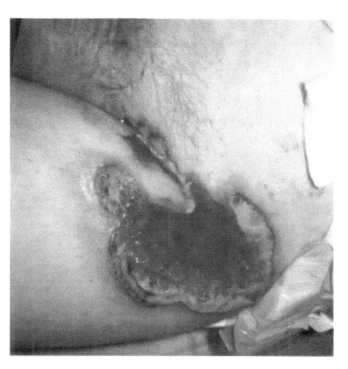

Figure 10.68. Pyoderma gangrenosum.

Pathology

Before diagnosis is made, infective causes of ulcers must be excluded. The histology is not diagnostic and not distinguishable from bacterial infection. The most characteristic feature is a dermal neutrophil-rich infiltrate with leukocytoclasis. Pseudoepitheliomatous hyperplasia, poorly formed granulomas and, at the advancing edge of the lesion, folliculitis may be subtle clues.

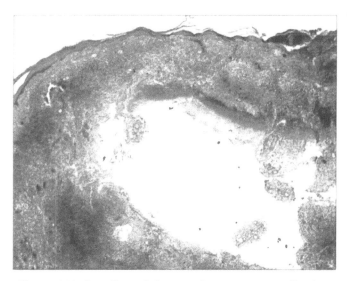

Figure 10.69. Ulcer of buttock due to pyoderma gangrenosum. The ulcer cavity undermines the epidermis.

Treatment

Treatment is often difficult. Corticosteroids, cyclosporin and other immunosuppressives (such as methotrexate) have all been used.

101. APHTHOUS ULCERATION

Aphthous (from the Greek for thrush) ulceration is usually thought of in relation to the mouth, where the ulcers, from time to time, affect a large minority of the population. Even though much less common on the vulva, they are most significant because of the distress they cause. One cause of this distress arises from diagnostic confusion with sexually transmitted infections, particularly herpes and syphilis. The cause of aphthous ulceration remains unknown. No infectious agent has been identified. Immune factors are probably relevant. Severe morbidity may arise from aphthous ulceration in HIV infected patients with CD4+ counts below 100/mm[3].

There is no good evidence to justify differentiating the Lipschutz ulcer (ulcus vulvae acutum) of the older texts from aphthous ulcers.

Aphthous ulcers are one of the main features of Behcet's disease (see below). However, patients should not be labelled as having Behcet's disease because of aphthous ulceration alone. When aphthous ulcers occur both in the mouth and vulva, the term 'complex aphthosis' should be used (not Behcet's syndrome).

Clinical features

Aphthosis may be minor (with one or more small ulcers resembling the common oral variety) or major. The latter applies when the ulcer, which may be solitary, is larger than 5mm in diameter. The ulcers may occur grouped in a form resembling herpesvirus infection and are then described as herpetiform.

Aphthous ulcers have a yellow slough base with an erythematous halo. They occur on the labia and vestibule and persist for a variable time, days or many weeks. Scarring with healing is an occasional feature of major aphthosis only. Inguinal lymphadenopathy is not a feature of this disorder.

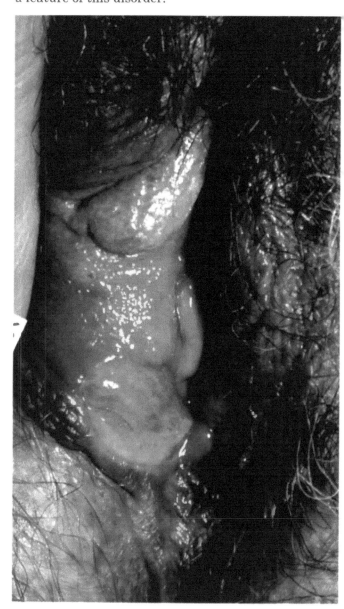

Figure 10.70. Major aphthosis.

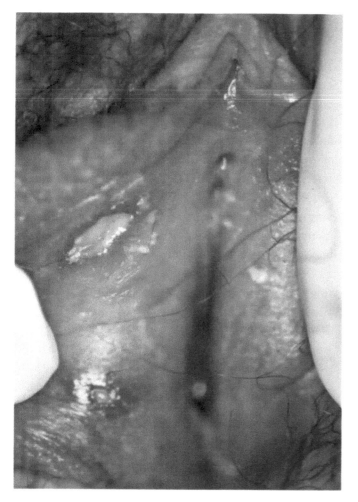

Figure 10.71. Aphthous ulceration.

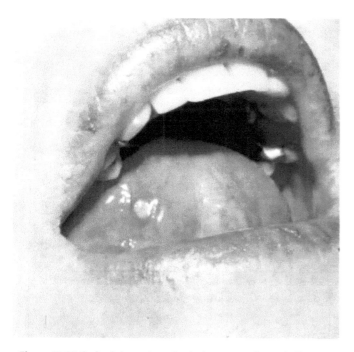

Figure 10.72. Oral aphthous ulceration in the same patient as in Fig. 10.71.

Pathology

If a sexually transmitted infection is possible, appropriate swabs and serology should be performed. Biopsy is indicated primarily to exclude the many other causes of genital ulceration. It can be convenient to take two biopsies, one (in formalin) for histology and the other (not in formalin) for microbiology.

The histological features of aphthous ulcers are not specific. They have a surface of fibrinopurulent debris overlying a predominantly lymphocytic infiltrate in which there are many activated lymphocytes. The activated lymphocytes may occasionally be so prominent as to cause confusion with non-Hodgkin's lymphoma.

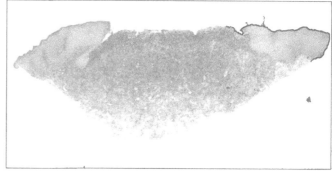

Figure 10.73. Aphthous ulcer of the vulva. A small, superficial ulcer with many inflammatory cells can be seen in the base.

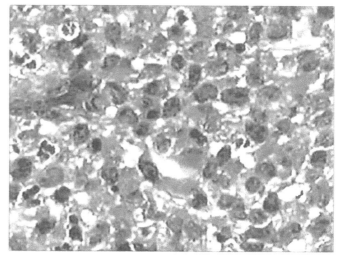

Figure 10.74. Aphthous ulcer of the vulva. Many large lymphocytes in the inflammatory infiltrate may mimic non-Hodgkin's lymphoma.

Treatment

As in the mouth, vulvar aphthous ulceration may be self-limiting. Major aphthosis is likely to require a course of prednisolone which can bring about healing in days.

102. BEHCET'S SYNDROME

In 1937, Behcet, a Turkish dermatologist, described a syndrome of recurrent aphthous stomatitis, genital ulceration and eye disease (especially iridocyclitis and retinal vasculitis). Its cause is unknown but it is a multisystem disease with underlying vasculitis and association with HLA B 51. Systemic disease includes thrombophlebitis, arthritis and gastrointestinal, cardiac and central nervous system involvement. Behcet's disease has been reported most commonly along the old silk road between Asia and Europe. Severe forms of the disease are found in Turkey and Japan. Ocular manifestations may progress to blindness. When major aphthous and genital ulcers occur without systemic disease, the term complex aphthosis is used.

Clinical features

Behcet's syndrome is rare. It can occur from childhood but the maximum age of onset is in the third decade. The vulva is affected by complex and major aphthosis, which characteristically relapses and remits. Ulcers are characteristically deep and painful and may lead to much tissue destruction, fibrosis and vulvar fenestration.

Pathology

The diagnosis is essentially clinical. There must be evidence of systemic involvement in addition to oral and genital aphthosis. This is usually ophthalmic inflammation. CNS and GIT involvement add strong supporting evidence. Pathergy, the appearance of a non-specific pustule 24-48 hours after needle prick, is characteristic of Behcet's disease.

The aphthous ulcers in Behcet's disease show similar histological features to those described above.

Treatment

Local and systemic corticosteroids can be very effective. Other drugs that may need to be tried include colchicine, cyclophosphamide, azathioprine, levamisole, dapsone, cyclosporin and thalidomide (if obtainable).

G. Other inflammatory disorders

103. FOX-FORDYCE DISEASE

Fox-Fordyce disease (FFD) is an uncommon, chronic, papular eruption confined to the apocrine areas of the body: axillae, breasts and anogenital area. The pathogenesis appears to be related to obstruction of apocrine gland bearing follicles but the cause of the obstruction is not clear. FFD is seen only in the reproductive age group and may improve with pregnancy or the oral contraceptive pill and worsen with menstruation, suggesting that it may have a hormonal basis. The presence of androgens seems necessary for FFD to develop but the severity of the disease is not related to the level of androgens.

Clinical features

Vulvar FFD is a pruritic, papular eruption which affects mons pubis and labia majora. The pruritus is worsened by conditions which cause sweating such as anxiety and heat. The papules are minute, perifollicular and flesh colored or darker. Lichenification from scratching may be apparent.

Pathology

The main features are lichen simplex chronicus and follicular cysts of apocrine gland bearing skin. Apocrine ducts and glands are dilated. It has been suggested that the diagnostic histological lesion is spongiosis and lymphocytosis at the junction of the apocrine duct and infundibulum of the hair follicle and that this can best be demonstrated by transverse (horizontal) sectioning.

Treatment

Topical corticosteroids may be successful but treatment is often unrewarding. Topical clindamycin or tretinoin cream is occasionally successful. It may be necessary to resort to physical methods of destruction of the papules with diathermy or laser or even excise the affected skin.

104. HIDRADENITIS SUPPURATIVA (ACNE INVERSA)

Hidradenitis suppurativa (HS), is a chronic inflammatory disorder of apocrine gland bearing skin. It is only seen after puberty, coincidental with the development of the apocrine sweat glands. The pathogenesis of HS is a defect of terminal follicular epithelium with follicular occlusion. Apocrine gland involvement is secondary. Inflammation and secondary bacterial infection cause extensive tissue destruction and scarring. The vulva is less commonly affected than the axilla but the clinical features are similar in the two sites. HS commonly occurs in otherwise healthy women. In particular, sex steroid levels are usually normal but improvement is reported in pregnancy. Obesity may be relevant.

Clinical features

The labia majora and genitocrural folds tend to be most affected. The lesions are chronic and relapsing. They begin with tender, red, subcutaneous areas of induration and swelling which extend and progress to discharging sinuses. The sinus discharge may be profuse and foul smelling, causing severe social inconvenience. Scarring and tissue distortion may occur. Pendulous masses of vulvar tissue forming large polyps, following long-standing localised lymphatic obstruction due to fibrosis, occur in the severe variant, HS polyposa, which may resemble Crohn's disease.

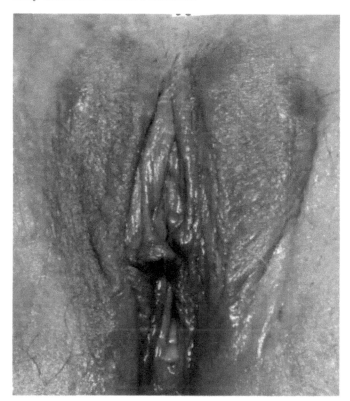

Figure 10.75. Acne inversa.

Pathology

The diagnosis is usually made clinically. When treated surgically, the specimen shows sinuses and cysts lined by squamous epithelium and/or inflamed granulation tissue, acute and chronic inflammation, edema and fibrosis. Unless granulomas are seen, the appearances may be indistinguishable from Crohn's disease.

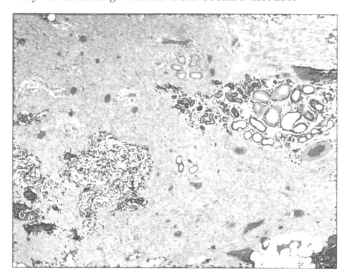

Figure 10.76. Hidradenitis suppurativa of the vulva with deep dermal fibrosis, inflammatory nodules and adjacent dilated apocrine glands.

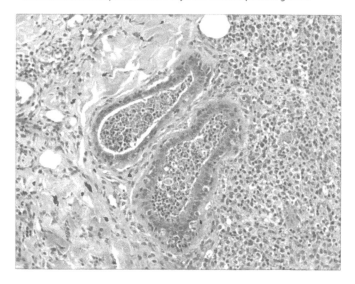

Figure 10.77. Hidradenitis suppurativa showing apocrine gland involvement.

Treatment

An attempt should be made to isolate the organism associated with the exacerbations so that appropriate antibiotic therapy can be used. Tetracyclines are used for their anti-inflammatory effect. Other forms of medication, including steroids, hormonal manipulation and retinoids, are generally disappointing. In severe cases when antibiotics fail, it is likely that excision of the affected skin will be undertaken. The excision may need to be extensive (down to the deep fascia). Plastic surgery may be required for closure but the procedure should prove curative. Laser surgery has been used.

105. PILONIDAL SINUS COMPLEX

Pilonidal sinus complex is characteristically a disease of the natal cleft of young, hairy males. Rarely, however, it may affect the vulva. The pathogenesis is uncertain. It may result from traumatic implantation of hair shafts, bacterial infection and abscess formation or an abnormality of ectodermal growth.

The hair beneath the skin surface results in an epithelial lined sinus presenting clinically as an abscess or painful sinus in a woman of reproductive age. The great majority of clinically significant pilonidal sinus complexes are found over the coccyx. Rarely, similar pathology is found on the vulva, usually close to the clitoris.

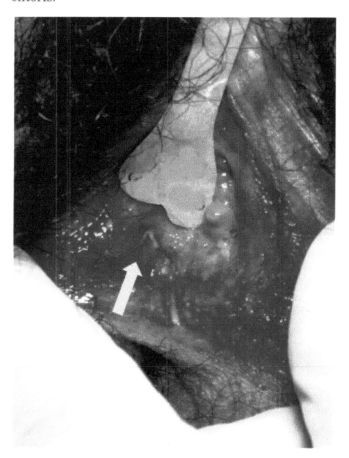

Figure 10.78. Pilonidal sinus. Note hair emerging from sinus indicated by arrow.

Pathology

There is a subcutaneous and dermal chronic abscess containing the diagnostic feature of hair shafts.

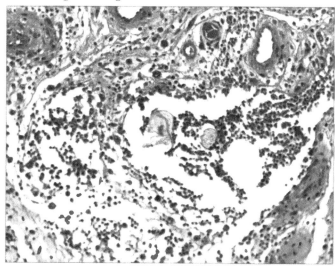

Figure 10.79. Vulvar pilonidal sinus containing a hair shaft and polymorphs.

Treatment

The entire sinus containing all of the hair must be excised to effect cure.

REFERENCES

Anhalt GJ. Paraneoplastic pemphigus - the role of tumours and drugs. Brit J Dermatol 2001; 144:1101-4.

Assman J et al Tacrolimus ointment for the treatment of vulvar lichen sclerosus J Am Acad Dermatol 2003; 48: 935-7

Attanoos RL, Appleton MA, Douglas-Jones AG The pathogenesis of hidradenitis suppurativa: a closer look at apocrine and apoeccrine glands. Br J Dermatol 1995; 133: 254-8

Batta K, Munday PE, Tatnall FM Pemphigus vulgaris localized to the vagina presenting as a chronic vaginal discharge Br J Dermatol 1999; 140: 945-7

Bell HK, Farrar CW, Curley RK Papular acantholytic dyskeratosis of the vulva. Clin Exp Deramatol 2001; 26: 386-8

Bickle K, Roark TR, Hsu S. Autoimmune bullous dermatoses: a review Am Fam Physician 2002; 65: 1861-70

Brenan J, Dennerstein G, Sfameni S, Drinkwater P, Marin G, Scurry J. Evaluation of patch testing in patients with chronic vulvar symptoms. Aust J Derm 1996; 37:40-43.

Brstryn JC. How should pemphigus be treated?. JEADV 2002; 16: 562-3.

Carlson JA, Grabowski R, Mu XC, Del Rosario A, Malfetano J, Slominski A Possible mechanisms of hypopigmentation in lichen sclerosus Am J Dermatopathol 2002; 24: 97-107

Chang TW Familial allergic seminal vulvovaginitis Am J Obstet Gynecol 1976; 1126: 442-4

Cooper PH Acantholytic dermatosis localized to the genitocrural area. J Cutan pathol 1989; 16: 81-4

Crone AM, Stewart EJ, Wojnarowska F, Powell SM Aetiological factors in vulvar dermatitis J Eur Acad Dermatol Venereol 2000; 14: 181-6

Edwards L. Hansen R. Reiter's syndrome of the vulva the psoriasis spectrum. Arch Dermatol 1992; 128:811-4

Egar CA, Lazarova Z, Darling TN, Yee C, Cote T, Yancey KB. Anti-epiligrin cicatricial pemphigoid and relative risk of cancer. Lancet 2001; 357:1850-1

Farrell AM, Kirtschig G, Dalziel KL, Allen J, Dootson G, Edwards S et al. Childhood vulval pemphigoid: a clinical and immunopathological study of five patients. Br J Dermatol 1999; 140: 308-12.

Feller ER, Ribaudo S, Jackson ND Gynecologic aspects of Crohn's disease Am Fam Physician 2001; 64: 1725-8.

Fischer GO. The commonest causes of symptomatic vulvar disease: a dermatologist's perspective. Aust J Dermatol 1996; 37: 12-8.

Fisler RE, Saeb M, Liang MG et al. Childhood bullous pemphigoid. Am J Dermatopathol 2003; 25(3):183-9.

Fleming TE, Korman NJ. Cicitricial pemphigoid. J Am Acad Dermatol 2000; 43:571-91.

Frirsch PO, Sidoroff A. Drug-induced Stevens-Johnson syndrome/toxic epidermal necrolysis. Am J Clin Dermatol 2000; 1: 349-60.

Ghate J, Jorizzo J. Behcet's disease and complex aphthosis. J Am Acad Dermatol 1999; 40:1-18.

Gimenez-Garcia R, Perez-Castrillon L. Lichen planus and hepatitis C virus infection. JEADV 2003; 17:291-5.

Girardi M, Lewis J, Glusac E, Filler RB, Geng L, Hayday AC, Tigelaar RE Resident skin-specific gamma-delta T cells provide local, nonredundant regulation of cutaneous inflammation. J Exp Med 2002; 195: 855-67

Grattan C, Sabroe R, Greaves M. Chronic urticaria. J Am Acad Dermatol 2002; 46: 645-57.

Halbert A, Chan J Anogenital and buttock ulceration in infancy Aust J Derm 2002; 43: 1-8

Harris B, Harris K, Penneys NS Demonstration by S-100 protein staining of increased numbers of nerves in the papillary dermis of patients with prurigo nodularis. J Am Acad Dermatol 1992; 26: 56-8

Howard A et al. Circulating basement membrane zone antibodies are found in lichen sclerosus of the vulva. Aust J Dermatol 2004; 45:12-15.

Iwahashi K, Miyazakin T, Kuji N, Yoshimura Y Successful pregnancy in a woman with a human seminal plasma allergy J Reprod Med 1999; 44: 391-3

Jansen T, Altmeyer, Plewig G. Acne inversa (alias hidradenitis suppurativa). JEADV 2001; 15:532-40.

Johnson M, Farmer E. Graft versus host reactions in dermatology. J Am Acad Dermatol 1998; 38:369-92.

Kamada A, Saga K, Jimbow K. Apoeccrine sweat duct obstruction as a cause for Fox-Fordyce disease. . J Am Acad Dermatol 2003; 48: 453-5

Kelly R. Cutaneous vasculitis and cutaneous vasculopathies. Aust J Dermatol 1995; 36:109-17

Kint B, Degreef H, Dooms-Goosens A. Combined allergy to human seminal plasma and latex: case report and review of the literature. Contact Dermatitis 1994; 30: 7-11

Klein PA, Appel J, Callen JP. Sarcoidosis of the vulva: a rare cutaneous manifestation. J Am Acad Dermatol 1998; 39: 281-3

Krishnan R et al Acantholytic dermatosis of the vulvovaginal area. CUTIS 2001; 67:217-9.

Lebwohl M, Ali Svad. Treatment of psoriasis: topical therapy. J Am Acad Dermatol 2001; 45:487-498.

Lee ES, Allen D, Scurry JP Pseudoepitheliomatous hyperplasia in lichen sclerosus of the vulva. Int J Gynecol Pathol. 2003 Jan;22(1):57-62

Lee LA Behcet disease Semin Cutan Med Surg 2001; 20: 53-7

Levin C, Zhai H, Bashir S, Chew AL, Anigbogu A, Stern R, Maibuch H. Efficacy of corticosteroids in acute experimental irritant contact dermatitis Skin Res Technol 2001; 7: 214-8

Liu Z, Diaz LA Bullous pemphigoid: end of the century overview J Dermatol 2001; 28: 647-50

Lotery HE, Galask RP, Seabury Stone M, Sontheimer RD. Ulcerative vulvitis in atypical Reiter's syndrome. J Am Acad Dermatol 2003; 48(4): 613-6.

Lynch PJ. Lichen simplex chronicus (atopic/ neurodermatitis) of the anogenital region.Dermatol Ther. 2004;17(1):8-19

Marren P, Wojnarowska F, Powell S. Allergic contact dermatitis and vulvar dermatoses. Brit J Derm 1992; 126: 52-56.

McCalmont CS, Lesbin B, White WL, Greiss FC Jr. Jorizzo JL Vulvar pyoderma gangrenosum Int J Gynaecol Obstet 1991; 35: 175-8

Mor F, Weinberger A, Cohen IR Identification of alpha-tropomyosin as a target self-antigen in Behcet's syndrome/ Eur J Immunol 2002; 32: 356-65

Mutasim DF. Management of autoimmune bullous diseases: pharmacology and therapeutics. J Am Acad Dermatol 2004; 51:6:859-77.

Muzyka BC, Glick M Major aphthous ulcers in patients with HIV disease. Oral Surg Oral Med Oral Pathol 1994; 77L 116-20

Najarian DJ, Gottlieb A. Connections between psoriasis and Crohn's disease. J Am Acad Dematol 2003; 48:805-21

Obuch M, Maurert T et al. Psoriasis and human immunodeficiency virus infection. J Am Acad Dermatol 1992; 27: 667-673.

Oyama et al. Autoantibodies to extracellular matrix protein 1 (ECMP 1) in lichen sclerosus. Lancet 2003; 362:118-123.

Powell F et al. Pyoderma gangrenosum - a review of 86 patients. Q J Med 1985; 55:173-86.

Prinz K The role of T cells in psoriasis J Eur Acad Dermatol Venereol 2003; 257-270

Rademaker M. Allergic contact dermatitis to a sanitary pad. Aust J Dermatol 2004; 234-5.

Rippke F, Schreiner V, Schwanitz HJ The acidic milieu of the horny layer: new findings on the physiology and pathophysiology of skin pH Am J Clin Dermatol 2002; 3: 261-72

Robinson N, Hashimoto T et al The new pemphigus variants. J Am Acad Dermatol 1999; 40: 649-671

Rogers RS 3rd Recurrent aphthous stomatitis in the diagnosis of Behcet's disease Yonsei Med J 1997; 38: 370-9

Rowan DM and Jones RW. Idiopathic granulomatous vulvitis. Aust J Dermatol 2004; 45:181-3.

Scurry J. Does lichen sclerosus play a central role in the pathogenesis of human papillomavirus negative vulvar squamous cell carcinoma? The itch-scratch-lichen sclerosus hypothesis. Int J Gynecol Cancer. 1999 Mar;9(2):89-97.

Scurry J, Dennerstein G, Brenan J, Oster A, Mason G, Dorevitch A. Vulvitis circumscripta plasmacellularis: a clinicopathological entity? J Reprod Med 1993; 38(1):14-18.

Smith HR, Basketter DA, McFadded JP Irritant dermatitis, irritancy and its role in allergic contact dermatitis. Clin Exp Dermatol 2002; 27: 138-46

Stashower ME, Krivda SJ, Turiansky GW Fox-Fordyce disease: diagnosis with transverse histologic sections. J Am Acad Dermatol 2000; 42: 89-91

Tanaka M, Aiba S, Matsumura N, Aoyama H, Tagami H Prurigo nodularis consists of two distinct forms: early onset atopic and late onset non-atopic Dermatology 1995; 190: 269-76

Thirar S, Deroux E, Dourov N, Evrad L, Peny MO, Simon P, Parent D Granulomatous vulvitis, granulomatous cheilitis: a single diagnosis? Dermatology 1998; 196: 455-8

Thomsen JS, Sonne M, Benfeldt E, Jensen SB, Serup J, Menne T Experimental itch in sodium sulphate-inflamed and normal skin in humans: a randomised, double-blind, placebo-controlled study of histamine and other inducers of itch. Br J Dermatol 2002; 146: 792-800

Understanding atopic dermatitis pathophysiology and etiology. Supplement to J Am Acad Dermatol 2001; 45:S51-568.

Urbanek M, Neill SM, McKee PH Vulval Crohn's disease: difficulties in diagnosis. Clin Exp Dermatol 1996; 21: 211-4

Van de Scheur et al. Ano-genital granulomatosis - the counterpart of oro-facial granulomatosis. JEADV 2003; 17:184-9.

Wollina W Treatment of bullous pemphigoid: what's new. J Eur Acad Dermatol Venereol 2003; 17: 623

Chapter 11

5. ENDOCRINE AND METABOLIC DISORDERS AND DISORDERS OF PIGMENTATION

106. ESTROGEN EXCESS - IATROGENIC

Estrogens are amongst the most frequently used medications, for contraception in the combined oral contraceptive pill and for hormone replacement therapy (HRT) in the postmenopausal or oophorectomized woman. The modern oral contraceptive has had its estrogen content reduced to the minimum required for ovulation suppression and cycle control and is seldom implicated in the disorders which follow. HRT, particularly when the estrogen dosage is greater than that required for replacement, is the usual cause of symptoms referrable to the lower genital tract from estrogen excess.

Clinical features

An increase in physiological secretions (5) and/or pruritus due to *Candida albicans* infection (37) are the commonest adverse vulvovaginal effects.

Diagnosis

A vaginal swab should be examined in every case. A serum estradiol and follicle stimulating hormone (FSH) are useful guides to the adequacy or otherwise of estrogen replacement. If the prescribed estrogen is other than estradiol, a misleadingly low estradiol result may be obtained because of the specificity of radioimmunoassay techniques used by most laboratories today. In such a case, the FSH will still be low.

Treatment

Reduction of HRT dosage is all that is required for the increased physiological discharge. The management of recurrent candidiasis (37) is described in Chapter 9. Where the excessive estrogen levels have resulted from the use of estradiol implants, recurrent candidiasis can be a problem for over a year while the levels fall, sometimes necessitating the use of long term oral azoles.

107. PRECOCIOUS PUBERTY

Precocious puberty (that is, isosexual precocity) is said to occur when secondary sexual characteristics become manifest before the age of 8 years. Most cases result from premature gonadotrophin production of uncertain cause. Occasionally, the cause is an ovarian tumor.

Breast development and menstruation are the usual manifestations likely to bring the girl to medical attention. As with iatrogenic causes above (which can apply in this group), there is the potential for excessive vaginal secretions and/or candidiasis.

108. ESTROGEN DEFICIENCY

Estrogen deficiency is a common cause for a woman's presentation to her medical practitioner and could therefore be considered an endocrine disease. Nevertheless, because the commonest cause of estrogen deficiency (6) are normal phases of a woman's life, this subject is fully discussed in Chapter 7.

109. ADRENOCORTICAL (VIRILIZING) SYNDROMES

The relevance of adrenal hyperactivity to the vulva is with regard to the increase in androgen activity causing virilization. In the infant, congenital adrenal hyperplasia may present with sexual ambiguity. Hirsutes, acne and/or alopecia are the likely causes of presentation in the older female but more pronounced virilization is associated with enlargement of the clitoris.

Adrenal insufficiency (Addison's disease) can cause pigmentation of the vulva and vagina. The macules may vary from honey brown to blue black, depending on the patient's complexion.

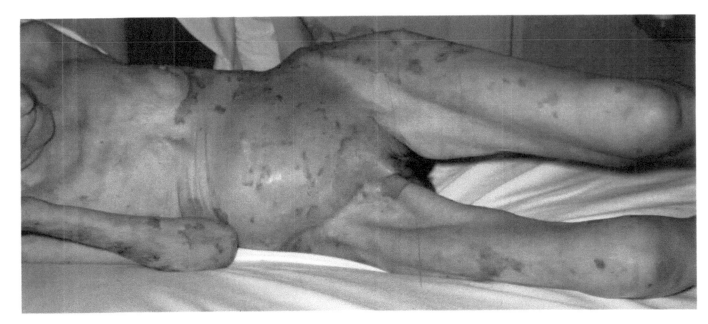

Figure 11.1. Glucagonoma.

Polycystic ovarian syndrome, the commonest endocrinopathy of women in the reproductive years, is associated with increased ovarian stromal production of androgen and decreased sex hormone binding globulin capacity. Women so affected often complain of hirsutes, acne and/or male pattern baldness rather than genital manifestations.

110. IATROGENIC VIRILIZATION

Systemic or topically administered androgenic drugs are potential causes of virilization. Thus, hirsutes, acne, clitoral enlargement, voice deepening and male pattern baldness may occur with prescribed androgens and other drugs with androgenic side effects such as danazol, diazoxide, minoxidil and phenytoin.

Testosterone ointment has been used in the past for the treatment of lichen sclerosus of the vulva and was occasionally associated with clitoral enlargement and discomfort.

111. GLUCAGONOMA SYNDROME

Necrolytic migratory erythema (NME), glucose intolerance and hyperglucagonemia constitute this syndrome, usually due to an alpha cell tumor of the pancreas. NME is rarely due to liver or other metabolic disease.

The characteristic lesions of NME occur between the lower abdomen and thighs inclusive, accentuated around the vulva and anus. They are red, blistered and crusted with annular lesions which spread in an irregular manner and coalesce. They may be painful. The woman is likely to be middle aged and also have wasting, anemia, glossitis and diarrhea. NME resembles the rash of zinc deficiency but zinc levels are normal.

Pathology

NME is a clinicopathological diagnosis. The pathological features overlap with those of acrodermatitis enteropathica. NME may be the first manifestation of a glucagonoma.

Skin biopsy shows confluent parakeratosis, confluent epidermal pallor or necrosis located to the upper part of the epidermis, mild interface change, papillary edema leading to bullae and a lymphohistiocytic infiltrate.

Treatment

The lesions resolve after removal of the pancreatic tumor -when this is the cause.

112. ACANTHOSIS NIGRICANS

Acanthosis nigricans (AN) is usually a cutaneous manifestation of insulin resistance. Hyperinsulinemia produces increased binding to insulin-like growth factor receptors on keratinocytes and fibroblasts producing the changes described below. Certain malignancies (adenocarcinoma of the stomach and lymphoma) may produce insulin-like cytokines resulting in AN with a normal plasma insulin.

Insulin resistance and hyperinsulinemia are associated with obesity and may occur with mutation of the insulin receptor gene (type A syndrome) or with antibodies against the insulin receptor in association with other autoimmune disease (type B syndrome). One of the major biochemical features of polycystic ovarian syndrome is insulin resistance with hyperandrogenism, obesity and sequelae including AN, type 2 diabetes mellitus, hyperlipidemia and cardiovascular disease.

Clinical features

AN affects axillae, neck, cubital fossae and groin as well as ano-genital skin. Orogenital involvement is usually associated with malignancy, when nail changes also occur, namely dystrophy and whiteness. The characteristic skin changes are pigmentation and thickening resulting in increased skin markings, folds and papilla formation.

Pathology

The diagnosis is clinicopathological. Investigations should include glucose tolerance, fasting plasma insulin and assessment for polycystic ovarian syndrome.

The histological changes of AN are hyperkeratosis, acanthosis, papillomatosis and, sometimes, horn cysts. These changes are not specific and may be indistinguishable from seborrheic keratosis. Clinical correlation is, therefore, required for interpretation of pathological findings. The pigmentation appears to be related to hyperkeratosis rather than increased melanin.

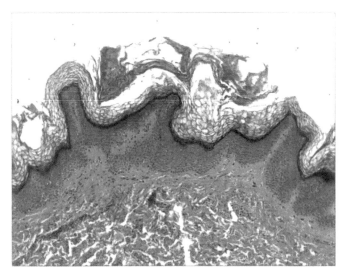

Figure 11.2. Acanthosis nigricans: hyperkeratosis and acanthosis.

Treatment

There is no treatment for the skin changes themselves. Therapeutic efforts must be aimed at the causes above, especially weight reduction and management of malignancy or autoimmune disease.

113. ZINC DEFICIENCY

Dermatitis enteropathica (DE), also known as **acrodermatitis enteropathica**, is an uncommon disorder occurring as a manifestation of zinc deficiency. It is a rare autosomal recessive condition in neonates. Zinc deficiency is also seen in breast fed premature infants whose mothers have low zinc levels in their milk. In adults, the zinc deficiency may be the result of malabsorption or malnutrition. Zinc deficiency shares many clinical and pathological features with NME (**111**) but a common underlying pathogenetic mechanism has not been found.

Zinc deficiency presents with a vesicular, crusted eruption on the hands and feet and well demarcated areas of periorificial crusted erythema also affecting the vulva. The lesions on the face and around the mouth produce a clown-like appearance. There is associated hair loss and diarrhoea

The diagnosis is confirmed by serum zinc estimation. The lesions resolve with zinc administration (zinc sulphate 2 mg/kg for adults, 0.3 mg/kg for the neonate).

114. AMYLOIDOSIS

Amyloidosis refers to a diverse family of diseases characterised by the extracellular deposition of amorphous eosinophilic material which have in common a beta-pleated sheet appearance on ultrastructure. The amyloidoses are classified according to the type of protein forming the amyloid. The main types of amyloid are derived from immunoglobulin light chains (as in multiple myeloma), SAA protein (a product of chronic inflammation) and sundry localised types.

Primary localised genitourinary amyloidosis localised to the urethra has been reported 40 times. It has been postulated to be associated with an idiopathic response to urethritis. Patients present with a lump, which may be confused with cancer.

Vulvar amyloidosis is rare. It is most commonly seen, incidentally, as a late manifestation of systemic amyloidosis, especially in multiple myeloma. In these cases, it is usually observed incidentally in biopsies taken for other reasons or associated with pruritic diseases such as lichen simplex or lichen sclerosus. Rarely, nodular cutaneous amyloidosis forms a clinical mass in the vulva. Amyloid is best seen in the walls of blood vessels and in sub cutaneous tissue. Confirmation with special stains such as Congo red is essential.

115. LIGNEOUS VAGINITIS

"Ligneous" inflammation of the lower female genital tract is so-named because of the firm "woody" nature of its tissue change. It is a rare chronic inflammatory condition, of unknown etiology, which affects mucous membranes. Vaginal disease may rarely precede or more commonly follow the more common ligneous conjunctivitis by a period of several years. Genital disease usually presents with vaginal discharge and inspection reveals necrotic lesions in the vagina and cervix. The skin of the vulva is not involved. A unique patient with infertility and dysmenorrhea also showed ligneous inflammation of the endometrium and fallopian tubes.

Pathology

The ulcerated areas show layers of inflammatory debris, inflamed granulation tissue, amorphous eosinophilic material and fibrosis. The diagnostic feature is the amorphous eosinophilic material, which superficially resembles amyloid. However, at least some of this material is fibrin. It does not stain with Congo red or any other amyloid stain.

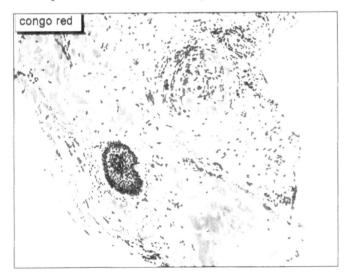

Figure 11.3. Amyloidosis of the vulva stained with Congo red. The stain is positive in the amorphous dermal material and thick-walled vessel.

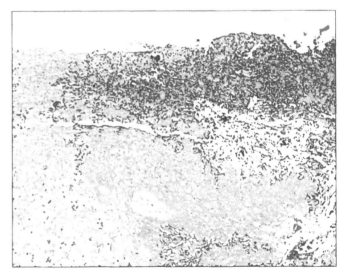

Figure 11.4. Ligneous vaginitis. The surface is ulcerated with an organizing fibrinous exudate.

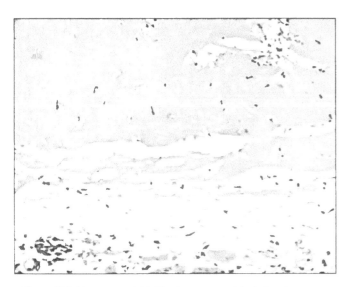

Figure 11.5. Ligneous vaginitis. The deep aspect of the lesion shows a dense mass of fibrin.

Treatment

Only symptomatic treatment can be offered as no specific treatment is known.

116. CALCINOSIS

Deposits of calcium phosphate may rarely be found in the skin of the vulva. Calcinosis cutis is calcium deposition in the skin and may be due to abnormal calcium or phosphorous metabolism (for example, renal or parathyroid disease), secondary to a local lesion, or idiopathic (in otherwise healthy women). Calcinosis is rare in the vulva and is mainly confined to the idiopathic form. It has been described in the vulvas of 7 children and 1 adult. By contrast, idiopathic scrotal calcinosis is fairly common. Recently, the idiopathic nature of scrotal calcinosis has been queried, with the description of various degrees of calcification in epidermal cysts.

The deposits appear as painless, white nodules only a few millimetres in diameter.

Pathology

The dermis shows nodules of amorphous basophilic material, which may not be able to be sectioned with the microtome because of their hardness.

117. VERRUCIFORM XANTHOMA

Verruciform xanthoma (VX) is a rare, benign, tumor-like lesion of uncertain pathogenesis demonstrating xanthoma cells in the dermis. The source of the lipid has been shown to be degenerating keratinocytes. A wide age range may be involved but adults are predominantly affected. VX is confined to sites where squamous epithelium is found. It is either sporadic or associated with a range of disorders, including lichen planus, acantholytic disorders, HIV, squamous cell carcinoma, Milroy's disease and the CHILD (congenital hemidysplasia with ichthyosiform erythroderma and limb defects) syndrome. The mouth is the commonest site, followed by the vulva and vagina. Only occasionally is extragenital skin affected.

Verruciform xanthoma appears as discrete single or multiple, red/pink, papillary/granular/verrucous growths.

Pathology

The squamous mucosa or epidermis shows parakeratosis, marked regular acanthosis and a marked neutrophilic infiltrate. The papillary dermis is filled with xanthoma cells. Beneath the xanthoma cells, there is a dense band-like infiltrate of plasma cells and marked vascularity.

Treatment

The lesions in themselves are harmless. If treatment is required, wide local excision has achieved success but wire loop electrosection, laser and x-ray therapy have failed.

HYPO-PIGMENTATION (HYPOMELANOSIS)

Loss of melanin is commonly seen as part of the pathology of vulvar dermatoses including lichen sclerosus and lichen planus. This contributes to the whiteness of these lesions. Depigmentation in the absence of other apparent skin pathology is the distinguishing feature of vitiligo.

118. VITILIGO

Vitiligo is an acquired patchy loss of melanin from the skin seen most often in the flexures, on the limbs and on genital skin. The appearance of vitiligo on the vulva can raise the suspicion of precancer but the condition is completely benign.

It affects about 1% of the population and there will be a family history of the condition in a quarter of these. Its cause is unknown but some evidence points to neuro-chemical mediators. Other possible causes are melanin destruction by toxic precursors and free radicals or an autoimmune basis. The latter is supported by association with other autoimmune diseases including pernicious anemia and thyroiditis.

Clinical features

There is no alteration of sensation with vitiligo and the presentation results from the concern of the patient or her doctor regarding the appearance of the lesions. They may occur at any age but usually appear before 20. The white patches are sharply demarcated, vary in size and are not raised at all. They tend to be symmetrical but may be unilateral or segmental. There may be an inflammatory border in the early stages. Hair growing in the patches of vitiligo becomes white.

Diagnosis

It should be possible to diagnose vitiligo clinically. If biopsy is performed, the features are an absence of melanocytes and melanin. The edge of an advancing lesion, particularly if clinically inflamed, will also show occasional lymphocytes adjacent to residual

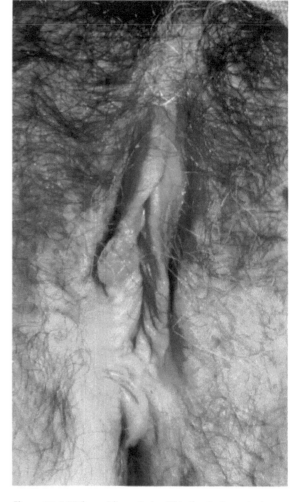

Figure 11.6. Vitiligo with psoriasis within the depigmented patches.

melanocytes within the basal layer of the epidermis. This is consistent with the view that vitiligo is due to a lymphocyte-directed apoptosis of melanocytes.

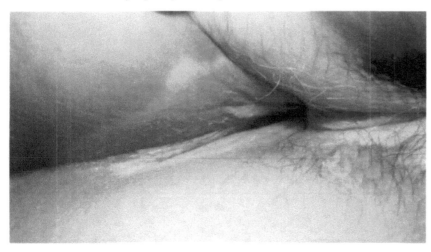

Figure 11.7. Natal cleft of the patient in Fig 11.6.

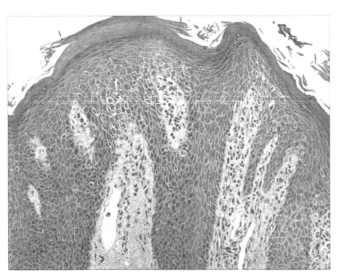

Figure 11.8. Biopsy from the labium majus of the patient in Fig. 11.6 The histology is dominated by a subacute spongiotic tissue reaction. The vitiligo appears as an absence of basal pigmentation and melanocytes, but requires an immunoperoxidase study for melanocytes to confirm the diagnosis.

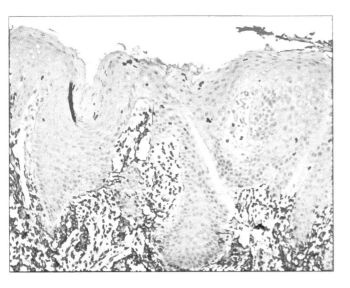

Figure 11.9. The biopsy in Fig. 11.8 stained with MART 1. It shows a complete absence of melanocytes (which would stain dark brown) at the dermo-epidermal junction. Normally, there is one melanocyte for approximately every 10 basal squamous cells.

Treatment

It should not be necessary to treat vulvar vitiligo. Topical corticosteroids, pimicrolimus and tacrolimus may be helpful if treatment is sought.

119. HYPER-PIGMENTATION (HYPERMELANOSIS)

Increased melanin deposition may be secondary to inflammatory dermatoses where there is basal layer damage. This phenomenon is known to the pathologist as pigment incontinence. It is seen, for example, in fixed drug eruptions, classically that caused by sulfonamides. Other drugs associated with hypermelanosis include minocycline, antimalarials and heavy metals. Hypermelanosis may be a physiological feature of pregnancy. It may also be a feature of acanthosis nigricans, Addison's disease, Cushing's disease, hyperthyroidism, acromegaly, HIV infection and hemochromatosis (bronze diabetes).

Melanocytic Macules (**157**), associated syndromes and pigmented nevi (moles **159**) are discussed in Chapter 13. Increased melanin deposition is a feature of differentiated (warty) vulvar intraepithelial neoplasia (previously called bowenoid papulosis) (**130**).

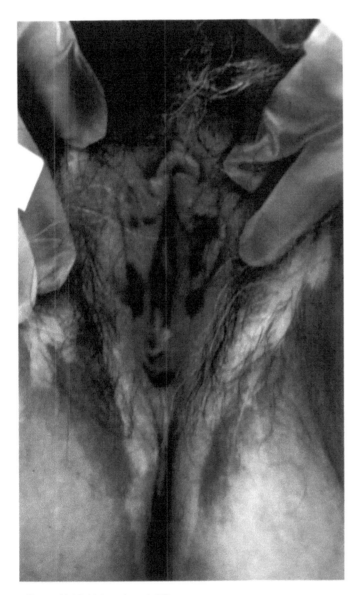

Figure 11.10. Melanosis and vitiligo.

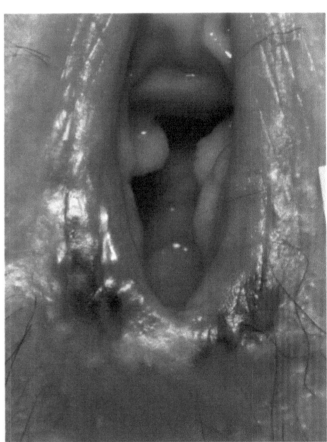

Figure 11.11. Melanosis.

REFERENCES

Bernardo BD, Huettner PC, Merritt DF, Ratts VS Idiopathic calcinosis cutis presenting as labial lesions in children: report of two cases with literature review. J Pediatr Adoles Gynecol 1999; 12: 157-60

Crook TJ, Koslowski M, Dyer JP, Bass P, Birch BR A case of amyloid of the urethra and review of this rare diagnosis, its natural history and management, with reference to the literature. Scand J Urol Nephrol 2002; 36: 481-6

Garcia Hidalgo L Dermatological complications of obesity. Am J Clin Dermatol 2002; 3: 497-506

Grasinger CC, Wild RA, Parker IJ Vulvar acanthosis nigricans: a marker of insulin resistance in hirsute women. Fertil Steril 1993; 59: 583-6

Hamidi Asl K, Liepnieks JJ, Bihrle R, Benson MD Local synthesis of amyloid fibril precursor in AL amyloidosis of the urinary tract. Amyloid 1998; 5: 49-54

Horejsi J Acquired clitoral enlargement: diagnosis and treatment. Ann N Y Acad Sci 1997; 17: 369-72

Konig A, Wennemuth G, Soyer HP, Hoffman R, Happle R, Krause W. Vulvar amyloidosis mimicking giant condylomata acuminata in a patient with multiple myeloma Eur J Dermatol 1999; 9: 29-31

Kovacs S. Vitiligo. J Am Acad Dermatol 1998; 38:647-66

Luxman D, Cohen JR, Gordon D, Wolman I, Wolf Y, David MP Unilateral vulvar edema associated with paracentesis in patients with severe ovarian hyperstimulation syndrome. A report of 9 cases. J Reprod Med 1996; 41: 771-4

Marinkovich MP, Botella R, Datloff J, Sangueza OP. Necrolytic migratory erythema without glucagonoma in patients with liver disease. J Am Acad Dermatol 1995; 32: 604-9

Northcutt AD, Vanover MJ. Nodular cutaneous amyloidosis involving the vulva. Case report and literature review. Arch Dermatol 1985; 121: 518-21

Ozcelik B, Serin IS, Basbug M, Ozturk F. Idiopathic calcinosis cutis of the vulva in an elderly woman. A case report. J Reprod Med 2002; 47: 597-9

Rapoport M, Yona R, Kaufman S, Segal M, Kornberg A Unusual bleeding manifestations of amyloidosis in patients with multiple myeloma. Clin Lab Haematol 1994; 16: 349-53

Remes-Troch JM et al. Necrolytic migratory erythema: a cutaneous clue to glucagonoma syndrome. J E A D V 2004; 18:591-5.

Chapter 12

6. TRAUMA

120. OBSTETRIC TRAUMA

The commonest cause of moderate or severe physical trauma to the vagina and vulva is childbirth. Most primigravidas and many parous women delivering vaginally at or near term will experience tearing of the lower vagina and/or vulva around the introitus unless the perineum is incised (episiotomy) to enlarge the introitus. In the milder cases these tears involve only skin, do not bleed excessively and will heal within a few days without suturing. In the severest cases, often when instrumental delivery has been performed in a suboptimal manner, lacerations can extend through deep tissue to involve adjacent structures, even bladder or rectum.

Clinical features

The primigravida with a fetus at or near term is most at risk. Labor is not necessarily prolonged and sometimes quite severe tearing is experienced when a normal delivery is relatively rapid. Signs of imminent tearing are blanching of the perineum, bleeding or tearing of the vulva in front of the presenting part. Maneuvers involving rotation of the presenting part may lacerate the vagina with relatively little trauma to the vulva.

The vulva should always be carefully inspected after any delivery. Gaping lacerations are most common around the fourchette, both sagittal and circumferential. Vestibule, labia minora and occasionally the clitoris may be involved. Tears involving the vagina may be associated with profuse bleeding because of the vascularity of this organ.

Vulvovaginal hematoma is a relatively uncommon result of obstetric trauma. It results from the shearing force of the fetal head passing down the vagina tearing blood vessels beneath the epithelium. It presents with a very painful swelling and possibly shock and/or urinary retention.

Fistulae are associated with suboptimal or absent obstetric care and difficult labor. They may present in the puerperium with true urinary incontinence (vesicovaginal, rarely ureterovaginal or urethrovaginal fistula) or fecal incontinence (perineal tear including anal sphincter or rectovaginal fistula). Vaginal prolapse is usually a late manifestation of obstetric trauma. Although more common after vaginal delivery, it is still seen in women who have only been delivered by caesarean section as a result of fascial stretching from pregnancy.

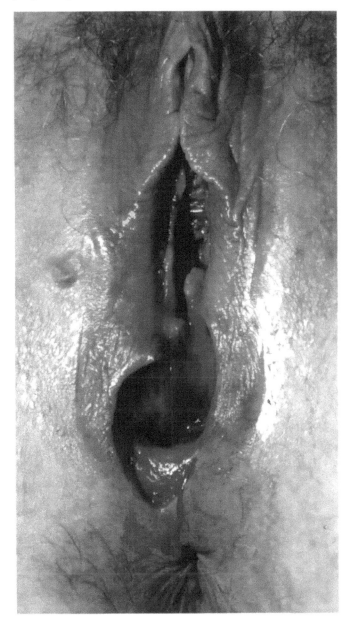

Figure 12.1. Episiotomy showing (intact) anal sphincter.

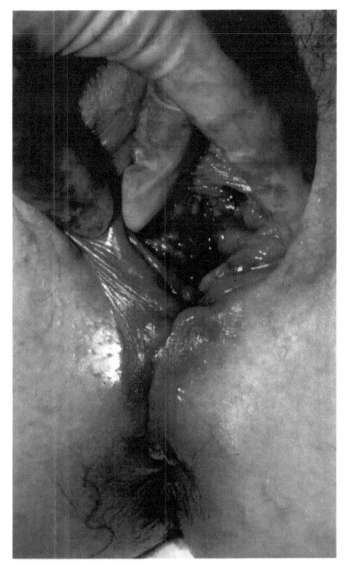

Figure 12.2. The episiotomy in Fig. 12.1 after repair.

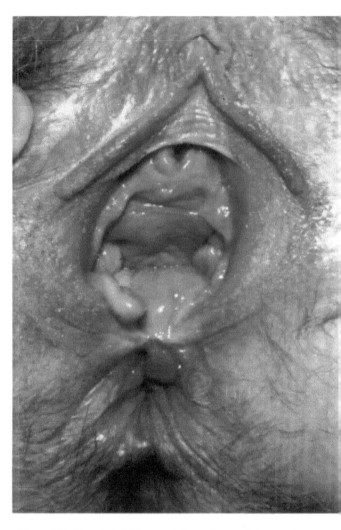

Figure 12.3. Complete dehiscence of the perineum that was not repaired shown one year after the (forceps) delivery. The mucosa of the anal canal is continuous with the epithelium of the vagina.

Treatment

Severe trauma to the vulva and vagina is best prevented by optimal management of the labor and delivery. The use of episiotomy continues to be the subject of debate. Available evidence suggests that episiotomy does not prevent urinary incontinence or influence the incidence of long term dyspareunia. There is, however, a paucity of randomized, controlled trials of episiotomy, a procedure that may vary from one operator to the next. Thus, the outcome is likely to be different between, say, a midline episiotomy with a 'hockey stick' posterior end to avoid the anal sphincter, no larger than necessary to prevent tearing, cut and repaired in layers by an experienced gynecologist and a laterally placed episiotomy cut at the wrong time and left unsutured.

Over 3 decades of obstetric and gynecologic practice has convinced this author that an appropriately cut and correctly repaired episiotomy will significantly reduce morbidity from obstetric trauma, particularly with regard to the preservation of normal anatomy. In general, episiotomies and vulvar lacerations that gape are best repaired in layers with absorbable sutures. Vaginal lacerations should only need to be sutured if they are bleeding significantly or are large.

A vulvovaginal hematoma should be incised and drained and any apparent bleeding vessels ligated. Vaginal packing and insertion of a urethral catheter will be necessary if the bleeding continues. Blood transfusion may be required.

The repair of obstetric fistulas involves relatively complex surgery and is the subject of text books on its own.

121. SEXUAL TRAUMA

Female genital sexual trauma can arise from attempting vaginal penetration with phallus, fingers or foreign object with or without the woman's consent. The commonest, clinically recognizable situation is tearing of the hymen with loss of virginity, the most serious is rape. The effects of sexual trauma are likely to be most severe in the prepubertal girl, the virgin, the postmenopausal, pregnant or postnatal woman or the woman who has undergone surgery involving the vagina such as hysterectomy or vaginal repair.

Where sexual trauma has arisen against the woman's wishes, the psychological sequelae are likely to be even greater and longer lasting than the organic. In the majority of rape cases, clinically recognizable genital trauma will not be apparent even when there are signs of extragenital trauma, for example bruising and abrasions of the limbs from struggling to resist. Patients in this regrettably common situation require communication and handling with particular care and sensitivity.

Clinical features

The vast majority of sexual trauma never comes to medical attention. When it does, it will be because of hemorrhage, pain or emotional distress with or without the likelihood of legal action. Rarely, the clinician will need to deal with a false allegation of rape arising from the need for an alibi, revenge or attention seeking behavior.

The hymen is not a particularly vascular or sensitive structure so its tearing with loss of virginity is seldom reported. Occasionally, a sizeable artery does run around the hymen and its tearing can result in considerable blood loss.

Coital injuries range from relatively minor tears and fissures of the fourchette and labial sulci (see also **273** arousal failure and **274** vaginismus) to lacerations of the vagina that can even extend into the pouch of Douglas, bladder or rectum, fortunately rarely. Perineal dehiscence and large hematomas are also described.

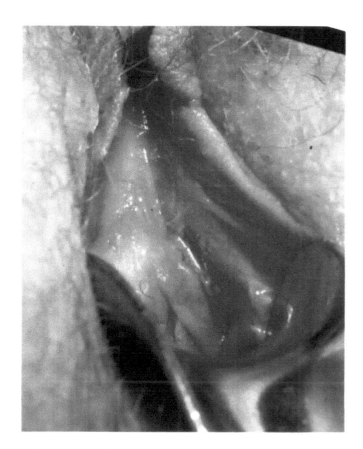

Figure 12.4. Coital tear in the anterior vestibule.

Diagnosis

When the patient is the victim of sexual assault, the examination needs to be much more detailed than a routine clinical examination. The reader is referred to the appropriate forensic texts for description of the clinical data and specimen collection and documentation required in such cases. These requirements may vary between countries or even states.

Treatment

When the injuries have arisen from consensual sex, management is likely to consist of examination, reassurance and instruction to avoid penetration for a couple of weeks to allow healing. The woman may require the advice given to the patient with arousal failure and vaginismus.

Examination may reveal lacerations that require suturing for hemostasis. Surgical repair may need to be extensive, particularly in assault cases

122. ACCIDENTAL TRAUMA

The genital region in the female is the least exposed body surface and rarely traumatized in accidents unless extensive extragenital injuries have been sustained. Most significant vulvar injuries arise from falls astride objects or as the result of being thrown against the handlebars of bicycles or motorcycles.

Where vulvar lacerations and hematomas indicate significant trauma, vaginal examination, if necessary under anesthesia, is imperative, searching for foreign bodies in the vagina, vaginal lacerations and penetration into bladder, rectum or peritoneal cavity.

Anatomical disruption and bleeding lacerations must be repaired, if necessary in layers, with absorbable sutures. A vaginal pack and urethral catheter may occasionally be necessary for hemostasis. The pack should be well soaked in an antibiotic cream (for example, clindamycin cream) and left in no longer than 24 hours. Bladder or rectal involvement requires surgery beyond the scope of this manual.

123. SELF-INDUCED TRAUMA

Although uncommon, significant trauma to the vulva and (less commonly) vagina, caused by the woman herself, can create diagnostic difficulty. By far the commonest form of self-induced vulvar trauma is excoriation from scratching pruritic epithelial disorders. These excoriations may present as vulvar ulcers and require biopsy for confirmation. The patient may or may not admit to this self-induced trauma upon direct questioning.

When self-induced genital trauma other than scratching pruritic lesions occurs, significant psychopathology is likely to be present adding to diagnostic difficulty. Factitial dermatitis, also known as dermatitis artefacta, is one form of such trauma. It can be caused by the fingernail, a sharp object or application of caustic chemicals. Patients who damage themselves in this manner are likely to pick sites more easily accessible than the vulva.

Clinical features

The patient may present with pain, bleeding or discharge or the lesions may be noticed incidentally during examination for some other reason.

Excoriations are tiny (a couple of millimeters only), usually superficial, weeping ulcers commonly seen on lichenified vulvar skin. They are most likely multiple and are all within easy reach of the fingernail. A solitary, deeper excoriation may mimic a more sinister lesion.

In the uncommon situation where self-mutilation has resulted from psychopathology, the lesions may take on any form, depending on the instrument used, but are likely to have a bizarre appearance and not mimic other genital disease (see also somatoform disorder 272).

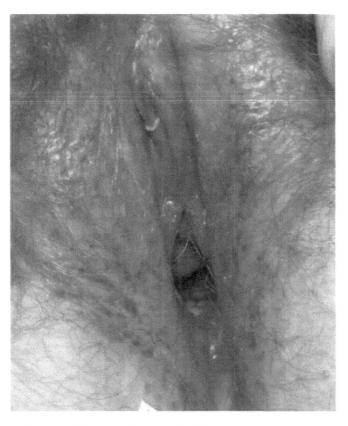

Figure 12.5. Multiple excoriations of the labia majora.

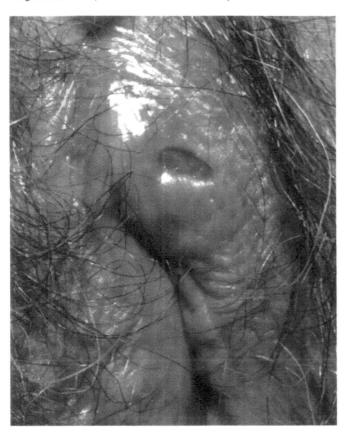

Figure 12.6. Excoriation presenting as a vulvar ulcer.

Diagnosis

Biopsy may be necessary to differentiate excoriation from other causes of epithelial loss. Excoriations occur on a background of the changes of an itchy dermatosis such as lichen simplex chronicus or lichen sclerosus. Excoriations, first and foremost, affect the stratum corneum, which may be partly or completely lost and show parakeratosis, edema, polymorphs and red blood cells, together forming a 'parakeratotic scale crust'. The prickle cell layer shows focal spongiosis, red blood cells and polymorphs A small amount of fibrin is seen beneath the basement membrane, associated with bleeding, polymorphs and later, an increased number of lymphocytes and plasma cells. Excoriations have an important differential diagnosis of fungal infection and psoriasis, which also produce a crust of parakeratosis and polymorphs. A PAS stain is mandatory but a negative stain does not exclude fungal infection.

A formal psychiatric examination may be necessary where self-mutilation is suspected.

Treatment

Excoriations will heal by themselves once the underlying pruritus is attended to. Sedation is likely to be necessary in addition to the appropriate topical therapy in the more severe case. The reader is also referred to the psychologist's approach (Chapter 4). The psychiatric management of self-mutilation is beyond the scope of this manual.

IATROGENIC TRAUMA

124. SURGICAL TRAUMA
Vulvar surgery is performed to treat neoplastic and pre-neoplastic lesions and for the correction of anatomical abnormalities, both congenital and acquired. Generally speaking, it is contraindicated in the treatment of inflammatory non-infections, non-neoplastic disorders and in the management of dyspareunia, which is functional in origin.

Cold knife, diathermy and laser are all used on the vulva and vagina. This folded epithelium with loose, vascular connective tissue does very well with excision, plastic procedures and repair with fine, absorbable sutures. The surface treatment of lesions (without excision and suture) with diathermy or laser, however, has the potential to produce chronic pain. Rarely, erosive lichen planus (including vulvitis circumscripta plasmacellularis) may occur at the site of previous laser treatment as a Kobner phenomenon. Laser is thus best restricted to situations such as extensive intraepithelial neoplasia, where excisional surgery may be relatively mutilating.

The use of non-absorbable mesh or tape beneath the vaginal epithelium, for example with incontinence surgery, is increasing. Its complications will be addressed under **foreign body**, below.

125. CHEMICAL TRAUMA
Clinical human papillomavirus infection and intraepithelial neoplasia are frequently treated with cytotoxic or caustic applications. These include podophyllin, 5-fluorouracil, trichloracetic acid and imiquimod. Imiquimod supposedly acts as an immune modulator but does have the potential in practice to produce a similar response to the others.

Particularly when used excessively, these applications can cause a severe inflammatory response sometimes going onto epithelial necrosis and ulceration. This damage will generally resolve within a couple of weeks of cessation of the applications. As with the surgical treatments above, such a response may leave the woman with chronic pain in the area.

126. IRRADIATION
The vulva and vagina tend to respond to irradiation in a worse manner than most skin elsewhere. This is most likely to be seen as a result of the use of radiotherapy in the treatment of uterine cancer by external beam or intracavity usage. Nevertheless, newer techniques now permit tumorocidal doses of radiation beneath the epithelium without producing the surface damage that has precluded, for example, radiotherapy for vulvar malignancy in the past.

Irradiation of the vulva or vagina results in a response ranging from some apparent mottling (poikiloderma), atrophy and telangiectasia through to complete epithelial loss usually associated with fibrosis. Cytological changes may persist for decades. These include lack of maturation (basal cells only), marked dyskaryosis with bizarre cell shapes, hyperchromasia and loss of the normal nuclear-cytoplasmic ratio.

The above effects will be exacerbated by estrogen lack. Topical or systemic estrogen replacement (in the postmenopausal or oophorectomized woman) and the use of vaginal dilators are the likely essentials of treatment.

127. FEMALE CIRCUMCISION AND RELATED PROCEDURES
Of the order of 100-126 million women and girls, mainly in Africa and the Middle East, have undergone some surgical procedure performed on the vulva for solely traditional reasons. These procedures, usually performed before puberty, vary between cultural groups. They range from nicking the foreskin of the clitoris through circumcision to removal of the clitoris, labia minora and closure of the introitus by incision and suture together of the labia minora. Closure of the introitus as described is referred to as infibulation and may be performed alone. Its intent is to ensure virginity prior to marriage. However, there are numerous other reasons for performing these procedures: they include rite of passage, group identification, hygiene beliefs and belief in psychosexual benefit. They are not confined to Islam and are not practiced by a large proportion of Muslims. They are performed by practitioners with no medical training and without any anesthesia

or attention to asepsis through to formal surgical procedures performed under general anesthesia by gynecologists.

The potential for complications arising from these practices is great. In the short term they include pain, hemorrhage, infection (tetanus, septicemia and others) and urinary retention. Death may result. In the longer term, there may be significant impairment of urinary and menstrual flow, clitoral and labial cyst formation, and the expected sexual dysfunction, both organic (from scarring) and psychogenic. It is intended that the infibulated vulva is reopened by the new husband with a knife or finger but this might be done incompletely with the potential for subsequent obstruction of delivery of the fetal presenting part and increased risk of major obstetric tears.

After the procedure is performed, emergency treatment may be required such as hemostasis, surgical repair and/or antibiotics and blood transfusion. Later, vulvoplasty may be indicated for sexual dysfunction and/or voiding difficulty. Where clitoral amputation has occurred, the clitoris can be restored to normal or near normal length by dissection and reattachment of its supports. This procedure is claimed to be associated with return of normal sexual response. Clitoral cysts may cause significant discomfort and require removal with or without a further plastic procedure. Finally, women may request a repeat infibulation with a change of partner.

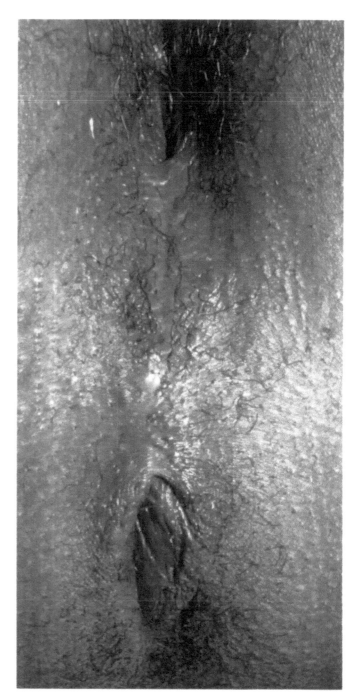

Figure 12.7. Ritual infibulation.

128. FOREIGN BODY

Retention of a foreign body within the vagina is of considerable clinical importance. In children, clinical disease will result from the presence within the vagina of pieces of toilet paper or more solid objects such as toys or other material inserted by the child herself. In the case of the adult, she is likely to present to her doctor because of retained tampon, objects used during sexual activity or pessaries used in the treatment of prolapse. Of increasing importance is erosion through the vaginal wall of non-absorbable tapes and mesh used in the treatment of stress incontinence and pelvic floor defects. A history of recent childbirth or gynecological surgery raises the possibility of retained packs or swabs. The repair of obstetric trauma carries a relatively high risk of retained pack. The risk is increased when the repair is not performed in an operating theatre, when lighting is inadequate and the procedure is left to relatively inexperienced staff assisted by nursing staff without operating room training (including the understanding of the need for pack and swab counts).

Clinical presentation

At any age, vaginal discharge is the commonest symptom of vaginal foreign body and is one of the reasons why speculum examination is a mandatory part of the management of this common symptom. In the prepubertal girl and postmenopausal, estrogen deficient woman, the atrophic epithelium will be relatively quickly inflamed and eroded by the foreign body so that the discharge may be blood stained. Vaginal foreign body in the child occasionally presents with recurrent urinary tract infection. Retained tampon produces a particularly offensive discharge. A common story is that the woman forgets that she has a tampon in the vagina and inserts another, thereby pushing the strings of the first tampon completely into the vagina. Thus, the finding of a retained tampon usually comes as a surprise to the patient.

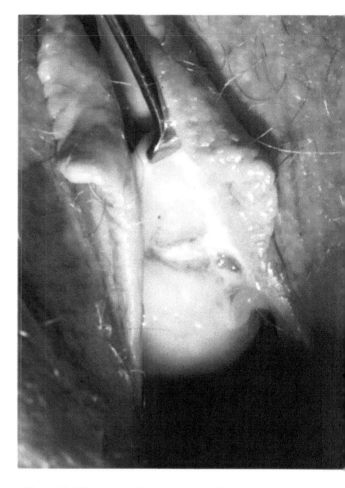

Figure 12.8. Tape inserted in the treatment of stress incontinence of urine eroding through vaginal wall.

Diagnosis

In the adult, the diagnosis is readily made on routine gynecological examination. However, in the case of erosion due to tape used in the treatment of stress incontinence, the diagnosis can be missed because of the elevation of the anterior vaginal wall produced by the procedure making its visualization very difficult. The affected area in these cases is best visualized with a Sims' speculum and dental mirror.

Speculum examination in the office is usually not possible in the case of the child, causing particular diagnostic difficulty. It is essential and should be possible to take a vaginal or at least introital swab under these circumstances. A finding of polymorphonuclear leucocytes in the presence of a normal flora should be considered an indication for examination under anesthesia.

Particularly with sharp objects, a careful search should be performed for laceration through to bladder or rectum. Erosion through to bladder or rectum has been reported with other than sharp objects such as surgical packs, pessaries and even a vibrator.

Treatment

Removal of the foreign object with sponge holding forceps at the time of the speculum examination will be the only treatment required in most cases. In the estrogen deficient patient, a couple of weeks usage of topical estrogen may hasten recovery and prevent adhesion formation.

Antibiotic therapy should only be necessary in the uncommon situation where ascending infection is present, most likely with tampons and packs long neglected. The decision to use antibiotics should be guided by clinical signs (fever, pelvic tenderness), the cervical swab and the white cell count.

Once tape or mesh erosion is detectable vaginally, the offending material will need to be removed. Complete removal vaginally may be very difficult. Sometimes the patient will be rendered free of symptoms with incomplete removal of the material (even if some remains).

REFERENCES

Bowyer L, Dalton ME. Rape and genital injuries. Br J Obstet Gynaecol 1997; 104: 617-620.

Buck P. Female Genital Mutilation. RCOG Statement No. 3 2003, May.

Ecker JL, Tan WM, Bansal RK, Bishop JT, Kilpatrick SJ. Is there a benefit to episiotomy at operative vaginal delivery? Observations over ten years in a stable population. Am J Obstet Gynecol 1997; 176(2): 411-414.

Fleming VEM, Hagen S, Niven C. Does perineal suturing make a difference? The SUNS trial. BJOG 2003; 110: 684-689

Fraunholz IB, Schopol B, Bottcher HD. Management of radiation injuries of vulva and vagina. Strahlentherapie und Onkologie 1998; 174 Suppl 3:90-2.

Heppenstall-Heger A, McConnell G, Ticson L, Guerra L, Lister J, Zaragoza T. Healing patterns in anogenital injuries: a longitudinal study of injuries associated with sexual abuse, accidental injuries, or genital surgery in the preadolescent child. Pediatrics 2003; 112(4): 829-37.

Hoffman RJ, Ganti S. Vaginal laceration and perforation resulting from first coitus. Pediatric Emergency Care 2001; 17(2):113-4.

Jensen PT, Groenvold M, Klee MC, Thanov I, Petersen MA, Machin D. Longitudinal study of sexual function and vaginal changes after radiotherapy for cervical cancer. International Journal of Radiation Oncology, Biology, Physics 2003; 56(4):937-49.

Jones JS, Rossman L, Wynn BN, Dunnuck C, Schwartz N. Comparative analysis of adult versus adolescent sexual assault: epidemiology and patterns of anogenital injury. Acad Emerg Med 2003; 10(8):872-7.

Penna C. Fallani MG. Fambrini M. Zipoli E. Marchionni M. Type III female genital mutilation: clinical implications and treatment by carbon dioxide laser surgery. American Journal of Obstetrics & Gynecology. 187(6):1550-4, 2002 Dec.

Pokorny SF. Long-term intravaginal presence of foreign bodies in children. A preliminary study. Journal of Reproductive Medicine 1994; 39(12):931-5.

Shah AN, Olah KS, Jackson R. Retained foreign bodies in the vagina. International Journal of Gynecology & Obstetrics 2003;81(2):221-2

Shield PW. Chronic radiation effects: a correlative study of smears and biopsies from the cervix and vagina. Diagnostic Cytopathology 1995; 13(2)107-19.

Sleep J, Grant A. West Berkshire perineal management trial: three year follow up. British Medical Journal Clinical ResearchEd. 1987. 295(6601): 749-51.

Smith YR, Berman DR, Quint EH. Premenarchal vaginal discharge: findings of procedures to rule out foreign bodies. Journal of Pediatric & Adolescent Gynecology 2002; 15(4):227-30.

Thabet SMA, Thabet ASMA. Defective sexuality and female circumcision: The cause and the possible management. J Obstet Gynecol Res 2003; 29(1):12-19.

Chapter 13

7. NEOPLASMS

A. Vulva

129. SEBORRHEIC KERATOSIS

The seborrheic keratosis (seborrheic or senile wart) is an extremely common benign squamous neoplasm of skin found all over the body except palms and soles, particularly from middle age onwards, and equally between genders. There is no special propensity to involve the vulva.

Clinical features

As elsewhere on the body, seborrheic keratoses appear as pigmented, friable, greasy, irregular, warty plaques, millimetres to centimetres in size. The usual sites of seborrheic keratoses are on the lateral vulva, mons, genitocrural fold and thigh. Growths resembling seborrheic keratoses, which contain HPV DNA, should be termed condylomas. Such warts are usually seen on the medial vulva in younger women compared to true seborrheic keratoses which usually occur on the lateral vulva in older women.

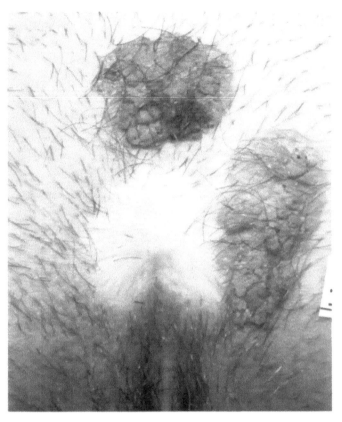

Figure 13.1. Large seborrheic keratoses. The white patch is the result of an attempted removal with diathermy.

Pathology

Seborrheic keratoses are neoplastic proliferations of benign squamous cells of the epidermis and follicular epithelium without atypia. They show various combinations of 4 cardinal features: acanthosis (proliferation of squamous cells), hyperkeratosis, horn cysts and papillomatosis. The squamous cells are generally basaloid, hence the alternative designation, "basaloid papilloma". They may be pigmented due to melanin production by non-neoplastic melanocytes.

Treatment

In view of the harmless nature of the lesions and occasional difficulties with eradication, they can be left untreated if the diagnosis is certain. They may be removed by excision and suture, cryotherapy or simple curettage and diathermy to the base.

VULVAR INTRAEPITHELIAL NEOPLASIA (VIN, SQUAMOUS DYSPLASIA, CARCINOMA IN SITU)

Squamous premalignant disease of the vulva is termed VIN and is synonymous with squamous dysplasia or carcinoma in situ. The term VIN has been widely adopted and replaces confusing terms such as erythroplasia of Queyrat, vulvar dystrophy with atypia, Bowen's disease and bowenoid papulosis. It is understood that VIN means only premalignant squamous cell disease on the vulva and excludes extramammary Paget's disease and intraepithelial melanoma. There are two clinicopathological types of VIN, the common form (warty basaloid), and differentiated. Warty basaloid VIN is the usual type. It is HPV related, while differentiated VIN usually develops on a background of lichen sclerosus.

130. VIN (COMMON FORM)

The common form of VIN is HPV-related and analogous to CIN and VAIN. It was previously thought that VIN was a fairly indolent disease compared to the cervical equivalent (CIN) but there is now evidence that high grade VIN treated conservatively, rather than with standard excision or ablative therapy, will progress to carcinoma in about 80% of cases. Spontaneous regression has been reported in selected cases.

Clinical features

The symptoms of VIN vary but commonly include pruritus and the finding of a lesion by the patient. The lesions vary in colour, size and shape and can be multifocal. There are no consistent colposcopic findings and any suspicious lesions should be biopsied.

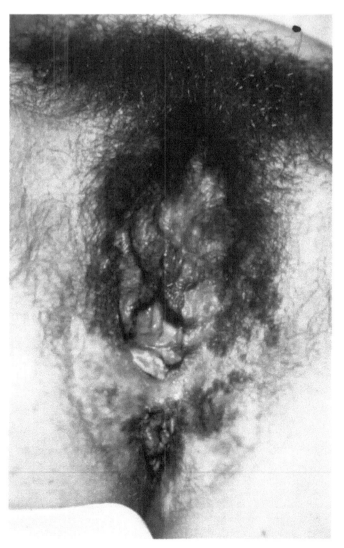

Figure 13.2. Vulvar intraepithelial neoplasia ('Bowenoid papulosis').

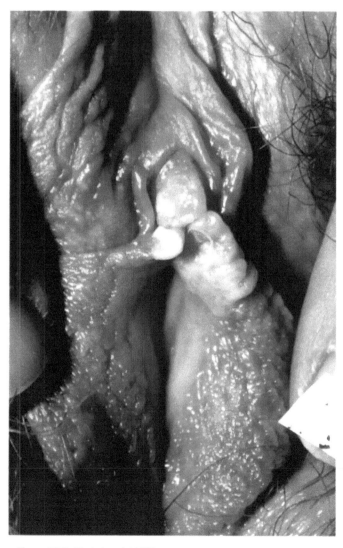

Figure 13.3 . Warty basaloid VIN.

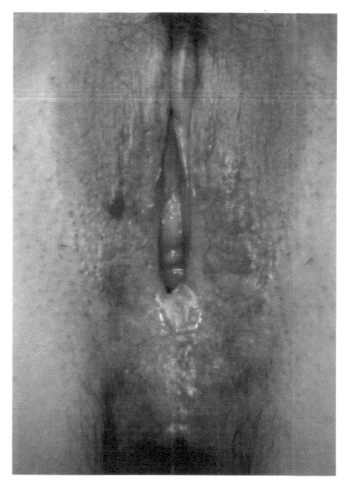

Figure 13.5. Warty basaloid VIN in a 19 year old.

Pathology

VIN is invariably hyperplastic. The architecture may be simple or quite complicated. A complicated appearance with apparently separated nests in the dermis may occur without implying invasion and results from one or more of an intrinsic irregular acanthosis associated with dysplasia, involvement of appendages and folding of the specimen (if it was not pinned out prior to fixation).

VIN usually shows parakeratosis on the surface, although, alternatively, there may be hyperkeratosis and hypergranulosis. In nearly all cases, a stromal lymphocytic infiltrate is seen in the dermis beneath the epithelium. The dysplastic epithelium shows delay in maturation, which manifests as immature cells extending above their usual place in the basal layers.

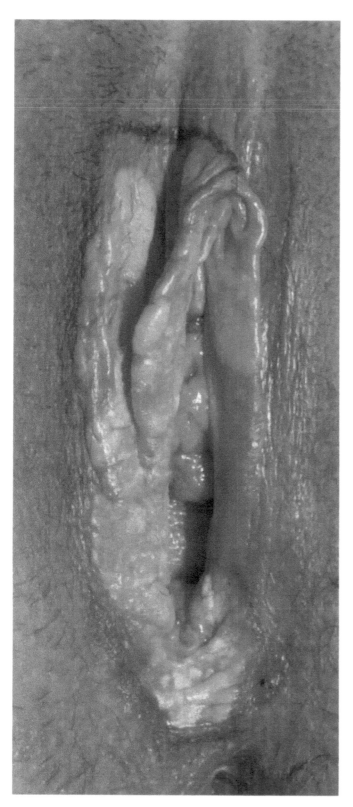

Figure 13.4. Warty basaloid VIN.

Mitosis and apoptosis are common, with usually one or more examples per high power field. Atypical mitoses, particularly lag-phase mitoses and polyploid mitoses are common.

The pathognomonic feature is squamous dysplasia. This is characterized by nuclear changes that correlate with aneuploidy. The best correlates are nuclear pleomorphism, hyperchromatism and enlargement, all of which must be seen in the basal layers to prevent confusion with koilocytosis. Koilocytosis may be seen on the surface, particularly in the lower grades of VIN.

As currently practiced, the grading of VIN depends primarily on the level at which atypical immature, vertically orientated basaloid cells flatten out as they mature into (abnormal) squamous cells. Three grades, VIN 1, 2 and 3 are defined depending on whether these cells are confined to the lower third (VIN 1), lower two thirds (VIN 2) and above the lower two thirds (VIN 3). These grades may alternatively be called mild, moderate and severe dysplasia.

Recently, it has been shown that VIN 1 is not a reproducible diagnosis, being confused with flat wart, inflammatory atypia (e.g., in lichen planus) and differentiated VIN (see below), and that VIN 2 and 3 are not clearly distinguished by pathologists. This may lead to some simplification of the VIN grading system. Already, some clinicians and pathologists tend to think in terms of low grade and high grade VIN. As a result, some pathologists grade VIN analogously to the Bethesda system for cervical smear reporting, that is, into low grade lesions corresponding to flat wart and VIN 1 and high grade lesions corresponding to VIN 2 and VIN 3.

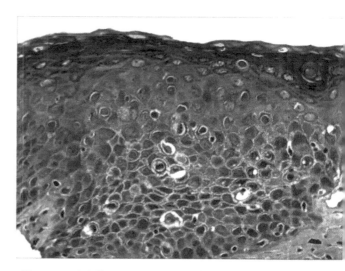

Figure 13.6. VIN. There is a mild degree of nuclear dysplasia and loss of maturation. Any degree of dysplasia is termed VIN.

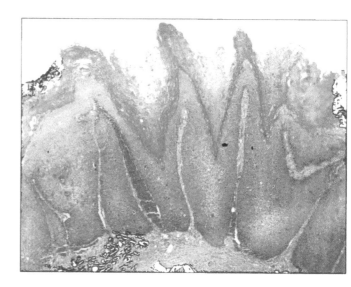

Figure 13.7. VIN, warty sub type, characterized by spiky acanthosis, parakeratosis and acanthosis.

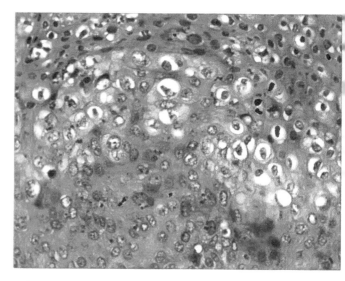

Figure 13.8. VIN, warty sub type. The surface shows koilocytosis.

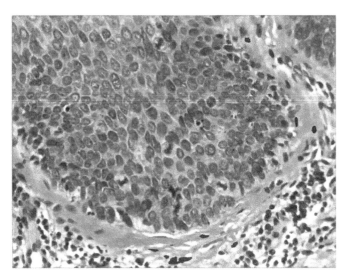
Figure 13.9. VIN, basaloid sub type. The epithelium is replaced by atypical immature cells.

Management

The active treatment of VIN is surgical excision or ablation. The CO2 laser can be used when early stromal invasion has been excluded in areas where surgical excision is difficult. VIN is best excised in hair-bearing areas because dysplastic epithelium can be found deeply placed around hair follicles. CO2 laser can be used in non-hair bearing areas, especially in the clitoral and peri-clitoral areas where a good therapeutic and cosmetic result can be obtained.

The recurrence rate of VIN can be as high as 30% and long-term follow-up is appropriate. Initially, this could be 6 monthly and then yearly. The follow-up examination should consist of thorough inspection with or without colposcopy and/or scrapings for cytology and/or biopsy of suspicious areas. Because of the higher incidence of other genital precancer in these women, inspection of the entire genital tract and Pap smear should be carried out at each visit.

It has been suggested that VIN in women with the following characteristics can be observed for 12 months to allow spontaneous regression prior to considering treatment: (1) Age under 30 years, (2) Lesions small, multifocal, pigmented, papular, (3) Race non-Caucasian, (4) Strong history of genital warts. Some of these characteristics remain controversial.

131. DIFFERENTIATED VIN (DVIN)

The immediate premalignant step of non-HPV vulvar squamous cell carcinoma has been postulated to be DVIN. The term 'differentiated' as applied to VIN is used in the sense of keratin production and does not imply low grade. DVIN is not seen very often before cancer. Explanations are that DVIN is a virulent form of VIN that rapidly transforms to invasive carcinoma or that its histological features are subtle and under-diagnosed.

DVIN is seen in three related settings: Most commonly, it is seen next to invasive SCC in excision specimens. Secondly, DVIN is frequent in the follow-up of women with the HPV negative vulvar squamous cell carcinoma. Thirdly, it may be seen in women, usually elderly, with lichen sclerosus and lichen simplex who do not have a history of squamous cell carcinoma. DVIN appears as a slightly raised pink area on a background of abnormal thickened and whitened skin. Any suspicious lesion should be biopsied in these settings or at least scraped for cytology. The latter investigation is more useful for areas of epithelial loss. A small, invasive carcinoma can seldom be clinically distinguished from DVIN because of the thickness of the epidermis.

Pathology

DVIN is subtler than the common (HPV-related) type of VIN. Like HPV-related VIN, the epidermis is thickened, shows parakeratosis on the surface and a lymphocytic infiltrate in the underlying stroma. A difference is that DVIN is often associated with dermal fibrosis or hyalinisation due to long standing lichen simplex and lichen sclerosus. Like HPV-related VIN, there may also be alterations in architecture, with elongated and frequently branched ridges. There may be involvement of hair follicles. Apparently separated nests of highly differentiated squamous cells may be seen in the papillary dermis raising the possibility of invasion.

In contrast to the common form of VIN, there is premature maturation with abundant intracytoplasmic keratin beginning in the suprabasilar layer. The abundant cytoplasmic keratin separates the nuclei. Under low power, this gives an orderly appearance.

However, despite the low-power orderly appearance, the squamous cells are abnormal. They are enlarged and their nuclei are enlarged and vesicular and contain macronucleoli. Intercellular bridges are prominent. Whorls of differentiated cells with or without keratin pearls may be seen and suggest imminent invasion. The basal cells are smaller and show more obvious nuclear atypia. Their nuclei are more hyperchromatic with irregular contours. The range of nuclear atypia is variable. Usually the atypia is slight to moderate in degree but is sometimes severe.

Mitoses are usually increased, but confined to the basal and suprabasal layers. Apoptotic cells may be seen at any level.

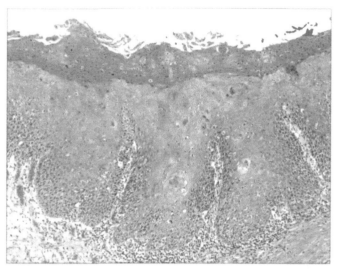

Figure 13.10. Differentiated VIN. The epithelium appears pink due to premature maturation of squamous cells. The dysplastic squamous cells are best seen in the basal layer. There are also parakeratosis, acanthosis and a dermal lymphocytic infiltrate-changes which are virtually always seen in DVIN.

P53 stains the basal layers.

Treatment
The treatment of DVIN is the same as for the common form (warty-basaloid) VIN.

132. SQUAMOUS CELL CARCINOMA (SCC)
Of all the vulvar malignancies, squamous cell carcinoma is the commonest histologic type. The histologic classification and incidence of vulvar malignancies is shown in Table 1.

Squamous cell carcinoma (SCC) of the vulva is a disease of significant clinical importance. It arises in the presence or absence of human papillomavirus (HPV). It accounts for up to 4% of female genital tract malignancies. It is a disease seen mainly in the older woman, between the ages of 60 and 90 years. However, in the last 3 decades there has been an increase in the

Table 1. Classification of vulvar cancers.
Squamous cell cancer (86%)
Melanoma (6%)
Adenocarcinoma (Bartholins gland) (4%)
Basal cell carcinoma (2%)
Sarcoma (2%)

frequency of HPV-related SCC in younger women.

Clinical features
Symptoms include a lump, ulcer, pruritus, pain and bleeding, with late symptoms including swelling of the leg and a groin mass. These tumors are often associated with an unpleasant odor and discharge. The different presenting cutaneous lesions (nodule, ulcer or cauliflower lesion) are shown in Figs. 13.10, 13.21 and 13.23. Most cancers occur on the labia majora. The next most common site is the periclitoral area but no site is exempt.

Locally the tumor extends progressively and directly to involve the vulva, vagina and peri-anal area. Lymphatic dissemination takes place from an early stage with involvement of inguinal and femoral nodes followed by pelvic nodes. Hematogenous spread to distant sites (lungs, liver, bone) is also seen.

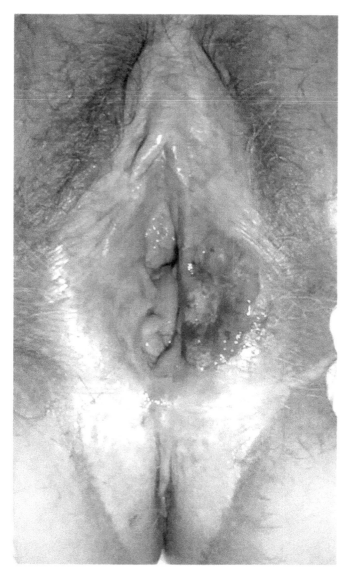

Figure 13.11. Lateral squamous cell carcinoma of the vulva.

Diagnosis

Diagnosis is made by punch or excision biopsy. The diagnosis is often delayed in patients with vulvar cancer and a biopsy should be performed early for any suspicious or persistent lesion. Examination should include palpation of the groin lymph nodes, Pap smear from the cervix, and colposcopy of the lower genital tract.

HPV has been detected in 25-33% of vulvar SCCs. The HPV-positive tumors occur in women on average 14 years younger when compared to HPV-negative vulvar cancers. They tend to be basaloid in appearance and arise from classical (warty-basaloid) vulvar intraepithelial neoplasia (VIN). The pathogenesis of HPV-negative cancers is less well understood but these cancers frequently arise on a background of lichen sclerosus, lichen simplex chronicus and differentiated VIN. These different clinicopathological features suggest that HPV-positive and negative cancers may be different diseases. Comparative genetic hybridization techniques have confirmed different genetic changes in HPV-positive and negative vulvar SCCs, which supports the clinicopathological data, indicating these are different cancer types.

Pathology

Vulvar squamous cell carcinomas are characterised by invasion. Invasion appears as a down growth into the dermis by irregular nodules, nests and tentacles of atypical squamous cells associated with an inflamed desmoplastic stroma. Superficial invasive squamous cell carcinoma needs to be distinguished from VIN when VIN shows a complicated architecture with apparently separated nests at the base. Tentacles, more abundant cytoplasm, larger, more vesicular nuclei and a desmoplastic reaction favor invasion.

There are two main subtypes of invasive vulvar squamous cell carcinoma: **keratinising** and **warty-basaloid**, depending on whether there is abundant extra- and intracellular keratin or not. Keratinising SCC is associated with DVIN and the absence of HPV DNA and warty-basaloid SCC with the HPV-related common form of VIN. There is, however, biological diversity, so that there is not a perfect correlation between the histological appearance and the presence or absence of HPV DNA. While there is some debate on whether keratinising or warty-basaloid types of SCC have different prognosis in the vulva, most studies have not found a significant difference.

Spindle cell SCC and giant cell SCC are variants of keratinising SCC, whose chief importance lies in their potential confusion with other tumors, particularly sarcomas. Two other squamous cell neoplasms: verrucous carcinoma and keratoacanthoma are described separately (see below).

The pathology report of an invasive squamous cell carcinoma should contain the following information of prognostic relevance.

Diameter: This is usually measured macroscopically.

Depth of invasion: This is measured from the top of the nearest normal dermal papilla. A depth of invasion equal to or less than 1mm deep (provided the diameter is less than 20mm), irrespective of whether lymph vascular space invasion is seen or not, is referred to as a superficial squamous cell carcinoma (stage 1a). Superficial squamous cell carcinoma has a minimal risk of lymph node metastasis.

Growth pattern: Examination of the advancing edge of the SCC will show either small separated nests or a broad, pushing front, respectively referred to as "spray" and "pushing" patterns. The spray pattern has the worse prognosis. While the growth pattern has prognostic relevance, a practical problem is that many SCC's appear mid-way between showing a purely spray or pushing pattern.

Grading: There have been many grading systems proposed. Most are based on the original Broders' system for grading SCC's in general. While these systems invariably work in a research setting, in practice they are often cumbersome and poorly reproducible. The key problem seems to be that the amount of intra- and extracellular keratin produced by the tumor is a parameter of grade in all systems, yet also relates to whether the carcinoma is keratinising or warty-basaloid type.

Lymph vascular space invasion: Lymph vascular space invasion is associated with a worse prognosis.

Perineural invasion: Perineural spread, as in other sites, is associated with an increased risk of recurrence.

Margins: There is an increased risk of recurrence with histological margins of less than 7mm (including the deep margin). A histological margin of 7mm equates to a clinical margin of 1cm, when shrinkage due to formalin fixation and skin elasticity is taken into account.

Adjacent premalignant disease: Keratinising SCC is associated with differentiated VIN, lichen simplex and lichen sclerosus. Warty-basaloid SCC is associated with the common form of VIN. The presence of adjacent changes should be recorded, particularly VIN. VIN seen at the margin is a predictor of recurrence.

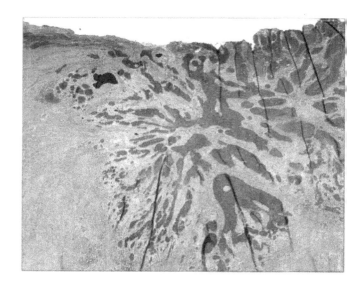

Figure 13.12. SCC, basaloid type. It is composed of basaloid cells with a spray pattern of growth and a depth of invasion of 4mm.

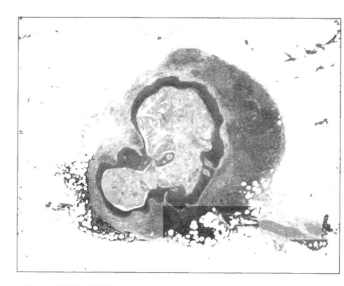

Figure 13.13. SCC. Metastasis in a groin lymph node from the cancer shown in Fig. 13.12.

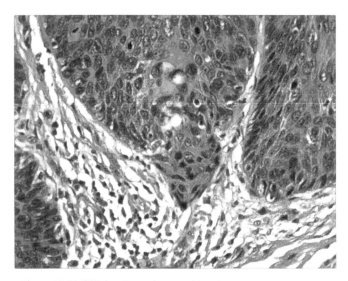

Figure 13.14. SCC showing early stromal invasion.

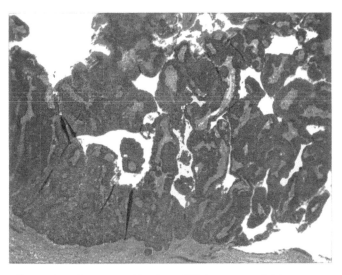

Figure 13.17. Squamotransitional type SCC shows a superficial resemblance to papillary transitional cell carcinoma of the bladder.

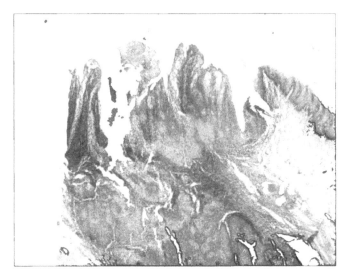

Figure 13.15. Warty (condylomatous) type SCC. This invasive SCC has a condylomatous surface.

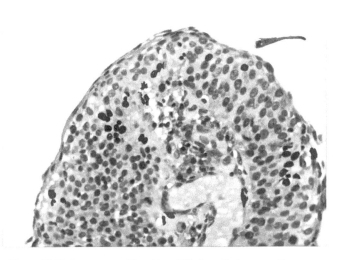

Figure 13.18. Squamotransitional type SCC. A papilla is covered by dysplastic epithelium.

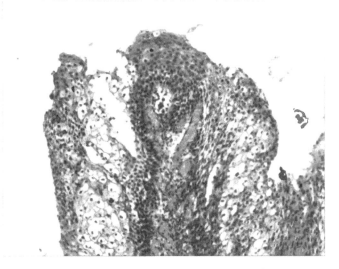

Figure 13.16. Condylomatous SCC. The exophytic portion of the tumor shows koilocytosis.

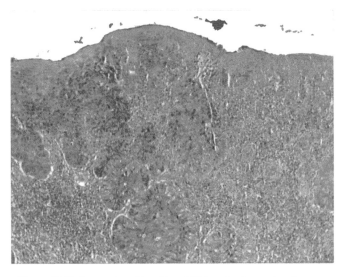

Figure 13.19. Squamotransitional type SCC. Invasive tumor showing basaloid cells forming lobules invading the lamina propria. The tumor has

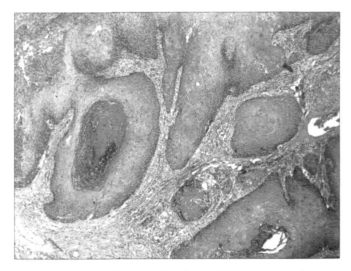

Figure 13.20. Well differentiated, keratinizing SCC. Large masses of eosinophilic tumor, with keratin pearls, invade the dermis.

Table 2. FIGO Staging for Vulvar Cancer (1994)

Stage I	Tumor (2 cm in greatest diameter, confined to the vulva or perineum; nodes are negative.
IA	As above with stromal invasion (1.0 mm
IB	As above with stromal invasion > 1 mm
Stage II	Tumor confined to the vulva and/or perineum, >2 cm in greatest dimension, nodes are negative.
Stage III	Tumor of any size with 1. Adjacent spread to the lower urethra and/or the vagina and/or the anus 2. Unilateral regional lymph node metastasis.
Stage IVA	Tumor invades any of the following: Upper urethra, bladder mucosa, rectal mucosa, pelvic bone or bilateral regional node metastasis.
Stage IVB	Any distant metastasis including pelvic lymph nodes.

Prognosis

Prognostic factors affecting patient survival include stage, tumor dimension (>2cm diameter), lymph node involvement (worse if 2 or more groin nodes and capsule breakthrough are found), lymph vascular space invasion and growth pattern (infiltrative or spray growth as opposed to a pushing growth pattern). The FIGO staging is surgical and is shown in Table 2. The 5-year survival rate for stage I disease is 90%, stage II 75%, stage III 50%, stage IV 15%. Most studies do not show a difference in prognosis between keratinising and basaloid SCC. Grading should be attempted but, while grading has been shown to be prognostically significant in studies, in practice it is cumbersome and poorly reproducible. The above mentioned growth pattern of the tumor is more reliable.

Treatment

The management of these cancers is essentially surgical. Radical vulvectomy and inguino-femoral lymphadenectomy is the standard procedure but is often modified according to the individual circumstances of the patient:

1). Stage IA tumors are treated with wide local excision down to deep fascia. Nodal dissection is not performed. In stage IA the depth of invasion is measured from the basement membrane of the most superficial adjacent dermal papilla and this must not exceed 1mm. The tumor should be excised with a 1cm margin (minimum 7mm on histology) to be adequate.

2). Lateral vulva lesions are treated with modified radical procedures usually involving unilateral vulvectomy and ipsilateral inguino-femoral lymphadenectomy. For a lesion to be considered lateral it should not be lower than a line drawn through the posterior fourchette or higher than a line drawn through the urethra.

3). Groin dissections are performed through separate incisions. This significantly reduces the rate of wound breakdown.

4). Sentinel lymph node biopsy can be performed in the groins, reducing the number of nodes removed and minimizing subsequent lymphedema. This technique involves Technetium-99m sulfur colloid being injected intradermally at the tumor margins, 90-180 minutes preoperatively. A similar injection of isosulfan blue dye 5-10 minutes before the groin dissection may also aid in the detection of the sentinel node. A handheld collimated gamma counter is employed to identify Tc-99m-labeled sentinel nodes. Clinical trials have shown the sentinel node to be an accurate predictor of metastatic disease to the inguinal nodal chain.

Wound breakdown (usually due to tissue tension in the wound and infection), lymphedema of the legs and psychosexual problems can be major complications. The modified procedures are aimed at reducing these problems.

Post-operative radiotherapy to the groins and pelvis may be necessary if the inguino-femoral nodes contain metastatic tumor. Vulvar radiotherapy may be necessary for close surgical margins (less than 7 mm). Large tumors can be treated surgically with primary closure if wide margins are not obtained. (Figures 4 and 5). This removes the unpleasant odor and discharge produced by these tumors and immediately makes the patient feel more comfortable. Radiotherapy can then follow.

Recurrent SCC of the vulva

High risk factors for recurrence include an infiltrative tumor pattern, extracapsular nodal spread in the groins and close surgical margins. Locally recurrent vulvar cancer can be simple to manage with further wide local excision if the lesion is small and no previous radiotherapy has been given to the site. Where large recurrences occur in previously radiated sites (Figure 13.23), large excisions are necessary to control the disease (Figure 13.24). Previous radiotherapy compromises wound healing, often necessitating musculo-cutaneous flaps or split skin grafts to obtain skin closure (Figure 13.25 and 13.26). Recurrence in the groin, regional lymph nodes or distally (for example, lung) is not easily treated and has a poor prognosis.

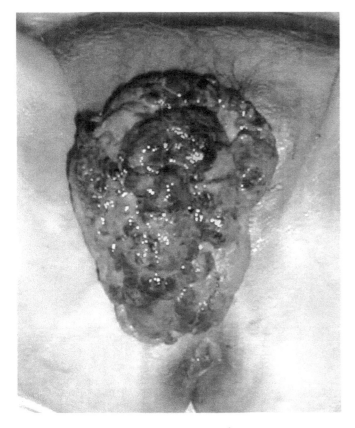

Figure 13.21. Large squamous cell carcinoma of the vulva.

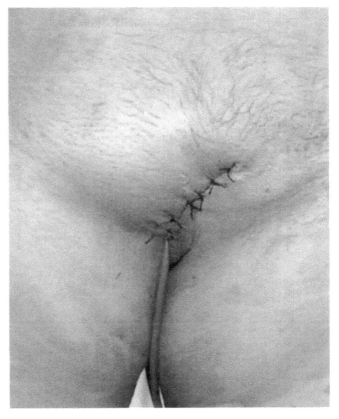

Figure 13.22. The patient in Fig. 13.21 after primary surgery.

Distinguishing between a local recurrence and a new primary may be academic. Pathologists should endeavour to distinguish the rarer event of local recurrence occurring as a dermal metastasis through lymphatic spread from a new primary occurring in a field of growth, as the former will have a worse prognosis. A lesion is more likely to be a new primary if it occurs more than 5 years after treatment of the previous tumor and is at a different site on the vulva.

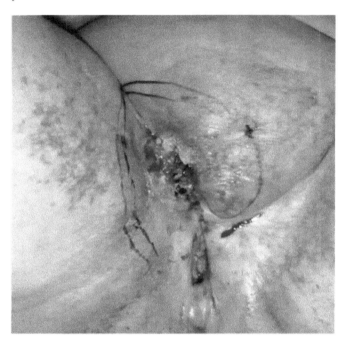

Figure 13.23. SCC recurring after surgery and radiotherapy.

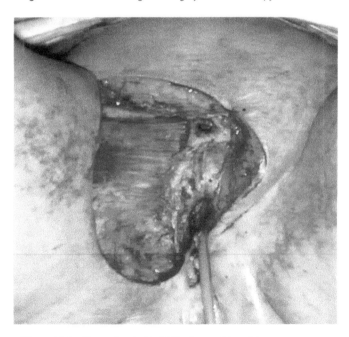

Figure 13.24. The patient in Fig. 13.23 after excision of the tumor.

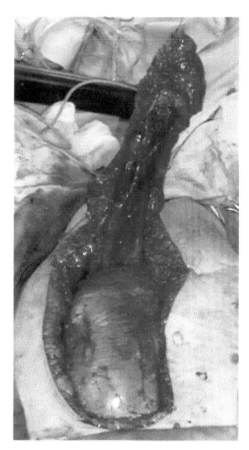

Figure 13.25. Dissection of a rectus flap to cover the defect in Fig. 13.24.

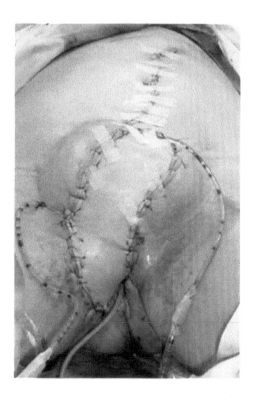

Figure 13.26. The patient in Fig. 13.23 after completion of surgery.

133. VERRUCOUS CARCINOMA

The term "verrucous carcinoma" (VC) was coined by the pathologist Lauren Ackerman in 1948 to describe a very well differentiated squamous neoplasm on the lip, which clinically and histologically shows some resemblance to a wart. Since then, VC has been described in sites wherever squamous epithelium is present. VC is most commonly described in the head and neck. The next most commonly reported sites in the female are the vulva, vagina and cervix. The name VC suggests a relationship with HPV. This is unfortunate, because only a minority of anogenital VC contain HPV DNA (usually types 6 or 11). Equally confusing, in 1926 Buschke and Loewenstein described large warty growths on the vulva as "giant condylomata" but these are now regarded as identical to verrucous carcinoma and not coalesced condylomata acuminata. We do not recommend the term "giant condyloma of Buschke-Lowenstein"

Clinical features

These vulvar tumors typically present in the 8th or 9th decade with a slow growing warty lesion, sometimes on a background of a chronic dermatosis such as lichen sclerosus. They may become large enough to obscure the entire vulva.

Pathology

The histological features are a thick covering of keratin, acanthosis with long blunt-ended ridges descending into the dermis and papillomatosis. There is no atypia in the usual sense or conventional invasion, although the tumor may push well into the dermis. The lack of conventional appearing atypia is testimony to the limitations of current histopathological criteria as these tumors show molecular changes consistent with premalignancy or malignancy. The features of VIN overlap those of DVIN and the dividing line between these two entities is not clearly marked but appears to be one of degree, with VC having longer ridges into the dermis. It is important for the pathologist to look hard for conventional invasion, which then places the tumor in the category of a usual type of SCC, no matter how well differentiated.

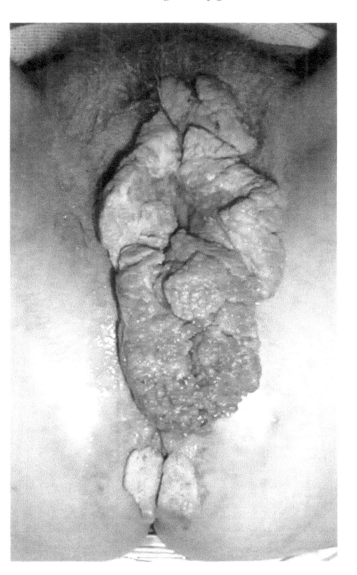

Figure 13.27. Verrucous carcinoma.

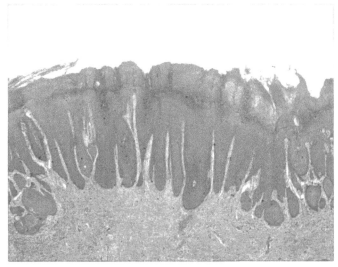

Figure 13.28. Verrucous SCC. A thick cover of parakeratosis overlies acanthosis composed of thick, blunt-ended ridges that resemble the "legs of baggy trousers". The epithelium is very eosinophilic.

Treatment

The treatment of VC is wide local excision. Involvement of the groin nodes is rare and lymphadenectomy is not routine, but clinically enlarged nodes should be biopsied. Radiotherapy is contraindicated because of reports of anaplastic transformation.

There is little data on the prognosis of VC of the vulva. It readily recurs if not excised with a wide margin and can transform into typical invasive SCC. Many of the tumors which appear to be verrucous carcinomas clinically, prove to be invasive pathologically and are thus classified as ordinary SCC.

134. KERATOACANTHOMA

The nature of keratoacanthoma (KA) is still controversial, but most regard it as a "self-healing SCC" rather than a reactive condition. It is rare on the vulva, with about one case found per 100 vulvar SCC's. The diagnosis is difficult. The history of a new rapid growth over the period of a few weeks is important, as is the appearance of a dimpled, raised keratotic nodule. Keratoacanthoma may be seen on a background of normal vulvar skin. If a KA is suspected clinically, then the lesion should be completely excised. The pathologist will not be able to diagnose KA with confidence by incisional biopsy. If the pathologist suspects KA by incisional biopsy for an assumed SCC, a request to the clinician to fully excise the lesion should be made before a diagnosis of KA is finalized. The histology of vulvar KA is similar to that of KA's of sun-exposed skin. The key feature is a crater-shaped keratotic lesion bordered by a proliferation of glassy keratinocytes.

135. BASAL CELL CARCINOMA (BCC)

BCC is the commonest human malignancy. It occurs almost exclusively on sun-damaged skin. Nevertheless, it rarely occurs on covered surfaces such as the vulva, where it accounts for 2% of malignancies.

Clinical features

Vulvar BCC typically occurs in the elderly (70-90 years). Its cause is generally unknown. Rarely, however, patients with one of the hereditary BCC syndromes (Gorlin's syndrome) may be afflicted with multiple vulvar BCCs at a young age.

BCCs are locally aggressive tumors but metastases to regional lymph nodes are so rare as to question the diagnosis when this occurs. BCCs present as long standing ulcers or nodules, usually less than 2 cm in diameter.

Pathology

The two main types of BCC, superficial multicentric and nodular, are the usual types seen on the vulva. The difference is that superficial BCCs do not invade the dermis, but nodular BCCs do. An important subtype of nodular BCC is morpheic BCC, characterized by very small groups of basal cells and abundant desmoplastic stroma. Morpheic BCC has a tendency for perineural invasion and an increased risk of recurrence. It has been reported on the vulva on rare occasions.

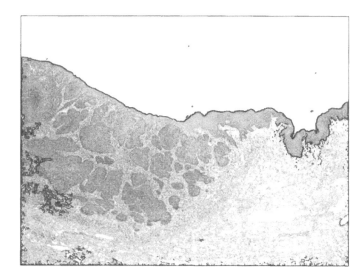

Figure 13.29. Nodular BCC. Note that the adjacent skin is normal.

Treatment

Treatment is wide local excision. Local recurrence occurs in about 20% of cases and re-excision is performed.

136. MERKEL CELL TUMOR

Merkel cell tumors (MCT) are highly malignant neuroendocrine carcinomas generally occurring on sun-exposed skin. Only a few cases have been reported on the vulva.

Pathology

MCT are typically dermal in location, despite the epidermal location of normal Merkel cells. MCT appear as small cell carcinomas. Sheets of small cells with necrosis, crush artefact and frequent mitoses and apoptosis are seen. The small size of the cell is due to the minimum amount of cytoplasm. The diagnosis can be confirmed by immunoperoxidase. This shows paranuclear dot positivity with keratin markers and positivity with one or more neuroendocrine markers such as synaptophysin and chromogranin.

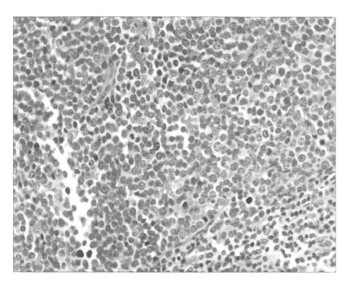

Figure 13.30. Merkel cell tumor. The tumor is composed of a sheet of markedly atypical, small round blue cells.

Treatment

Local excision followed by chemotherapy (cisplatin) is the treatment of choice. They metastasize widely and are associated with a poor prognosis

137. SYRINGOMA

Syringomas are common benign growths showing eccrine sweat duct differentiation. They appear as small yellow subepidermal papules, a few millimeters in diameter. There is a marked female preponderance. Adolescence is the commonest time of presentation. Most frequent sites of involvement include the lower eyelids and malar areas, but vulvar involvement is also common. The lesions may present with vulvar pruritus, but are often asymptomatic. Tiny syringomas may be found incidentally in vulvar biopsies done for other reasons. There is a rare eruptive form characterised by the simultaneous appearance of innumerable lesions. Exacerbation may occur in pregnancy.

Pathology

Syringomas are unencapsulated proliferations of tubules and nests in the dermis. Comma and tadpole shapes are characteristic. The cells have pale cytoplasm and well defined cell borders and there may be PAS positive luminal secretion.

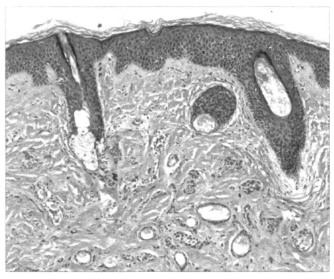

Figure 13.31. Syringoma. This common vulvar tumor is composed of small tubules and nests in the dermis.

Treatment

Syringomas may be excised if symptomatic or if the clinical diagnosis is unsure. They may be safely left, particularly if multiple and asymptomatic.

138. PLEOMORPHIC ADENOMA

These tumors, which are the most common salivary gland tumors, occur only rarely on the vulva and vagina. They appear to originate from two different tissues in the vulva and vagina: either mucinous glands (Bartholin's, Skene's or minor vestibular) or eccrine glands of the skin of the hair bearing vulva.

They are composed of sheets and strands of spindle-shaped or polygonal cells

Immunohistochemical studies show keratin and cytokeratin positive, whereas, S-100 protein, glial fibrillary acidic protein, vimentin, secretory component, and lysozyme are negative.

Treatment is by local excision.

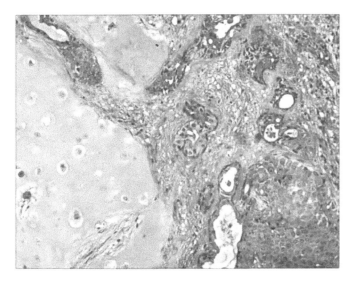

Figure 13.32. Pleomorphic adenoma. It consists of glands, nests, solid epithelial sheets and stroma which includes cartilage.

139. MICROCYSTIC ADNEXAL CARCINOMA

These eccrine gland carcinomas, similar to those seen on other sites of the body, have been rarely recorded on the vulva. Indolent localized growth is usual, with regional spread in 11% and metastases in 3%.

140. HIDRADENOMA PAPILLIFERUM

Hidradenoma papilliferum is a common benign apocrine tumor of the vulva, only rarely seen outside the anogenital area. Hidradenomas appear in women, usually of reproductive age, as bluish dermal nodules a few millimeters to a centimeter or more in diameter. They are usually found on the apocrine (hair-bearing) area of the vulva but may be seen on hairless vulva where apocrine glands are not found.

Pathology

Hidradenomas occur in the dermis as unencapsulated tumors showing glandular, cystic and papillary growth patterns. There are two layers of epithelial cells, large luminal columnar cells showing apocrine differentiation and, beneath these, small basaloid cells. Apocrine

differentiation appears as cells showing decapitate secretion (apical snouts) and abundant eosinophilic cytoplasm.

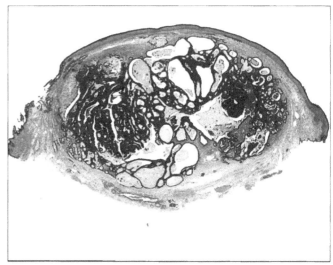

Figure 13.33. Hidradenoma papilliferum. A well circumscribed dermal cystic and glandular tumor.

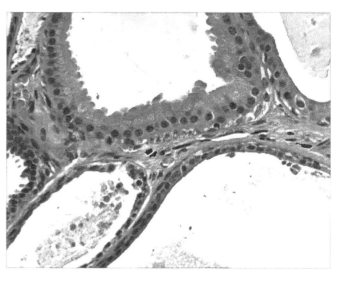

Figure 13.34. Hidradenoma papilliferum. Cystic spaces are lined by double layered apocrine epithelium, with an outer layer of eosinophilic cells with apical snouts and an inner layer of cuboidal cells.

Treatment

Complete excision of the lump suffices.

BREAST-LIKE TUMORS

Rarely, neoplasms, tumor-like lesions and lactating tissue identical to ectopic breast may be found in the vulva (258). The neoplasms include (141) **fibroadenoma, primary breast-like carcinoma** and (142) **cystosarcoma phyllodes.** Fibrocystic disease and the so-called "lactating adenoma" seen in lactating mothers, are probably associated non-neoplastic lesions. These breast-like lesions are found in the labium majus. There is current debate whether these lesions are, together with extramammary Paget's disease and possibly hidradenoma papilliferum, derived from purported specialized apoeccrine glands (mammary-like glands), remnants of the embryological milk-line from axilla to thigh or from portions of the apocrine gland and duct. Distinguishing between a primary breast-like carcinoma of the vulva and a metastasis from a carcinoma of ectopic breast has great prognostic significance.

Pathology

The pathology of these lesions resembles those of eutopic (ie. normally situated) breast.

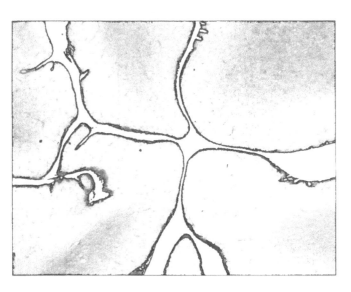

Figure 13.35. Cystoscarcoma phyllodes of the labium majus showing leaf-like protruberances of surface epithelium and proliferating stroma.

143. EXTRAMAMMARY PAGET'S DISEASE (EMPD)

Paget's disease is marked by the presence of large, neoplastic glandular cells with pale cytoplasm in the epidermis and skin appendages and is therefore a form of adenocarcinoma *in situ* of the skin. While first described on the nipple by James Paget in 1874, it has subsequently been found to occur on other sites, particularly where apocrine glands are present. Foremost among these sites of EMPD is the vulva. Vulvar Paget's disease can be classified according to site of origin of the abnormal cells and whether there is an invasive carcinoma arising from the Paget's or whether there is an associated sweat gland carcinoma (Table 3).

Table 3. Classification of Paget's disease of the vulva (Brown and Wilkinson)

1. Primary
   a. Intraepithelial only
   b. With stromal invasion
   c. With underlying skin appendage or vulvar subcutaneous gland carcinoma
2. Secondary
   a. Anorectal carcinoma
   b. Urothelial carcinoma
   c. Other carcinomas

PREMALIGNANT PAGET'S DISEASE

When compared to VIN (squamous dysplasia), Paget's disease accounts for only a small percentage of premalignant conditions of the vulva. No cause or predisposing factors are known.

Clinical features

The median age is approximately 70 years. Most commonly, the disease presents with irritation and itching.

Early disease usually first appears on the hair bearing area of the labia majora but spreads in all directions to involve the perianal region, genitocrural and inguinal folds and labia minora and vestibule. The lesions can vary in size but often have a reddish, raised, eczematoid appearance. Early Paget's disease appears as well demarcated velvety, soft, red or bright pink areas with scattered white islands of hyperkeratosis. Later the lesions become erythematous, plaque like and desquamative. The lesion can extend to involve the mons pubis, thigh or buttock. (Fig. 13.37).

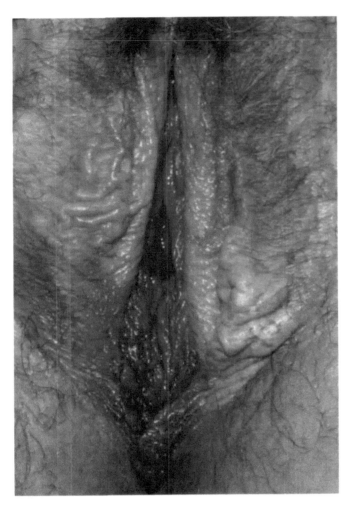

Figure 13.36. Paget's disease.

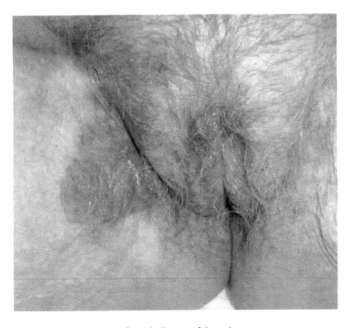

Figure 13.37. Extensive Paget's disease of the vulva.

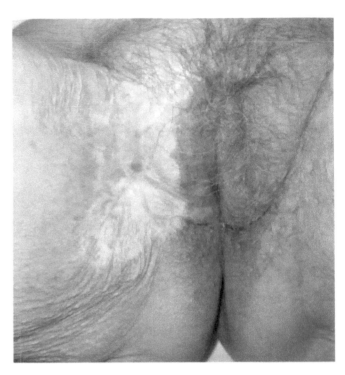

Figure 13.38. The patient in Fig. 13.37 after excision of the lesion and closure with a skin graft.

Pathology

Paget's cells are present mostly in the basal layer of the epithelium and are found singly or grouped into nests. The cells are large and contain abundant pale, finely granular cytoplasm, often with secretory vacuoles that stain positively for mucin. The nucleus may be hyperchromatic with a prominent nucleolus. Mitoses are usually seen. The diagnosis of EMPD can usually be made by the typical appearances of the cells and the demonstration of mucin in the cytoplasm. Occasionally an immunoperoxidase panel may be required. While there is no specific antibody for EMPD, primary cases usually stain with GCDFP 15, CEA and low molecular weight keratins such as CAM 5.2 and cytokeratin 7 and are negative for the melanocyte markers S100, HMB 45 and MART 1.

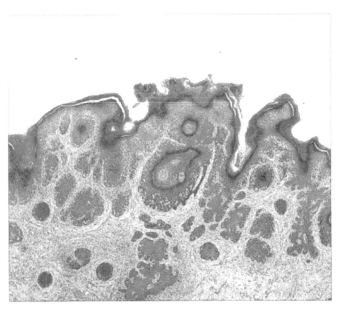

Figure 13.39. Extramammary Paget's disease showing hyperkeratosis, acanthosis and papillomatosis.

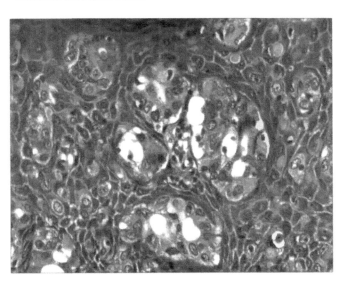

Figure 13.40. Extramammary Paget's disease characterized by intraepithelial nests and acini of large atypical glandular cells.

Treatment

The treatment for intraepithelial Paget's disease is wide local excision, with a margin of 1-2 cm. For the excision of large lesions the use of split skin grafts may be required.

Recurrences are common, as clear margins can be difficult to achieve. The high rate of positive margins is due to the microscopic involvement extending past the macroscopic lesion. Positive histological margins should be observed and not immediately re-excised. Recurrence occurs in 50% or more if the margin is involved histologically but also occurs in 15-20% in cases with negative margins. These cases are believed to be false negative histological margins due to the difficulty of determining histological margins in very irregular specimens and the occurrence of skip lesions. Recurrences are usually within 18 months and may be multiple.

Further wide local excision is indicated for clinically recurrent disease. The use of topical 5% imiquimod has been reported. There is no proven role for adjuvant therapy.

144. INVASIVE CARCINOMA ARISING FROM INTRAEPITHELIAL PAGET'S DISEASE

Intraepithelial Paget's disease extending into the dermis is rare. However, there is a study that reports that Paget's disease may progress to be invasive in up to 12% of cases. Some authors report this as an indolent disease and others report it as a disease which metastasizes early. Stromal invasion may occur initially or with recurrences during long term follow up and is seen particularly with large areas of Paget's disease. Pain, bleeding or a tumor suggest invasive disease.

There is a 4% incidence of vulvar adenocarcinoma associated with Paget's disease. The treatment is as for SCC of the vulva.

Primary Paget's disease also needs to be distinguished from pagetoid spread from a primary adenocarcinoma of the rectum, cervix, vagina or vulvar apocrine glands or transitional carcinoma of the bladder. Periurethral and perianal lesions may indicate secondary involvement of skin by a non-cutaneous internal neoplasm. Continuity with the primary site is the key but immunoperoxidase markers are also helpful in diagnosing "secondary Paget's disease". Bowel carcinomas are usually cytokeratin 20 positive and bladder carcinomas mark with uroplakin III and usually cytokeratin 20. Both these markers are negative in the primary form of Paget's disease.

Synchronous neoplasms involving the breast, rectum, bladder, urethra, cervix or ovary are reported in up to 30% of patients. Much was made of this alarming statistic in the older literature in terms of the need to systemically investigate patients with Paget's disease. However, after exclusion of spread from local neoplasms, the age-adjusted incidence for coincidental carcinomas is no more than that in the general population.

145. PRIMARY BREAST-LIKE CARCINOMA

This is mentioned above (Breast-like tumors).

146. TRICHOFOLLICULOMA

Trichofolliculoma is an uncommon, benign cutaneous adnexal neoplasm most frequently occurring on the head and neck. It is very rare on the vulva. Local excision is required.

147. SEBACEOUS CARCINOMA

Extraocular sebaceous carcinoma is an uncommon skin neoplasm usually localised to the head and neck. Sebaceous glands are abundant on the vulva, but vulvar sebaceous carcinoma is a very uncommon neoplasm with only a handful of cases reported. In some of these, sebaceous carcinoma appears to have arisen from vulvar intraepithelial neoplasia.

ENDOMETRIOSIS-DERIVED EPITHELIAL NEOPLASMS

Rarely, primary (148) **endometrioid carcinoma, endometrioid stromal sarcoma** and (149) **clear cell carcinoma** have been reported, apparently arising in endometriotic tissue in the vulva.

TUMORS OF MUCINOUS GLANDS

Mucinous glands of the vulvovaginal region comprise the major mucinous glands (Bartholin's glands), paraurethral glands (Skene's glands) and minor vestibular glands. Tumors may arise from any of these glands. Bartholin's and vestibular gland tumors will be discussed in this section. Tumors of the paraurethral glands appear under urethral tumors.

150. BENIGN MIXED TUMOR (PLEOMORPHIC ADENOMA)

Benign mixed tumor (chondroid syringoma) most commonly occurs in the parotid salivary gland but they may be seen arising from sweat glands of the skin or mucinous glands from any site. Vulvar benign mixed tumors are rare tumors that may arise from Bartholin's

glands, minor vestibular glands or skin eccrine glands. They present as discrete, firm masses and show the same pathology as elsewhere on the body. Very rarely, carcinoma may arise within a vulvar benign mixed tumor, a well-recognised complication of benign mixed tumor in the parotid.

BARTHOLIN'S GLAND CARCINOMA

Bartholin's gland carcinomas account for about 5% of vulvar malignancies. The criteria for a tumor to be included as a Bartholin's were defined by Honan in 1897: 1) Bartholin's gland elements next to the carcinoma, 2) a transition from normal to neoplastic, 3) a tumor type histologically compatible with origin from the gland, 4) no other genital primary and, 5) covering epithelium should be intact. The cause of Bartholin's gland carcinomas is largely unknown. However, recently there have been several reports of carcinoma in situ of squamous epithelium of Bartholin's duct containing HPV DNA and associated with VIN.

Clinical features

Bartholin's gland carcinomas present as nodules in the deep tissue of the Bartholin's area of the labium majus. They may be associated with an abscess, but show a poor response to antibiotics. In the older literature, the mean age of occurrence is 50-62.

Pathology

Bartholin's gland carcinomas are typically squamous, adeno or adenosquamous carcinomas. Less commonly, transitional cell and anaplastic carcinomas may be found.

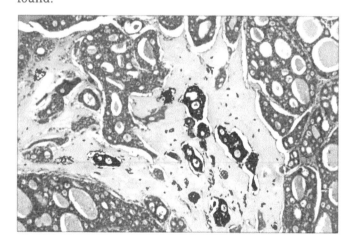

Figure 13.41. Adenoid cystic carcinoma of Bartholin's gland showing cribriform nests of epithelium and hyaline stroma.

151. SQUAMOUS CELL CARCINOMA

Squamous cell carcinoma is the commonest type of carcinoma occurring in Bartholin's gland and accounts for more than 50% of cases in recent series. It is associated with HPV 16 or 18 in most cases where HPV DNA has been looked for. Squamous cell carcinoma in situ (high grade squamous intraepithelial lesion) has been described in Bartholin's duct and in a Bartholin's cyst, providing an explanation of the pathogenesis of a squamous cell carcinoma in a gland that does not contain squamous epithelium.

152. ADENOCARCINOMA

There are a variety of adenocarcinomas arising in Bartholin's gland. All are rare. The most commonly reported is **(154) adenoid cystic carcinoma**, of which only 46 were identified in the literature in a review in 1996. Like its salivary gland counterpart, it appears as a glandular and solid nested proliferation of epithelial and myoepithelial cells and myxohyaline stroma. It has a propensity for perineural invasion and recurrence. Other types include adenocarcinomas which do not show any special features, **(153) mucinous adenocarcinoma, (155) prostatic type** and clear cell carcinoma.

156. TRANSITIONAL CELL CARCINOMA

Transitional cell carcinoma is another rare type of Bartholin's gland carcinoma. Like SCC, it appears related to HPV infection.

Small cell carcinoma

This is a rarely reported type of Bartholin's gland carcinoma.

Metastatic carcinoma

There are rare reports of metastases to Bartholin's gland from distant primaries such as breast and kidney

Treatment and Prognosis.

The treatment of Bartholin's gland carcinoma is radical local excision. Ipsilateral lymphadenectomy is often performed. Nodal metastases are seen in 1/3 of cases at the time of diagnosis and indicate a poor prognosis.

In these situations, postoperative radiation to the vulva, groins and pelvis will decrease the chance of recurrence.

MELANOCYTIC DISEASES

Discrete, pigmented lesions can be found on the vulvas of some 10% of women. Many have been overtreated in the past because of the fear they may predispose to malignant melanoma. It is now believed that most melanomas arise de novo. A full range of melanocytic lesions occurs on the vulva. While common moles, similar to those seen elsewhere on the body, are the most frequent, there are also several melanocytic lesions which show site-specific features. These include genital melanocytic macule, atypical genital melanocytic nevus and melanoma in situ.

157. GENITAL MELANOTIC MACULES (VULVOVAGINAL MELANOSIS)

Genital melanocytic macules (vulvovaginal melanosis) are discrete patches of vulvovaginal hyperpigmentation. The cause is unknown. The clinical significance of genital macules is twofold. Firstly, although perfectly benign, they may closely resemble in situ (or early invasive) malignant melanoma. Secondly, they may be part of Carney's complex, with myxomas of the skin and heart, or Peutz-Jeghers syndrome, which includes hamartomatous intestinal polyps and some specific neoplasms.

Clinical features

Brown or black patches with a sharp outline are noted by the patient or her doctor on examination. They vary in size up to 2 cm. and may be multiple. There is no thickening or sensory change. Take away the pigmentation and the vulva appears entirely normal. They tend to be found in or adjacent to the vestibule and occasionally in the vagina or (rarely) on the cervix. These macules tend to occur in the reproductive years, often when the patient is in her 20's or late teens, compared to vulvar melanoma which gradually increases in incidence with age and is very rare under the age of 30 years.

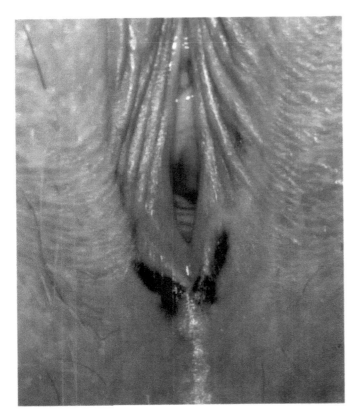

Figure 13.42. Melanosis.

Pathology

Melanosis appears as hyperpigmentation of the basal layer. The number of melanocytes is usually increased but may be normal or even reduced. The melanocytes are never confluent (strips of single junctional melanocytes touching each other), nested or atypical. Unlike lentigoes, genital melanotoc macules do not show acanthosis. The dermis may show melanin within macrophages (pigment incontinence), but there is no dermal melanocytic proliferation.

Diagnosis

Regular examination or biopsy is usually required to exclude melanoma. There are a number of reports in the literature testifying that melanosis cannot be distinguished clinically from melanoma in situ. Less commonly, it is claimed that melanosis may rarely precede melanoma in situ. In our experience, cases that progressed, showed atypical melanocytes at the outset and should not have been diagnosed as genital melanocytic macules. Biopsy is indicated for any changing or otherwise suspiscious lesions. Investigation

for cardiocutaneous or Peutz-Jeghers syndromes should also be considered.

Treatment

Provided the condition is diagnosed correctly, only reassurance is required. Although no treatment is required for melanosis, in practice, excision biopsy is commonly undertaken for patient (and/or doctor) anxiety or cosmetic reasons.

158. LENTIGO

Lentigoes are common, benign, pigmented lesions occurring on skin all over the body, including the vulva. They usually appear as small, slightly raised, well-demarcated, very darkly pigmented papules no more that a few millimeters in diameter. Their slightly raised nature, due to acanthosis, distinguishes them from vulvar melanosis, which, if the pigment could be removed, would look like normal vulva. Histologically, there is basal hyperpigmentation, increased single, non-atypical melanocytes of the junction and acanthosis. Lentigoes carry no malignant potential.

159. MELANOCYTIC NEVUS (MOLE)

Nevi are common on the vulva. They may only be distinguished from melanocytic macules by the presence of nests of melanocytes in the nevus after biopsy. Nevi involve the vulva in 2% of Caucasian women. They are acquired collections of melanocytes which have lost their dendritic processes. They begin as junctional nevi and then undergo maturation as melanocytes drop off into the dermis to become compound nevi with both junctional and dermal components. Eventually, nevi become purely intradermal. Vulvar nevi are clinically and histologically similar to extragenital nevi apart from one type, the atypical melanocytic nevus of the genital tract, which will be considered separately. Genital nevi are slow to mature which led to the myth that they all should be excised because of the risk of malignant change.

There is a rare genetic "dysplastic nevus syndrome" with a high incidence of melanomas which led Wallace Clark to describe similar histologic features in acquired dysplastic nevi. This term has been very controversial as it is implied a high incidence of malignancy with these lesions. A recent NIH consensus conference suggested that the term be dropped and replaced by atypical or Clark's nevus.

Congenital nevi are present at birth and giant lesions may have a large 'bathing trunk' distribution. There is an increased risk of malignancy with giant nevi, but the risk with small congenital nevi is controversial.

Clinical features

Nevi vary from flesh coloured to brown or black. They are uniform in shape and colour and may be flat, dome shaped, or have a warty surface. The junctional nevus tends to be flat and uniformly pigmented. The compound nevus is thicker with a central black area and surrounding brown skin. The intradermal nevus may be flesh coloured or dark and just appear as a lump. Nevi may eventually disappear spontaneously.

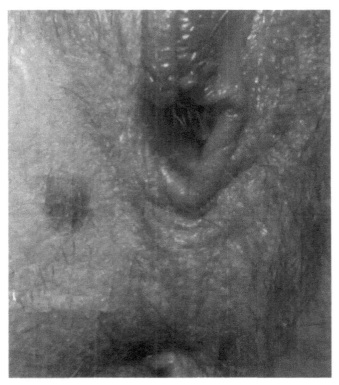

Figure 13.43. Benign pigmented nevus.

Pathology

Nevi are benign proliferations of melanocytes and are divided into junctional, compound and dermal according to where the melanocytic proliferation is located. They are distinguished from lentigo by the finding of nests of melanocytes. Nevi are symmetrical and, while single melanocytes are also seen as well as nests, there is no confluence (strips of single melanocytes touching each other at the junction), no upward spread into the prickle cell layer (except in certain well defined situations) and no atypia. The dermal component shows maturation (smaller neval cells in the depth of the lesion), less or absent pigmentation in the deeper melanocytes and an absence of mitoses.

Treatment

Congenital and acquired nevi require no treatment unless there is a change in shape or color when they need excision for histology.

160. ATYPICAL MELANOCYTIC NEVUS OF GENITAL TRACT

Atypical melanocytic nevus of the genital tract (AMNGT) is a distinct clinicopathological entity that has features which simulate melanoma. These uncommon nevi present in young women where they are seen mostly on the labia minora and clitoral regions but may be found anywhere on the vulva.

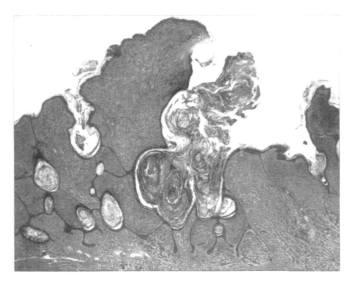

Figure 13.44. Papillomatous dermal nevus of the mons. Papillomatosis and a dermal proliferation of neval cells are seen.

Pathology

AMNGT shows a "nested and dyshesive" pattern, characterised by the confluence of enlarged nests with variation in size, shape and position at the dermo-epidermal junction and by the diminished cohesion of melanocytes, which show nuclear enlargement and prominent nucleoli. There may also be upward (pagetoid) spread, but this lacks cytologic atypia. There is a dermal component in about half the cases. Symmetry and lack of single melanocyte confluence are helpful features that distinguish AMNGT from melanoma.

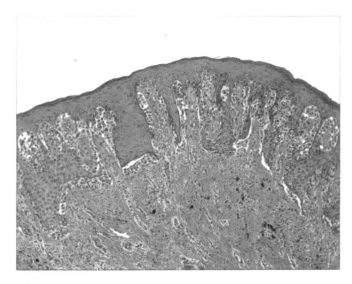

Figure 13.45. Atypical melanocytic genital tract nevus showing regular acanthosis with extensive junctional proliferation of melanocytes.

Treatment
Excision is curative.

161. MELANOMA IN SITU
Melanoma in situ usually presents on the vulva and vagina as a large, irregularly pigmented and shaped macule. Melanoma in situ may not be distinguishable clinically from the more common vulvovaginal melanosis, although a young age and multiple lesions points towards a benign lesion. Biopsy is required to distinguish the two conditions with certainty.

Pathology
Melanoma in situ is most frequently of the acral lentigenous type, with a linear, junctional confluent proliferation of atypical melanocytes.

Treatment
The treatment is local excision. The lesions may be poorly defined histologically and difficult to excise completely. They have a propensity to recur and eventually invade.

162. MALIGNANT MELANOMA
Vulvar malignant melanoma accounts for about 3% of all malignant melanomas and 10% of vulvar malignancies. It is the second commonest vulvar malignancy after squamous cell carcinoma. Along with the anus and urethra, the genital tract (vulva, vagina and cervix in that order) is the site of predilection for malignant melanoma occurring on covered areas.

Clinical features
Malignant melanoma shows a gradually increasing incidence with age and the mean is 55 years. They have not been recorded in prepubertal girls. The first symptoms noticed by patients are usually a lump, bleeding or pruritus. Other presentations include a mass in the groin and a change in a pigmented lesion. About 75% of vulvar malignant melanomas occur centrally on the labia minora and clitoral region. The clinical differential diagnosis comprises other pigmented skin lesions, particularly melanosis and nevus.

Pathology
Melanomas are diagnosed using the same guidelines as for cutaneous melanomas elsewhere. Acknowledging that there is decreasing emphasis on typing melanomas, mucosal lentigenous type followed by nodular melanomas are the most common. Pathologists usually use Clark's levels to stage melanomas. This depends on the tissue plane to which the tumor invades. However, because of different histology on the vulva and vagina, this is usually inappropriate. Most pathologists measure the melanoma thickness according to Breslow and state the figure in their report. The Breslow system describes tumor thickness as measured from the surface of the epithelium (see table 4). Chung's levels are a modification of the Clark levels as measured from granular layer. Breslow's depth alone should suffice for vulvovaginal melanomas.

Table 4. Tumor thickness and survival.

Breslow level (tumor thickness from epithelium surface)		
≤1.50mm	100% 5 year survival	60% 10 year survival
>1.50≤3.0mm	40% 5 year survival	40% 10 year survival
>3.0mm	20% 5 year survival	20% 10 year survival

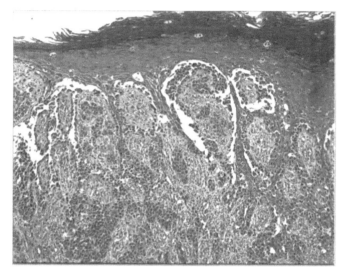

Figure 13.46. Invasive melanoma. Nests of atypical melanocytes invade the dermis.

Treatment and prognosis

Treatment has become more conservative in recent years. Wide local excision with or without groin node dissection is recommended. Most investigators propose complete excision for melanomas thinner than 1mm and wide excision for thicker melanomas. Although the place of inguino-femoral lymphadenectomy is not yet clearly defined, some studies have shown an improvement in 5 year survival if lymphadenectomy is performed. Adjuvant chemotherapy is not effective. Interferon alfa-2b use has shown an increase in relapse-free and overall survival.

Prognosis overall is poor. Survival rates depend on tumor thickness and/or infiltration level. The important cut-off is 1mm depth of invasion. For thin melanomas (less than 1mm), several series have shown 100%

survival. At the other end of the scale, lymph node metastases are associated with a 0-30% 5-year survival.

163. SUPERFICIAL ANGIOMYXOMA

These are a recently described benign skin tumor which may be associated with Carney's syndrome. While a wide range of sites may be involved, a recent series of 17 cases on the labia of young women, mean age 21 years, raises the possibility that the vulva may be a site of predilection. Tumors are usually small, less than 50mm in diameter, and present as polyps or apparent cysts. So far, none of our patients with vulvar cutaneous myxomas have had Carney's syndrome.

Pathology

The tumor is an atypical myxoma composed of a low density population of spindle cells in a myxoid matrix with delicate thin walled, capillary sized vessels. There are always a few inflammatory cells, including polymorphs, which are a helpful pointer to diagnosis. Tumor cells are invariably CD34 positive but S100, factor XIIIa and hormone receptor negative. There are conflicting reports on whether smooth muscle actin is positive.

Treatment

Wide local excision is recommended. There is a recurrence rate of 30-40%, further indicating that the lesions should be completely excised with a clear margin.

164. CELLULAR ANGIOFIBROMA

Cellular angiofibroma is a recently described, uncommon benign spindle cell neoplasm which occurs virtually exclusively in women in the vulvovaginal region. Patients are usually in the second half of reproductive life and present with a medium sized mass, mean 3cm, often preoperatively diagnosed as a labial or Bartholin's cyst.

Pathology

The tumor is a well circumscribed spindle cell neoplasm with three components: an hypercellular component of uniform, bland, spindle cells (resembling the cells in spindle cell lipoma), numerous thick-walled and often hyalinized vessels (which distinguishes the lesion from spindle cell lipoma) and a scarce component of mature adipocytes. Stromal cells negative for actin, desmin, CD34 and S100, suggesting that, by default, they are fibroblasts.

Treatment
Local excision is adequate. While only a few cases have been reported, the behaviour of the tumor appears entirely benign. No case has recurred or metastasised.

165. ANGIOMYOFIBROBLASTOMA
Angiomyofibroblastoma is a benign mesenchymal tumor, which occurs almost exclusively in women in the vulvovaginal area. Women, most often in their 30's and 40's, present with a mass, usually less than 5cm (up to 12cm has been recorded), which is often preoperatively misdiagnosed as a Bartholin's cyst.

Pathology
Angiomyofibroblastomas are well-circumscribed tumors composed of mesenchymal cells and numerous blood vessels. There are hyper- and hypocellular areas. The mesenchymal cells are mainly spindle cells, but there are desmin-positive epithelioid cells with eosinophilic cytoplasm around blood vessels. The blood vessels are mainly small to medium sized capillaries.

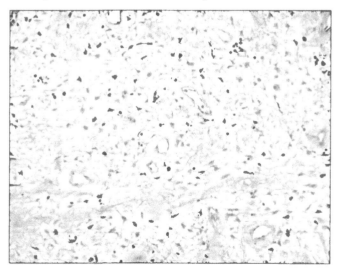

Figure 13.47. Angiomyofibroblastoma. There is proliferation of plump spindle cells and thick walled vessels.

Treatment
Local excision is adequate. The prognosis is excellent, with a low recurrence rate after complete excision. A single case of transformation to sarcoma has been described.

166. AGGRESSIVE ANGIOMYXOMA
Aggressive angiomyxoma (AAM) is an uncommon, distinctive soft tissue tumor of disputed fibroblastic or myofibroblastic histogenesis which occurs almost exclusively in the pelvis of adult women. Most cases occur between the ages of 21 and 38 years. Patients present with a vulvar, vaginal or perineal mass. The tumor appears as a large, gelatinous mass which permeates the pelvic tissues.

Pathology
The tumor is composed of abundant myxoid stroma with sparse spindle cells without atypia. There are numerous medium to large, thick walled and often hyalinized blood vessels and delicate capillaries present, often with evidence of recent or old bleeding. Areas of smooth muscle differentiation may be seen, particularly around vessels. A minority of cases show angiomyofibroblastoma (AMFB)-like areas. Smooth muscle antigen and, in most cases, desmin reactivity are seen. However, these markers are also seen in AMFB making them unhelpful in distinguishing the two tumors and forming the basis of the suggestion that the two tumors are the poles of a spectrum. Nevertheless, it is important to distinguish AAM from AMFB as, unlike AAM, AMFB has little tendency to recur after local excision.

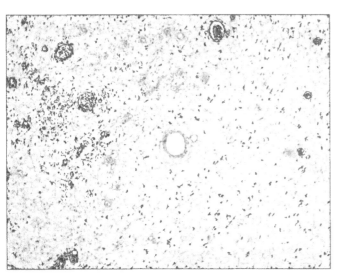

Figure 13.48. Aggressive angiomyxoma. This low power view shows lowly cellular myxoid tissue with frequent blood vessels.

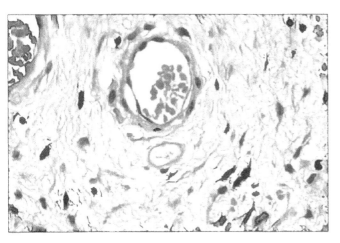

Figure 13.49. Aggressive angiomyxoma. Bland spindle cells in a myxoid matrix with small blood vessels are seen in this high power view.

Treatment.

Surgical excision. Obtaining clear surgical margins is virtually an impossibility.

Aggressive angiomyxoma has a high recurrence rate of 30-50% but no metastatic potential.

167. DERMATOFIBROSARCOMA PROTRUBERANS (DFSP)

This is an uncommon fibrous tumor of the dermis of intermediate grade malignancy, with a tendency for local recurrence, although it rarely metastasises. The trunk and extremities are the usual sites for DFSP. However, within the rare group of vulvar

sarcomas, DFSP is one of the commonest types. It occurs predominantly in the fourth to sixth decades as a slowly growing mass, several centimeters in diameter, on the outer hair-bearing vulva.

Pathology

The histology is of a dermal tumor, with inevitable involvement of the subcutis, composed of bland spindle cells with oval to wavy nuclei in tight storiform pattern. It may be associated with fibrosarcomatous areas. The tumor is CD 34 positive and shows characteristic cytogenetic features.

Figure 13.50. Dermatofibrosarcoma protruberans. Low power view showing densely cellular, storiform (matted) proliferation of spindle cells.

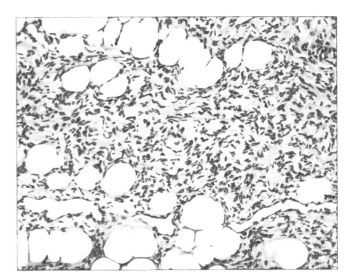

Figure 13.51. Dermatofibrosarcoma protruberans. High power view of spindle cells invading fat.

Treatment

Excision with a wide clear surgical margin of 3cm is recommended to minimise recurrence. Survival rates range from 91-100% and local recurrence rates of 20-49%. Close follow-up is recommended.

169. KAPOSI'S SARCOMA

Kaposi's sarcoma of the vulva is a rare vascular lesion associated with the aquired immunodeficiency syndrome (AIDS). It is caused by infection with Herpes hominis 8 virus. It presents initially as a patch, developing into a plaque then a nodule. The nature of Kaposi's sarcoma is still being debated. It has been variously regarded as a multifocal infection, a neoplasm, or binomial. That is, it begins as a non-neoplastic condition in the patch stage and progresses into a neoplasm.

Pathology

Kaposi's sarcomas show various stages and can be quite difficult to diagnosis in the early (patch) stage. The key features are a spindle cell proliferation with extravasated red blood cells and eosinophilic globules and telangiectatic vessels with atypical endothelial cells.

170. ANGIOSARCOMA

Angiosarcomas are malignant endothelial cell proliferations that mainly occur in several clinical situations. One of these, prior radiotherapy, applies to the vulvovaginal area. Five cases of vaginal angiosarcoma of the vagina have been reported. Three have followed radiotherapy for other malignancies. However, since angiosarcoma after radiotherapy is so rare, multimodality therapy for lower genital tract malignancies should not be withheld for fear of this complication.

171. LEIOMYOMA (MYXOID AND EPITHELIOID)

While infrequent compared to the incidence in the uterus, smooth muscle tumors are one of the commonest types of soft tissue tumors of the vagina, vulva and urethra. They are most commonly seen in the fourth and fifth decades. In terms of behavior, they are less predictable than uterine tumors and therefore form their own category. A rare variant, vulvar leiomyomatosis presents as single or multiple skin or mucosa-based superficial nodules of benign smooth muscle. This rare condition may be associated with smooth muscle tumors elsewhere in the body. There is an association with Alport's syndrome, a disease with deficiency of type IV collagen, a major component of basement membrane.

Pathology

The vulvovaginal smooth muscle tumors are believed to form a biologic continuum, rather than distinct benign and malignant categories. This view necessitates different terminology to describe smooth muscle tumors in this location. Specifically, as well as benign (leiomyoma) and malignant (leiomyosarcoma), there is a group with intermediate histological features termed "atypical smooth muscle tumor" which has an increased risk of recurrence. The histological patterns described are spindled (comparable to uterine leiomyoma), epithelioid (plump cells with increased amounts of eosinophilic or clear cytoplasm) and myxohyaline (myxoid or hyaline matrix between tumor cells). Myxoid change invariably occurs in younger women and may be associated with pregnancy. Vulvar leiomyomatosis consists of benign smooth muscle.

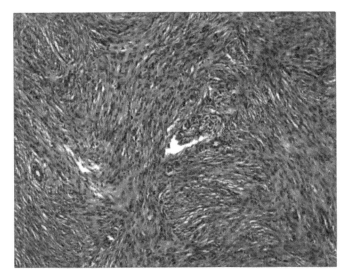

Figure 13.52. Vulvar leiomyoma. Dense proliferation of smooth muscle cells is seen, without atypia or mitoses.

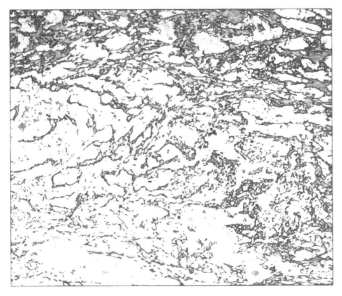

Figure 13.53. Leiomyoma. Myxohyaline change is frequent in vulvar leiomyomas.

Treatment

For well circumscribed tumors that clinically appear to be benign, simple surgical excision is advised. Excision is the only certain method of excluding a malignancy.

172. SMOOTH MUSCLE TUMOR OF INTERMEDIATE DIFFERENTIATION (ATYPICAL LEIOMYOMA)

These are defined as having at least one of mitoses, nuclear atypia or an invasive margin, and show a propensity for recurrence. As recurrence may occur many years after the primary tumor has been excised, long term follow up is recommended for this group. The recurrence is often more histologically worrying than the primary.

173. LEIOMYOSARCOMA

These tumors present as single or multiple nodules on the vulva or vagina. They are most commonly seen in the labium majus and can be difficult to clinically distinguish from benign smooth muscle tumors.

Pathology

Clinically malignant smooth muscle tumors are diagnosed using the following criteria: 1) >50mm size, 2) infiltrative margins, 3) >5 mitoses per 10 HPF, 4) moderate to severe cytological atypia are required and, 5) coagulative necrosis associated with any one of the other criteria.

Treatment

Wide surgical excision with a margin of 1-2 cm is the treatment of choice. Radiation may be used as adjuvant treatment for high-grade lesions or for local recurrences.

174. RHABDOMYOSARCOMA (SARCOMA BOTRYOIDES)

This is very rare on the vulva and occurs more commonly (although still rarely) on the vagina. See rhabdomyosarcoma of vagina (**220**).

175. NEUROFIBROMA (NEUROFIBROMATOSIS)

Although neurofibromas (NF) are one of the commonest benign mesenchymal tumors of skin, they are fairly infrequent on the vulva. They may be solitary, but are more often seen as part of neurofibromatosis. They form soft skin coloured papules and may be pedunculated. NF may become manifest for the first time in pregnancy. Clitoral involvement with NF usually presents with clitoromegaly, may be congenital and may be the first sign of the disease.

Pathology

NF are unencapsulated spindle cell lesions composed of cells with wavy or angulated nuclei and fibrillary eosinophilic cytoplasm, that mark with S100. They do not show atypia or mitoses.

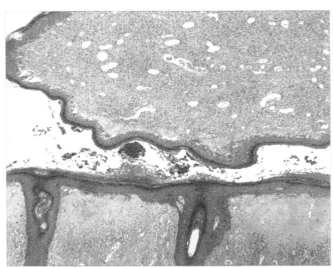

Figure 13.54. Clitoral neurofibroma in a patient with neurofibromatosis. A polypoid neurofibroma lies apparently disconnected from the epidermis. There is coexistent lichen sclerosus.

176. SCHWANNOMA

Schwannoma is another widely distributed benign peripheral nerve sheath tumor but is less common than neurofibroma. A few cases have been reported on the vulva and these appeared similar to those seen elsewhere macroscopically and microscopically.

177. GRANULAR CELL TUMOR

Granular cell tumors are uncommon nerve-sheath derived benign tumors seen in skin and mucosa. The oral cavity is the most common site but there also appears to be a predilection for the vulva where, rarely, they may be multiple. The tumor appears as dermal or subcutaneous nodules up to 3 cm in diameter (usually much smaller) and may ulcerate.

Pathology

There is a reactive epidermal hyperplasia overlying an unencapsulated dermal and subcutaneous tumor with an infiltrative border, The tumor is composed of large cells with very distinctive, abundant, eosinophilic granular cytoplasm and small, round, regular nuclei. A close association with nerves and S100 positive staining are evidence of their nerve origin.

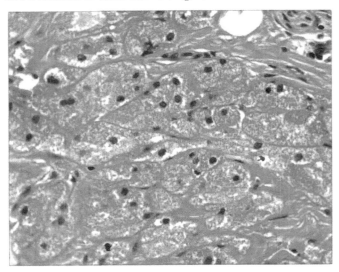

Figure 13.55. Granular cell tumor. There are nests of large, eosinophilic granular cells with small, central, pyknotic nuclei.

Treatment

The treatment is local excision. Because the lesion is subcutaneous and locally infiltrative, complete excision may be difficult.

178. MALIGNANT PERIPHERAL NERVE SHEATH TUMOR

Malignant peripheral nerve sheath tumor (previously termed neurofibrosarcoma) is the malignant counterpart of neurofibroma. Most patients have neurofibromatosis. A handful of primary vulvar malignant peripheral nerve sheath tumors have been reported. It is treated by surgical excision.

Pathology

Malignant peripheral nerve sheath tumors are sarcomas with atypia and mitoses that show some histological or immunohistochemical evidence of peripheral nerve differentiation. Paradoxically, immunoperoxidase characteristically shows only weak and focal staining with neural markers like S100 and strong staining should lead to a questioning of the diagnosis. Occasionally, high-grade spindle cell tumors arising in the setting of neurofibromatosis are negative for all diagnostic markers.

179. MALIGNANT GRANULAR CELL TUMOR

A single case of a vulvar granular cell tumor with clinical and histological features of malignancy has been described. Wide excision is recommended.

LIPOMA AND VARIANTS

Fatty tumors are relatively uncommon on the vulva compared to their incidence on the trunk and limbs. When they do occur on the vulva, they tend to show a higher incidence of histological variants.

Lipomas appear as soft, subcutaneous, rounded or pedunculated masses in the fatty areas of the vulvas of adult women, particularly in the labium majus.

Pathology

Lipomas are composed of mature fat, often with a component of fibrous tissue (181) (fibrolipoma). Variants found in the vulva include (180) spindle cell lipoma and hibernoma. Spindle cell lipoma has overlapping features with cellular angiofibroma but is distinguished by the lesser numbers of thick walled vessels.

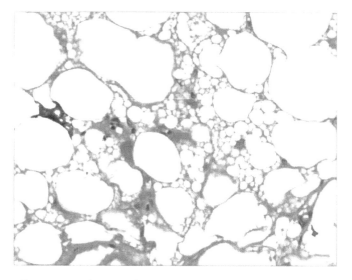

Figure 13.56. Hibernoma characterized by multivacuolar brown fat cells with mildly enlarged nuclei.

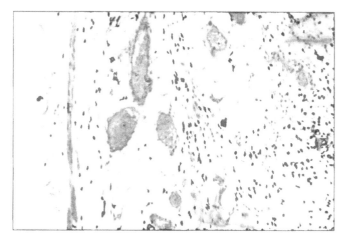

Figure 13.57. Spindle cell lipoma in the labium majus of a 19 year old girl. The tumor is well circumscribed and composed of mature fat, spindle cells and blood vessels.

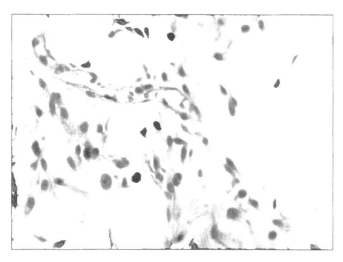

Figure 13.58. Spindle cell lipoma showing bland spindle cells and mature fat cells.

Treatment

They are treated by simple excision.

182. LIPOSARCOMA

For a long time, it was believed that liposarcomas did not occur in the vulva. Recently, however, 6 cases of atypical lipomatous tumors/well differentiated liposarcoma have been reported. The tumors occurred in women with a mean age of 52 years.

Pathology

Four cases in the series mentioned above had the usual appearance of lipoma-like lesions, but with variation in size and nuclear atypia of adipocytes and occasional lipoblasts. The other two cases had an unusual appearance with numerous, mainly bivacuolar, lipoblasts.

Treatment

Local excision is the treatment of choice. The prognosis is good. In the above series only one patient had a recurrence, 10 years after being incompletely excised. There are no reports of the tumor metastasising.

183. SYNOVIAL SARCOMA

Two cases of synovial sarcoma on the vulva have been reported. One tumor recurred. Both were young, aged 30 and 37 years. The tumors were fairly small. The tumors showed the classical biphasic growth pattern of epithelial and spindle components, marking with keratin and vimentin respectively.

184. RHABDOID TUMOR

Rhabdoid tumors are rare but aggressive neoplasms, so named for their histological resemblance to rhabdomyosarcoma. They are found in many organs, sometimes developing within various other tumors. Eight cases have been reported on the vulva, of which only one has been a long term survivor. Local recurrences are common and the appearance of distant metastases is almost invariably fatal. Chemotherapy and radiotherapy do not appear effective in controlling the disease. Initial surgical removal may offer the best chance of cure.

Histologically, rhabdoid cells have an abundant eosinophilic cytoplasm containing paranuclear inclusions and vesicular nuclei with a centrally located prominent nucleolus. There are no cross striations. Ultrastructurally, the cytoplasmic inclusions are composed of whorled filaments. Immunohistochemically, rhabdoid tumors co-express vimentin and cytokeratins, but not desmin or myoglobin.

185. EPITHELIOID SARCOMA

Epithelioid sarcoma is a rare tumor occuring at a younger age than most other sarcomas. Fifteen cases on the vulva have been reported. Histology shows sheets and nodules, often with characteristic central necrosis, of high grade malignant cells with eosinophilic cytoplasm. They may be confused on superficial examination with an inflammatory granulomatous process like granuloma annulare. Radical vulvectomy or extensive local excision with inguinal lymphadenectomy at the time of diagnosis is recommended as the treatment of choice.

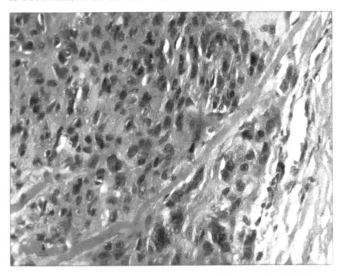

Figure 13.59. Epithelioid sarcoma characterised by atypical, spindled epithelioid cells.

186. ALVEOLAR SOFT PARTS SARCOMA

A few cases of alveolar soft parts sarcoma (ASPS) have been reported on the vulva. ASPS are rare high grade sarcomas of uncertain histogenesis, but with a distinctive histology characterized by solid and alveolar-like structures formed by cells with eosinophilic granular cytoplasm and infrequent mitoses. Most of the tumors contain intracytoplasmic PAS-positive, diastase resistant, rod-shaped crystals. Treatment is wide local excision.

187. LANGERHANS' CELL HISTIOCYTOSIS

This condition is due to a proliferation of a clonal population of Langerhans' cells with multiple organ involvement and may occur at any age. Flexures are usually involved with erythema, scaling and purpura. It may present with erosive intertrigo of the vulva and anal area. The lymph nodes, spleen, liver, lung and bone are often involved. It can present as Letterer-Siwe syndrome in infants. The Hand-Schuller-Christian syndrome presents with diabetes insipidus, exophthalmos and bone defect (mainly in the skull), and can occur at any age.

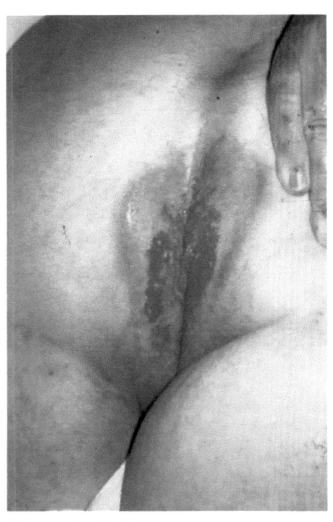

Figure 13.60. Langerhans' cell histiocytosis.

Pathology

The dermis shows an unencapsulated tumor. There is no Grenz zone and epidermal involvement is the rule. The tumor cells are a monomorphous population of cells with large, bean-shaped, grooved, pale nuclei with a visible nucleolus and pale cytoplasm. These Langerhans' cells mark with S100 and CD1a. There are typically admixed eosinophils.

Treatment

This consists mainly of corticosteroids, with or without chemotherapy.

189. NON HODGKIN'S LYMPHOMA

While non-Hodgkin's lymphoma is rare on the vulva, a wide range of vulvar lymphomas have been reported. These are classified into B and T cell types (with many subtypes) and staged similarly to lymphomas occurring elsewhere on the body.

B-cell lymphoma

B-cell lymphomas appear as purple to red, dermal or subcutaneous masses on the vulva. About half are stage 1E, that is, confined to the vulva, and half are secondary involvement from a systemic lymphoma. Most are diffuse large cell B-cell lymphomas.

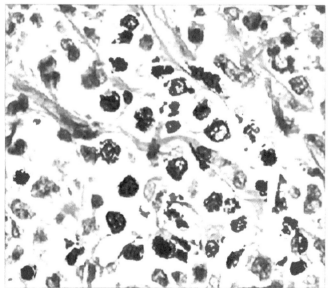

Figure 13.61. Non-Hodgkin's lymphoma. This large cell B-cell tumor of the vulva was part of a systemic lymphoma.

Treatment

Local excision biopsy followed by chemotherapy is the treatment of choice. Radiotherapy may also play a role.

Prognosis

Stage 1E lymphomas may be curable with local treatment. Systemic lymphomas generally respond to chemotherapy, but are incurable.

192. T CELL LYMPHOMA

Apart from exceedingly rare case reports of systemic lymphomas, the only T cell lymphoma to involve the vulva is cutaneous T cell lymphoma (CTCL, mycosis fungoides).

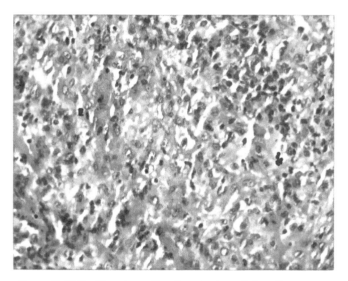

Figure 13.62. T cell lymphoma. There is a mixed population of large convoluted lymphocytes, small round lymphocytes and histiocytes.

193. CUTANEOUS T CELL LYMPHOMA (MYCOSIS FUNGOIDES)

This can present on the vulva. There are 2 disease types: mycosis fungoides (90%) and Sezary syndrome (10%). Mycosis fungoides presents initially around the buttocks, thighs, breasts and perineum. The skin lesions present as patches which are pink, scaly and wrinkled and progress to thickened plaques which eventually ulcerate. They may be hypopigmented in dark skins. It is a disease of older people with 75% presenting after the age of 50 years. In most cases the disease is confined to the skin and the prognosis is excellent. In about 5% of cases the disease becomes aggressive with involvement of lymph nodes, lungs, liver, spleen and gastro-intestinal tract. Sezary syndrome presents with erythroderma, pruritis, lympadenopathy and abnormal T4 lymphocytes in peripheral blood (Sezary cells).

Pathology

CTCL is characterized by a papillary dermal and epidermal lymphocytic infiltrate of neoplastic T helper (CD4+) lymphocytes. The neoplastic lymphocytes are atypical. They have larger and more convoluted nuclei. The atypia is more prominent in the epidermal lymphocytes. Atypia, however, is often minimal in early (patch) stage CTCL, making the diagnosis very difficult. T cell gene rearrangement (TCR), which indicates monoclonality, has been used in an effort to substantiate a diagnosis of early CTCL, although monoclonality does not always equate to clinical MF.

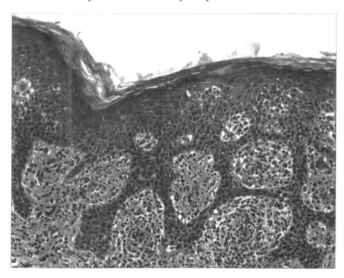

Figure 13.63. Mycosis fungoides. A dense infiltrate of lymphocytes is seen in the epidermis and dermis.

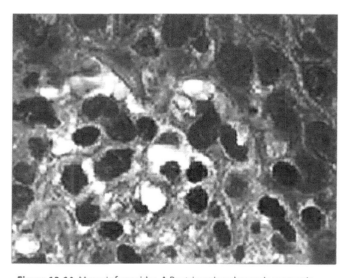

Figure 13.64. Mycosis fungoides. A Pautrier microabscess is present in the epidermis: the atypical lymphocytes with a clear space.

Treatment

Treatment of early patch stage disease is with topical corticosteroids which has a 96% response and 72% remission rate. Other treatments are topical nitrogen mustard and UV therapy. Advanced cases can be treated with bexarotene, denileukin diftitox, radiotherapy and chemotherapy.

194, 195. SECONDARY TUMORS OF THE VULVA

Less than 10% of vulvar tumors are metastatic. The most frequent primary sites are cervix, urethra, vagina, endometrium, breast, ovary, rectum and lymphoma. Patients with vulvar metastases tend to be younger (mean age 55) than those with primary vulvar carcinoma (mean age 73). Vulvar metastases often occur late in the course of the disease and are associated with a high rate of recurrence at the primary site and metastasis to other sites.

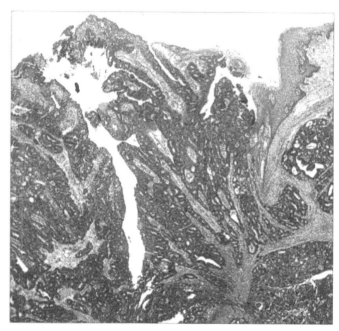

Figure 13.65. Metastatic carcinoma of the colon to the vagina. Irregular masses of complex glands are eroding through vaginal epithelium.

B. Vagina

196. VAGINAL INTRAEPITHELIAL NEOPLASIA (VAIN, SQUAMOUS DYSPLASIA/CARCINOMA IN SITU)

VAIN means squamous dysplasia and carcinoma in situ of the vagina. Women with a prior history of cervical intra-epithelial neoplasia (CIN) or vulva intra-epithelial neoplasia (VIN) are at increased risk of VAIN, representing a 'field effect' in the lower genital tract. VAIN is much rarer than CIN and occurs in patients of mean age 50-55, a decade older than those with CIN. There are no symptoms for VAIN and an abnormal cervical or vaginal vault smear should result in a colposcopic examination. When performing the colposcopy, the whole lower genital tract should always be examined. Colposcopic findings may include aceto-white epithelium after the application of 4% acetic acid or an iodine negative area after the application of Lugol iodine. The upper vagina is involved in 90% of cases and the lesions are often multifocal. A punch biopsy should be taken from these or any other suspicious areas. VAIN is almost certainly a precursor to vaginal cancer, with 3-10% of patients progressing to SCC.

Pathology

The pathology of VAIN is analogous to CIN and can be described as an HPV-related warty-basaloid type of dysplasia. The pathognomonic feature is squamous dysplasia. This is characterized by nuclear changes which correlate with aneuploidy. The best of these are basal nuclear pleomorphism, hyperchromatism and enlargement and atypical mitoses. The grading of VAIN depends primarily on the level at which atypical, immature, vertically orientated basaloid cells flatten out as they mature into (abnormal) squamous cells. Three grades, VAIN 1, 2 and 3 are defined, depending on whether these cells are confined to the lower third (VAIN 1), lower two thirds (VAIN 2) and above the lower two thirds (VAIN 3). These grades may alternatively be called mild, moderate and severe dysplasia. There may be koilocytosis on the surface, particularly with lower degrees of VAIN. Pathologists may also grade according to the Bethesda system for cervical smear reporting. That is, into LGSIL (low grade squamous intraepithelial lesion) corresponding to wart virus infection and VAIN 1 and HGSIL (high grade squamous intraepithelial lesion) corresponding to VAIN 2 and VAIN 3.

Treatment

Treatment may include excision, CO_2 laser ablation or diathermy of the area. If a high grade VAIN is confirmed at the vaginal vault after a previous hysterectomy, the vaginal vault together with the abnormal area is surgically excised. This prevents missing any abnormal tissue buried by the closure of the vault at the time of hysterectomy. Invasive lesions are found in 28% of patients undergoing upper vaginectomy for VAIN 3. The continued cytological surveillance of women after hysterectomy is to be encouraged if there is a history of lower genital tract neoplasia.

VAGINAL CANCER

Primary vaginal cancers are a heterogenous group and account for 1-2% of cancers of the female genital tract. Squamous cell carcinomas (SCC) account for 90% of vaginal cancers but are much rarer than cervical SCC. The mean age of women with vaginal SCC is about 60 years, about a decade older than those with cervical SCC. Nevertheless, 10% of patients with vaginal SCC are under 40 years. Most patients present with the symptoms of vaginal bleeding and discharge and are diagnosed with advanced disease. Patients (up to 30%) may also be asymptomatic and be detected by routine examination or vaginal cytology. The most common site for these cancers is the upper third of the vagina.

Table 5. Classification of primary vaginal cancers: Histopathology.

Infancy
    Endodermal sinus tumor
    Embryonal rhabdomyosarcoma
Adolescence/Young adult
    Clear cell carcinoma
Later adult life
    Squamous cell carcinoma
    Adenocarcinoma
    Melanoma
    Sarcoma

SQUAMOUS CELL CARCINOMA OF VAGINA
Pathology

Vaginal squamous cell carcinomas resemble cervical carcinomas in histological appearance. The great majority are associated with HPV infection. Most are non-keratinising (warty-basaloid), but may be keratinising. A very small subgroup of keratinising SCC, appearing in old women, are HPV negative and may be related to chronic inflammation, such as associated with the long-term wearing of pessaries. Stage is the most important prognostic factor. Where a resection has been performed, size, the depth and level of invasion, type, grade and lymphovascular invasion should be assessed.

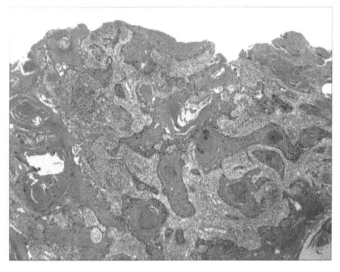

Figure 13.66. Keratinizing type SCC of the vagina in an octogenarian who wore a vaginal ring pessary for many years.

Treatment

Most vaginal cancers (squamous cell carcinomas) are treated with radiotherapy (external beam and brachytherapy, including implantation) because of the site of the tumors and because most patients are elderly. Early lesions may be suitable for surgery. Lesions close to the cervix can be treated with radical hysterectomy, partial upper vaginectomy and pelvic lymphadenectomy. Lesions close to the vulva can be treated with radical vulvectomy, partial lower vulvectomy and inguino-femoral lymphadenectomy. Surgical procedures are modified to suit individual circumstances.

Table 6. Carcinoma of the Vagina: FIGO stages

Stage I	The carcinoma is limited to the vaginal wall
Stage II	The carcinoma has involved the subvaginal tissue but has not extended to pelvic wall
Stage III	The carcinoma has extended to the pelvic wall
Stage IV	The carcinoma has extended beyond the true pelvis or has involved the mucosa of the bladder or rectum; bullous edema as such does not permit a case to be allotted to stage IV
IVA	Tumor invades bladder and/or rectal mucosa and/or direct extension beyond the true pelvis
IVB	Spread to distant organs.

197. PAPILLARY SQUAMOTRANSITIONAL CELL CARCINOMA

Papillary carcinomas of the cervix are rare tumors that show a variable mixture of squamous and transitional cell like differentiation. The papillary architecture is the key histological feature, as the tumors appear to behave similarly whether the cell type looks squamous, transitional or a mixture. The exophytic portion of the tumor consists of papillae with stromal cores which are covered by squamous or transitional-like epithelium resembling that of high grade VAIN or papillary urinary tract carcinoma. A few such tumors have been described in the vagina. There is a wide age range but, on average, the patients are older than conventional squamous cell carcinoma. Unlike transitional cell carcinoma of the urinary tract, the tumors are characteristically HPV 16 and cytokeratin 7 positive and cytokeratin 20 negative. These features are more akin to HPV-related genital tract squamous tumors rather than urinary tract neoplasms.

A key prognostic feature is whether there is stromal invasion of the base, as a minority of cases appear to be in situ. Often, the biopsy is too superficial to assess stromal invasion. To avoid an assumption of invasion and possible overtreatment in these cases, the pathologist should ask for a deeper biopsy. There have been too few cases to determine whether the tumor has a better or worse prognosis than conventional squamous cell carcinoma.

198. VERRUCOUS CARCINOMA

Verrucous carcinomas, similar clinically and pathologically to those seen in the vulva, may occur in the vagina. Patients are usually old and have a large wart-like tumor. These very well differentiated squamous tumors do not show atypia in the conventional sense and may invite a wrong diagnosis of "benign squamous papilloma" or condyloma acuminatum. However, like verrucous carcinomas elsewhere, these tumors readily recur and transform into conventionally invasive squamous cell carcinomas.

199. MULLERIAN PAPILLOMA

These are rare, benign glandular tumors of the cervix, and rarely the vagina, that occur almost exclusively in children, usually 2-4 years old. They show a fibrous stromal core, typically edematous and inflamed, covered by a single layer of bland columnar epithelium with eosinophilic cytoplasm.

200. BENIGN MIXED TUMOR (PLEOMORPHIC ADENOMA)

Benign mixed tumors are uncommon and typically seen around the menopause.

They are firm, well circumscribed submucosal tumors, usually several centimeters in diameter and are found near the hymenal ring, most commonly incidentally during pelvic examination. They are composed of bland spindle cells interrupted by bland epithelium which is usually squamous but may have a glandular component, which appears non-specific or mucinous. Treatment is simple excision.

201. ADENOCARCINOMA IN SITU (CERVIX-LIKE)

Rarely, adenocarcinoma in situ (ACIS) may occur in the vagina. In a few women, the squamocolumnar junction appears to be located in the vagina rather than its normal position in the cervix. When women with this anatomical variant develop ACIS, it involves the vagina. Women with vaginal adenosis also have an increased risk of developing premalignant disease, usually squamous (VAIN), but rarely ACIS in the vagina. It is treated by excision.

ADENOCARCINOMA

Up to 10% of primary vaginal cancers are adenocarcinomas. The mean age at presentation (51 years) is about 10 years earlier than the squamous cell carcinomas of the vagina. They may be non-specific in appearance (common type), show adenosquamous differentiation, or be endometrioid, clear cell or mucinous carcinomas or carcinosarcomas (malignant mixed mullerian tumor). The clinical presentation and treatment is as for SCC of the vagina.

COMMON TYPE

These adenocarcinomas may resemble those of the colon or be non-specific in appearance.

202. CLEAR CELL CARCINOMA

The clear cell adenocarcinomas may be associated with in utero exposure to diethylstilbestrol (DES). DES was first used in the 1940s and ceased a few years after the publication of the paper by Herbst and Scully in 1970 associating in utero exposure to DES with vaginal adenosis and clear cell adenocarcinomas. Most of these tumors occur at an early age between 18-24 years. Most are located in the upper vagina and present with abnormal vaginal bleeding or discharge. Prognosis is determined by the stage of the disease at diagnosis. Stage I disease is treated with wide local excision and staging laparotomy including retroperitoneal lymphadenectomy. This is followed by radiotherapy, both local and pelvic as required. More advanced stage disease is treated with radiotherapy alone.

203. ENDOMETRIOID CARCINOMA

The endometrioid carcinomas are associated with endometriosis or adenosis and resemble the common endometrioid carcinoma of the endometrium.

204. MUCINOUS CARCINOMA

Occasional primary mucinous carcinomas of the vagina have been reported. Some of these have been associated with some prior long-standing abnormality such as cloacal remnant, retrovaginal fistula or a neovagina fashioned from colon.

205. ADENOSQUAMOUS CARCINOMA

A few primary vaginal carcinomas are adenosquamous carcinomas, like those seen in the cervix.

206. CARCINOSARCOMA

A handful of primary carcinosarcomas (malignant mixed mullerian tumors) have been described. They look and behave like carcinosarcomas of other sites in the genital tract.

207. SMALL CELL CARCINOMA

The vagina may rarely harbor small cell carcinomas analogous to those seen in the cervix. Like small cell carcinomas elsewhere, these are aggressive tumors that grow and disseminate quickly and, despite being chemo- and radiotherapy-sensitive, have a poor prognosis.

Pathology

Histopathology is similar to small cell carcinoma of the cervix. The tumor consists of undifferentiated sheets of closely packed small cells, with hyperchromatic nuclei, without visible nucleoli and a minimal amount of cytoplasm. Nuclear moulding, apoptosis, a high mitotic count, necrosis and the deposition of basophilic material (the Azzopardi phenomenon) are features. Most cases show immunohistochemical evidence of neuroendocrine differentiation, with at least one of synaptophysin or chromogranin positive, although this is not necessary as diagnosis is made on routine hematoxylin and eosin stains.

Treatment

Excision of the lesion followed by chemotherapy is the treatment of choice. Radiotherapy may also be used. Although the prognosis remains poor, chemotherapy and radiotherapy increase tumor-free survival.

208. GENITAL MELANOCYTIC MACULE

Melanosis affects the vagina much less commonly than the vulva (157).

209. MELANOMA IN SITU

Pigmented macules in the vagina, analogous to those in the vulva, usually show melanosis (157) but occasionally show melanoma in situ and even invasive melanoma. Biopsy is required for diagnosis. Occasional cases of melanoma in situ may be very extensive or multifocal.

Pathology

In contrast to melanosis, where hyperpigmentation of the basal layer is not associated with a significant melanocytic proliferation, melanoma in situ shows confluence (melanocytes so closely packed as to form a continuous proliferation), nests, upward spread into the prickle cell layer and atypia.

Treatment

Treatment is by surgical excision. Clear margins may be difficult to obtain and lesions may recur repeatedly and ultimately develop into invasive malignant melanomas, sometimes after a period of many years.

210. MALIGNANT MELANOMA

Although more than 150 cases have been reported in the literature, vaginal malignant melanomas are rare and account for less than 1% of the vaginal malignancies. The main presenting symptoms are vaginal bleeding, vaginal discharge, and the presence of a mass. On examination they are seen as dark lesions that can be ulcerated. Tumors are predominantly located in the lower one-third and in the anterolateral aspect of the vagina.

Pathology

Invasive vaginal malignant melanomas arise from melanoma in situ and appear as sheets and nests of atypical melanocytes invading stroma. Spindle, epithelioid nevoid cell types occur and the cells may be pigmented. S100, HMB 45 and MART I provide evidence of melanocytic differentiation.

Treatment

No standard management is described, but local excision followed by radiotherapy or chemotherapy is often used. The depth of invasion as measured from the surface of the epithelium (analogous to Breslow's depth) provides prognostic information (see vulva melanoma section). The prognosis is generally poor, with a mean reported survival time of 15 months.

212. ANGIOMYOFIBROBLASTOMA

Angiomyofibroblastoma (AMFB) may be found in paravaginal soft tissue, as well as the vulva. In a recent series of 12 cases of AMFB, 9 were vulvar and 3 vaginal.

213. AGGRESSIVE ANGIOMYXOMA

Aggressive angiomyxoma may be found in paravaginal and pelvic soft tissue as well as vulva, although most cases present as vulvar masses.

214. KAPOSI'S SARCOMA

Kaposi's sarcoma may rarely be seen in the vagina in women with AIDS

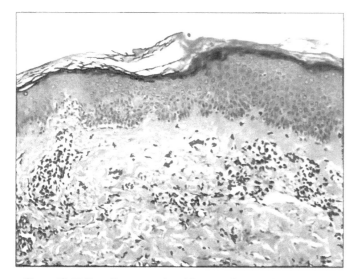

Figure 13.67. Kaposi's sarcoma. A proliferation of endothelial cells is seen in the cracks between coarse collagen fibres, extravasated red cells and lymphocytes.

215. ANGIOSARCOMA

Angiosarcoma is a rarely reported malignant tumor of the vagina. Most cases have been associated with previous therapeutic irradiation, particularly for cervical carcinoma.

216. LEIOMYOMA

Leiomyoma of the vagina is rare. Only about 300 cases have been reported in the literature. It generally presents in the second half of reproductive life with a slow growing mass within the vaginal wall. For a vaginal smooth muscle tumor to be called a leiomyoma, unlike uterine tumors, no mitoses, atypia or invasion should be tolerated. Surgical excision is recommended. Occasionally, tumors designated as vaginal leiomyomas in the literature have recurred, although it is not known whether these cases showed any histological features suggesting intermediate differentiation at the outset.

217. SMOOTH MUSCLE TUMOR, INTERMEDIATE DIFFERENTIATION

Vaginal smooth muscle tumors, if they show at least one of mitoses, nuclear atypia or an invasive margin, should be termed smooth muscle tumors of intermediate differentiation, to indicate that they have an increased risk of recurrence. Recurrences may occur years later and tend to show more aggressive histology.

218. LEIOMYOSARCOMA

Primary vaginal leiomyosarcomas represent 2-3% of all vaginal malignancies. More than 60 cases have been reported in the literature. The tumor size ranges from 2 to over 10 cm. Clinically malignant smooth muscle tumors are diagnosed using similar criteria to their vulvar counterparts with the following criteria: 1) >50mm size, 2) infiltrative margins, 3) >5 mitoses per 10 HPF, 4) moderate to severe cytological atypia are required and, 5) coagulative necrosis associated with any one of the other criteria. Wide surgical resection with a margin of 1-2cm is recommended as the primary treatment. Radiation may be used as adjuvant treatment for high-grade lesions or for local recurrences. There is an overall 5 year survival rate of 40%.

219. RHABDOMYOMA

While there is skeletal muscle deep to the labium majus, there is none in the vagina. Vulvovaginal skeletal muscle tumors occur predominantly in the subepithelial stroma of the vagina. Genital rhabdomyomas are rare polypoid tumors occurring during the reproductive age group. The tumors are typically less than 3cm in diameter. The vagina rather than the vulva is typically involved, although vulvar lesions have been reported.

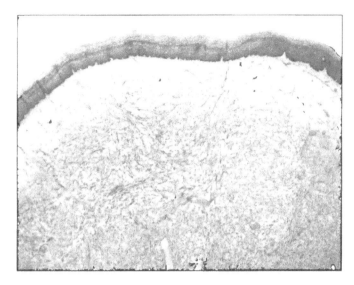

Figure 13.68. Rhabdomyoma of the vagina. An unencapsulated tumor is present in the lamina propria.

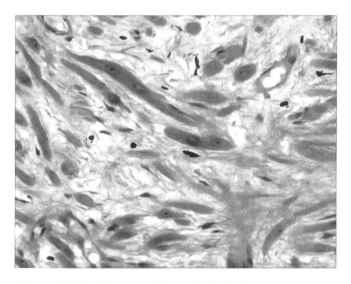

Figure 13.69. Rhabdomyoma of the vagina showing large strap cells with abundant eosinophilic cytoplasm.

Pathology

Rhabdomyomas are tumors composed of mature skeletal muscle cells with prominent cross-striations and no evidence of nuclear atypia.

Treatment

Local excision will suffice. Recurrences are not recorded.

220. RHABDOMYOSARCOMA (SARCOMA BOTRYOIDES)

Rhabdomyosarcoma (RMS), although rare, is the usual form of genital tract sarcoma in girls and young women. The tumor may originate in the vagina, cervix, or vulva. Cervical RMS mainly presents in teenagers, while vulvar and vaginal RMS characteristically occur in prepubertal girls and infants.

Pathology.

The characteristic features are those of embryonal rhabdomyosarcoma as seen in other sites. The tumor appears as a polypoid mass, either covered by normal mucosa or ulcerated. There may be edema and low cellularity imparting a false low power impression of benignity. However, there is a conspicuous increase in cellularity beneath the mucosa (the so called "cambium" layer) and around vessels. The tumor forms a discohesive spindle cell population, with pleomorphic and hyperchromatic nuclei and a variable amount of eosinophilic cytoplasm. Longitudinal and cross striations may be seen. However, cross striations are only seen in about half the cases and are not required for diagnosis. Immunoperoxidase stains will usually show positive muscle markers.

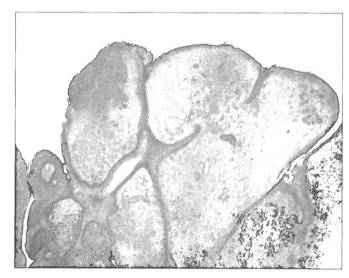

Figure 13.70. Sarcoma botryoides of the vagina. Lobules of edematous tumor are covered by normal squamous epithelium.

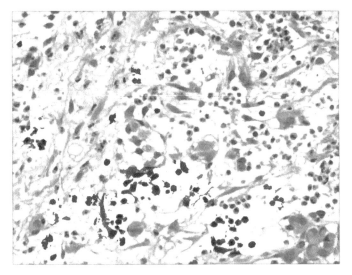

Figure 13.71. Sarcoma botryoides of the vagina showing small round blue and larger cells with eosinophilic cytoplasm and edematous matrix.

Treatment

Along with other pediatric sarcomas, there have been great improvements in survival and tissue conservation with multimodality therapy. Current protocols are to give chemotherapy either alone or, if not completely effective, followed by local treatment (radiotherapy or surgery) for a residual mass of viable tumor or clinical relapse. Only a minority of girls end up having radical surgery. Girls with non-metastatic RMS of the genital tract now have an excellent survival rate of over 90% 5 year survival and 78% overall survival.

221. NEUROFIBROMA

Vaginal neurofibromas, particularly if large, are rare. If a vaginal neurofibroma is found, a search should be made for other sites of Recklinghausen's disease. On first principles, it has been recommended that large tumors be removed surgically to avoid risk of progression to malignancy.

222. SCHWANNOMA

Schwannomas of the female genital tract are very rare, and a case reported in 1992 claimed to be first example reported in the vagina. The patient was a 37-year-old woman with a cellular schwannoma. Schwannomas, however, may occur in soft tissue of any site, and rare examples have been reported in the rectovaginal septum, retrovesical soft tissue and paracolpos.

223. GRANULAR CELL TUMOR

A single case of a vaginal granular cell tumor in a woman aged 58 years, has been reported.

224. ENDOMETRIAL STROMAL SARCOMA

While metastatic endometrial stromal sarcoma (ESS) to the vagina is not rare in the follow up of uterine ESS, primary vaginal ESS is extremely rare and appears to have been reported in the vagina on only two occasions, one occurring in endometriosis and one without.

225. MULLERIAN ADENOSARCOMA

Metastatic vaginal mullerian adenosarcoma (MA) occurs in a minority of cases during the follow up of uterine MA. Primary MA of the vagina has also been recorded extremely rarely occurring in endometriosis.

226. NON-HODGKIN'S LYMPHOMA

More than 30 non-Hodgkins' lymphomas of the vagina have been reported. The commonest symptom is vaginal bleeding. **Diffuse large cell B cell lymphoma** accounts for the great majority of cases but there is a wide variety of rare types that have been reported on one or two occasions. About half the patients have disease apparently localized to the vagina. These patients are younger (mean age about 40 years) than women with systemic lymphoma (mean age about 65 years), and have a better survival. There are very rare case reports of **T cell lymphoma** occurring in the vagina.

Local surgical excision is followed by chemotherapy and radiotherapy. About 60% of patients can expect long-term survival

227. YOLK SAC TUMOR

Yolk sac tumors histologically and immunohistologically similar to those found in the ovary may rarely be extragonadal. When these occur in the female genital tract, the vagina accounts for the great majority. Vaginal yolk sac tumors occur in infants and young girls less than 3 years old and present with bleeding, discharge or a mass. The tumors are located anywhere in the vagina, are typically exophytic and several centimetres in diameter. The prognosis has improved greatly with the use of chemotherapy after excision.

228. SECONDARY TUMORS OF THE VAGINA

Metastatic carcinomas to the vagina are more frequent than primary tumors, with spread from cervical, endometrial, ovarian, vulvar, colorectal and urological cancers and gestational trophoblastic disease. Metastases from kidney, breast and pancreas are also described. Spread to the vagina via the blood or lymphatics can occur in gestational trophoblastic disease and endometrial cancer and directly in the case of cervix, vulva, colorectal, urological and ovary cancers.

C. Urethra

229. INTRAEPITHELIAL NEOPLASIA
(DYSPLASIA/CARCINOMA IN SITU) OF URETHRA

Premalignant conditions of squamous cell, transitional cell and glandular epithelial cells and melanocytes are seen only infrequently. The squamous covered distal urethra is easily exposed to HPV and may be involved with HPV-type squamous dysplasia, usually as part of a more extensive VIN and VAIN. Premalignant conditions of the urethra provide a treatment challenge because of the importance of conserving urethral function.

MALIGNANT TUMORS OF URETHRA

Cancer of the female urethra is uncommon and accounts for only 0.02% of all cancers found in women. However, it is the only urinary tract neoplasm that has a predilection for women, with a sex ratio incidence of 4:1. The commonest malignancies are (230) **squamous cell carcinoma**, (235) **transitional cell carcinoma**, adenocarcinoma and malignant melanoma. Malignancies usually occur in middle-aged to elderly females. Urethral carcinomas present with a variety of symptoms referable to the urinary or lower genital tracts, namely hematuria, urethral or vaginal bleeding, dysuria, frequency, incontinence, retention, pain, dyspareunia or the finding of a mass.

Examination findings depend on the site. Meatal tumors most frequently look like caruncles. More proximal tumors form deeper masses. Direct spread is to the vestibule and labia, vagina, bladder neck and peri-urethral tissues. The type of lymph node spread depends on site. Distal tumors tend to spread to the inguinal nodes (like vulvar tumors), while proximal tumors tend to involve external and internal iliac nodes, obturator and presacral nodes. Hematogenous spread occurs late. Urethral malignancies tend to be high stage and have a poor prognosis. Surgery alone is used for early stage tumors and multimodality therapy for advanced stage tumors.

Adenocarcinoma of the female urethra accounts for only 10% of all urethral cancers but are a heterogenous group. There appear to be at least 3 main types. The commonest are those (232) **resembling colonic carcinomas**. The other two groups are (233) **clear cell** and (236) **prostatic type adenocarcinomas**. Colonic-type adenocarcinomas may be associated with a (231) **villous adenoma** and arise in the upper urethra. They include subtypes of mucinous and signet ring carcinomas. Clear cell carcinoma of the urethra resembles clear cell carcinoma of the endometrium, ovary and genitourinary tract. It has a particular female predilection and in one study of the disease, 18 of the 19 patients were female. It also has a marked tendency to arise in urethral diverticula. The age range is 35-80 and the mean age 58 years. A small group of urethral carcinomas resemble (236) **prostatic carcinoma,** with positive prostate specific antigen (PSA) staining.

240. MALIGNANT MELANOMA

Though an uncommon urethral malignancy, the urethra is the commonest site in the urinary tract for this malignancy. Urethral malignant melanomas occur in middle to old age. There is a predilection for women. Typically, the distal urethra is involved by a polypoid mass, which may or may not be pigmented. The tumors have been reported from 0.8 to 6cm in maximum dimension and showed 2 to 17mm depth of invasion. They have a poor prognosis. Conventional prognostic factors such as depth of invasion and tumor stage do not seem to be as important as the site.

241. LEIOMYOMA

Leiomyomas, although rare, are the most common mesenchymal neoplasms of the urethra, where they occur predominantly in females.

242. RHABDOMYOSARCOMA

A small proportion of childhood rhabdomyosarcoma botryoides of the urinary tract begin in the urethra.

243. LYMPHOMA

Malignant lymphoma rarely affects the urethra, When it does, localised disease needs to be distinguished from disseminated disease. A literature review found in 18 cases, one-year survival rate was 91% for local stage and less than 35% for disseminated stage (Inuzuka et al) . The authors concluded it appeared therapy, including excision, radiation and chemotherapy, is effective for patients with local stage but not for patients with disseminated disease.

244. PLASMACYTOMA

Plasmacytomas are unusual soft-tissue collection of neoplastic monoclonal plasma cells that must be distinguished from the much more common multiple myeloma. The most common sites of plasmacytoma are the upper respiratory tract and skin, although any site of disease is theoretically possible. Five cases of primary urethral plasmacytomas have been reported, including a patient with a 12 year follow up with no recurrence after local radiation as definitive treatment.

245. METASTATIC AND DIRECT SPREAD TO THE URETHRA

These tumors are rare. They include metastases from the urinary tract, particularly the bladder, genital tract (both lower and upper) and from distant sites.

REFERENCES.

Al-Ghamdi A, Freedman D, Miller D, Poh C, Rosin M, Zhang L, Gilks CB. Vulvar squamous cell carcinoma in young women: a clinicopathologic study of 21 cases. Gynecol Oncol 2002; 84: 94-101

Amin MB, Young RH Primary carcinomas of the urethra. Semin Diagn Pathol 1997; 14: 147-60

Andersen ES, Sorensen IM Verrucous carcinoma of the female genital tract: report of a case and review of the literature. Gynecol Oncol 1988; 30: 427-30 2003; 34: 559-64

Bai H, Cviko A, Granter S, Yuan L, Betensky RA, Crum CP. Immunophenotypic and viral (human papillomavirus) correlates of vulvar seborrheic keratosis. Hum Pathol 2003; 34: 559-64

Battles OE, Page DL, Johnson JE Cytokeratins, CEA, and mucin histochemistry in the diagnosis and characterization of extramammary Paget's disease Am J Clin Pathol 1997; 108: 6-12

Borazjani G, Prem KA, Okagaki T, Twiggs LB, Adcock LL. Primary malignant melanoma of the vagina: a clinicopathological analysis of 10 cases. Gynecol Oncol. 1990 May;37(2):264-7

Brainard JA, Hart WR Proliferative epidermal lesions associated with anogenital Paget's disease Am J Surg Pathol 2000; 24: 543-52

Brand A, Covert A. Malignant rhabdoid tumour of the vulva: case report and review of the literature with emphasis on clinical management and outcome. Gynecol Oncol 2001; 80: 99-103

Brown HM, Wilkinson EJ Uroplakin-III to distinguish primary vulvar Paget disease from Paget disease secondary to urothelial carcinoma. Hum Pathol 2002; 33: 545-8

Bruckner AL, Frieden IJ Hemangiomas of infancy J Am Acad Dermatol 2003; 48: 477-493

Buhl A, Landow S, Lee YC, Holcomb K, Heilman E, Abulafia O Microcystic adnexal carcinoma of the vulva. Gynecol Oncol 2001; 82: 571-4

Buonaguro FM et al Kaposi's sarcoma: aetiopathogenesis, histology and clinical features. JEADV 2003; 17: 138-54

Cardosi RJ, Speights A, Fiorica JV, Grendys EC Jr, Hakam A, Hoffman MS. Bartholin's gland carcinoma: a 15 year experience. Gynecol Oncol 2001; 82: 247-51

Carlson JW, McGlennen RC, Gomez R, Longbella C, Carter J, Carson LF Sebaceous carcinoma of the vulva: a case report and review of the literature. Gynecol Oncol 1996; 60: 489-91

Chen YH, Wong TW, Lee JY Depigmented genital extramammary Paget's disease: a possible histogenetic link to Toker's clear cells and clear cell papulosis J Cutan Pathol 2001; 28: 105-8

Chu T Langerhans cell histiocytosis Aust J Derm (2001) 42: 237-242

Chulia MT, Paya A, Nivero M, Ceballos S, Aranda FI. Phyllodes tumor in ectopic breast tissue of the vulva. Int J Surg Pathol 2001; 9: 81-3

Ciaravino G, Kapp DS, Vela AM, Fulton RS, Lum BL, Teng NN, Roberts JA. Primary leiomyosarcoma of the vagina. A case report and literature review. Int J Gynecol Cancer. 2000 Jul;10(4):340-347

Clark WH Jr, Hood AF, Tucker MA, Jampel RM Atypical melanocytic nevi of the genital type with a discussion of reciprocal parenchymal-stromal interactions in the biology of neoplasia. Hum Pathol 1998; 29: Suppl (1): S1-24

Curtin JP, Saigo P, Slucher B, Venkatraman ES, Mychalazak B, Hoskins WJ Soft tissue sarcoma of the vagina and vulva: a clinicopathologic study. Obstet Gynecol 1995: 86: 269-72

Davis G, Wentworth J, Richard J Self-administered topical imiquimod treatment of vulvar intraepithelial neoplasia. A report of four cases.. J Reprod Med 2000; 45: 619-23.

Dennerstein G. Cytology of the vulva. J Reprod Med 1988 Aug;33(8):703-4.

DePasquale SE, McGuiness TB, Mangan CE, Husson M, Woodland MB. Adenoid cystic carcinoma of Bartholin's gland: a review of the literature and report of a patient. Gynecol Oncol 1996; 61: 122-5.

Dinh TV, Powell LC jr, Hannigan EV, Yang HL, Wirt DP, Yandell RB. Simultaneously occurring condylomata acuminata, carcinoma in situ and verrucous carcinoma of the vulva and carcinoma in situ of the cervix in a young woman. A case report. J Reprod Med 1988; 33: 510-3.

Dodson MK, Cliby WA, Pettavel PP, Keeney GL, Podratz KC. Female urethral carcinomas: evidence for more than one tissue of origin? Gynecol Oncol 1995; 59: 352-7

Doss LL Simultaneous extramedullary plasmacytomas of the vagina and vulva: a case report and review of the literature Cancer 1978; 41: 2468-74

Duray PH, Merino MJ, Axiotix C Warty dyskeratoma of the vulva. Int J Gynecol Pathol 1983; 2: 286-93

Escalonilla P, Grilli R, Cananero M, Soriano ML, Farina MC, Manzarbeitia F, Sainz R, Matsukura T, Requena L. Sebaceous carcinoma of the vulva. Am J Dermatopathol 1999; 21: 468-72

Fanning J, Lambert HC, Hale TM, Morris PC, Schuerch C. Paget's disease of the vulva: prevalence of associated vulvar adenocarcinoma, invasive Paget's disease, and recurrence after surgical excision. Am J Obstet Gynecol. 1999 Jan;180(1 Pt 1):24-7

Feakins RM, Lowe DG Basal cell carcinoma of the vulva: a clinicopathologic study of 45 cases. Int J Gynecol Pathol 1997; 16: 319-24

Fetsch JF, Laskin WB, Tavassoli FA Superficial angiomyxoma (cutaneous myxoma): a clinicopathologic study of 17 cases arising in the genital area. Int J Gynecol Pathol 1997; 16: 325-34

Flanagan CW, Parker JR, Mannel RS, Min KW, Kida M Primary endodermal sinus tumor of the vulva: a case report and review of the literature. Gynecol Oncol. 1997 Sep;66(3):515-8.

Frega A, Stentella P, Tinari A, Vecchione A, Marchionni M Giant condyloma or Buschke-Lowenstein tumor: review of the literature and report of 3 cases treated by CO2 laser surgery. A long tern follow-up. Anticancer Res 2002; 22: 1201-4

Fujiwaki R, Takahashi K, Nishiki Y, Ryuko K, Kitao M. Rare case of transitional cell carcinoma originating in Bartholin's gland duct. Gynecol Obstet Invest 1995; 40: 278-80.

Fukunaga M, Endo Y, Ishikawa E, Ushigome S Mixed tumor of the vagina. Histopathology 1996; 28: 457-6

Ghamande SA, Kasznica J, Griffiths CT, Finkler NJ, Hamid AM. Mucinous adenocarcinomas of the vulva. Gynecol Oncol 1995; 57: 117-20

Ghorbani RP, Malpica A, Ayala AG Dermatofibrosarcoma protruberans of the vulva: clinicopathologic and immunohistochemical analysis of four cases, one with fibrosarcomatous change and review of the literature. Int J Gynecol Pathol 1999; 18: 366-73

Gibson GE, Ahmed I Perianal and genital basal cell carcinoma: a clinicopathologic review of 51 cases. J Am Acad Dermatol 2001; 45: 68-71

Gilbey S, Moore DH, Look KY and Sutton GP Vulvar keratoacanthoma.Obstet Gynecol. 1997 May;89(5 Pt 2):848-50

Gilcrease MZ, Delgado R, Vuitch F, Albores-Saavedra J. Clear cell adenocarcinoma and nephrogenic adenoma of the urethra and urinary bladder: a histopathologic and immunohistochemical comparison. Hum Pathol 1998; 29: 1451-6

Gokden N, Dehner LP, Zhu X, Pfeifer JD Dermatofibrosarcoma protruberans of the vulva

Granter SR, Nucci MR, Fletcher CD Aggressive angiomyxoma: reappraisal of its relationship to angiomyofibroblastoma in a series of 16 cases. Histopathology 1997; 30: 3-10

Hart WR. Vulvar intraepithelial neoplasia. Historical aspects and current status. Int J Gynaecol Pathol. 2001; 20: 16-30

Hierro I, Blanes A, Matilla A, Munoz S, Vicioso L, Nogales FF Merkel cell (neuroendocrine) carcinoma of the vulva. A case report with immunohistochemical and ultrastructural findings and review of the literature. Pathol Res Pract. 2000;196(7):503-9

Hierro I, Blanes A, Matilla A, Munoz S, Vicioso L, Nogales FF Merkel cell (neuroendocrine) carcinoma of the vulva. A case report with immunohistochemical and ultrastructural findings and review of the literature. Pathol Res Pract. 2000;196(7):503-9

Huang YH, Chuang YH, Kuo TT, Yang LC, Hong HS Vulvar syringoma: a clinicopathologic and immunohistologic study of 18 patients and results of treatment. J Am Acad Dermatol 2003; 48: 735-9

Hyde S, Uitterhoeve LJ, Schilthuis MS, ten Kate FJ, van der Velden J. Sarcoma in association with multimodality management of vulvar cancer: two case reports. Gynecol Oncol 2001: 81: 320-3

Inizuka S, Koga S, Imanishi D, Matsuo T, Kametake H. Primary malignant lymphoma of the female urethra. Anticancer Res 2003; 23: 2925-7

Jensen K, Kohler S, Rouse RV Cytokeratin staining in Merkel cell carcinoma: an immunohistochemical study of cytokeratins 5/6, 7, 17, and 20. Appl Immunohistochem Mol Morphol 2000; 8: 310-5

Jones RW Vulval intraepithelial neoplasia: current perspectives. Eur J Gynaecol Oncol 2001; 22: 393-402

Jones RW, Baranyai J, Stables S. Trends in squamous cell carcinoma of the vulva: the influence of vulvar intraepithelial neoplasia. Obstet Gynecol 1997; 90: 448-52.

Jones RW, Rowan DM. Vulvar Intraepithelial Neoplasia III: A Clinical Study of the Outcome in 113 Cases With Relation to the Later Development of Invasive Vulvar Carcinoma. Obset Gynecol 1994; 84:5:741-5.

Jones RW, Rowan DM Spontaneous regression of vulvar intraepithelial neoplasia 2-3 Obstet Gynecol 2000; 96: 470-2

Kajiwara H, Yasuda M, Yahata G, Yamauchi I, Satoh S, Hirasawa T,Osamura RY Myxoid leiomyoma of the vulva: a case report Tokai J Exp Clin Med 2002; 27: 57-64

Kaminski JM, Anderson PR, Han AC, Mitra RK, Rosenblum NG, Edelson MI. Primary small cell carcinoma of the vagina. Gynecol Oncol 2003; 88: 451-5

Kasamatsu T, Hasegawa T, Tsuda H, Okada S, Sawada M, Yamada T, Tsunematsu R, Ohmi K, Mizuguchi K, Kawana T. Primary epithelioid sarcoma of the vulva. Int J Gynecol Cancer 2001; 11: 316-20

Kazakov DV, Burg G, Kempf W. Clinicopathological spectrum of mycosis fungoides. J E A D V 2004; 18:397-415.

Koenig C, Turnicky RP, Kankam CF, Tavassoli FA Papillary squamotransitional cell carcinoma of the cervix: a report of 32 cases. Am J Surg Pathol 1997: 21: 915-21

Kuan SF, Montag AG, Hart J, Krausz T, Recant W Differential expression of mucin genes in mammary and extramammary Paget's disease. Am J Surg Pathol 2001; 25: 1469-77

Kuo TT, Chan HL, Hsueh S Clear cell papulosis of the skin. A new entity with histogenetic implications for cutaneous Paget's disease. Am J Surg Pathol 1987; 11: 827-34

Lane JE, Walker AN, Mullis EN Jr, Etheridge JG. Cellular angiofibroma of the vulva. Gynecol Oncol. 2001 May;81(2):326-9

Lehane P, Keane O et al. Genital melanotic macules J Am Acad Dermatol 1998; 38: 647-66

Lelle RJ, Davis KP, Roberts JA. Adenoid cystic carcinoma of the Bartholin's gland: the University of Michigan experience. Int J Gynecol Cancer 1994; 4: 145-9

Levitan Z, Kaplan AL, Kaufman RH. Advanced squamous cell carcinoma of the vulva after treatment for verrucous carcinoma. A case report J Reprod Med 1992; 37: 889-92

Li J, Ackerman AB "Seborrheic keratoses" that contain human papillomavirus are condylomata acuminata. Am J Dermatopathol 1994; 16: 398-405

Liu L, Davidson S, Singh M Mullerian adenosarcoma of vagina arising in persistent endometriosis: report of a case and review of the literature. Gynecol Oncol 2003; 90: 486-90

Logani s, Lu D, Quint WG, Ellenson LH, Pirog EC Low-grade vulvar and vaginal intraepithelial neoplasia: correlation of histologic features with human papillomavirus DNA detection and MIB-1 immunostaining Mod Pathol 2003; 16: 735-41

Lundquist K, Kohler S, Rouse RV Intraepidermal cytokeratin 7 expression is not restricted to Paget cells but is also seen in Toker cells and Merkel cells. Am J Surg Pathol 1999; 23: 212-9

Martelli H, Oberlin O, Rey A, Godzinski J, Spicer RD, Bouvet N et al. Conservative treatment for girls with non-metastatic rhabdomyosarcoma of the genital tract: A report from the Study Committee of the International Society of Pediatric Oncology J Clin Oncol 1999; 17: 2117-22

McAdam JA, Stewart F, Reid R Vaginal epithelioid angiosarcoma. J Clin Pathol 1998; 51: 928-30

Micheletti L, Barbero M, Preti M, Zanotto Valentino MC, Chirughello B, Pippione M. Vulva intraepithelial neoplasia of low grade: a challenging diagnosis. Eur J Gynecol Oncol 1994; 15: 70-4.

Micheletti L, Preti M, Zota P, Zanotto Valentino MC, Bocci C, Bogliatto F. A proposed glossary of terminology related to the surgical treatment of vulvar carcinoma. Cancer 1998; 83: 1369-75

Miles Prince H et al. Management of the primary cutaneous lymphomas. Aust J Derm 2003; 44: 227-42

Miliaras D Breast-like cancer of the vulva: primary or metastatic A case report and review of the literature. Eur J Gynecol Oncol 2002; 23: 350-2

Miranda JJ, Shahabi S, Salih S, Bahtiyar OM. Vulvar syringoma, report of a case and review of the literature. Yale J Biol Med. 2002 Jul-Aug;75(4):207-10

Moodley M. Moodley J Dermatofibrosarcoma protruberans of the vulva: a case report and review of the literature. Gynecol Oncol 2000; 78: 74-5

Moore RG, DePasquale SE, Steinhoff MM, Gajewski W, Steller M, Noto R, Falkenberry S. Sentinel node identification and the ability to detect metastatic tumor to inguinal lymph nodes in squamous cell cancer of the vulva. Gynecol Oncol. 2003 Jun;89(3):475-9

Mordkin RM, Skinner DG, Levine AM Long-term disease free survival after plasmacytoma of the urethra: a case report and review of the literature. Urology 1996; 48: 149-150

Mordkin RM, Skinner DG, Levine AM. Long term disease free survival after plasmacytoma of the urethra: a case report and review of the literature. Urology 1996; 48: 149-50

Mulayim N, Foster Silver D, Tolgay Ocal I, Babalola E. Vulvar basal cell carcinoma: two unusual presentations and review of the literature. Gynecol Oncol 2002; 85: 532-7

Nakamura S, Kato M, Ichimura K, Yatabe Y, Kagami Y, Suzuki R, Taji H, Kondo E, Asakura S, Kojima M, Murakami S, Yamao K, Tsuzuki T, Adachi GK, Miwa A, Yoshidai T. Peripheral T/natural killer-cell lymphoma involving the female genital tract: a clinopatholgical study of 5 cases. Int J Hematol 2001; 73: 108-114

Nascimento AF, Granter SR, Cviko A, Yuan L, Hecht JL, Crum CP. Vulvar acanthosis with altered differentiation. A precursor to verrucous carcinoma? Am J Surg Pathol 2004; 28: 638-643

Nasu K, Fujisawa K, Takai N, Miyakawa I. Angiomyofibroblastoma of the vulva. Int J Gynecol Cancer. 2002 Mar-Apr;12(2):228-31.

Nielsen GP, Shaw PA, Rosenberg AE, Dickersin GR, Young RH, Scully RE. Synovial sarcoma of the vulva: a report of two cases. Mod Pathol 1996; 9: 970-4

Nielsen GP, Young RH Mesenchymal tumors and tumor-like lesions of the female genital tract: a selective review with emphasis on recently described entities Int J Gynecol Pathol 2001; 20: 105-27

Nielsen GP, Young RH, Dickersin GR, Rosenberg AE Angiomyofibroblastoma of the vulva with sarcomatous transformation ("angiomyofibrosarcoma") Am J Surg Pathol 1997: 21: 1104-8

Nucci MR, Fletcher CD Liposarcoma (atypical lipomatous tumors) of the vulva: a clinicopathologic study of six cases. Int J Gynecol Pathol 1998; 17: 17-23

Nucci MR, Fletcher CDM Vulvovaginal soft tissue tumours: update and review. Histopathol 2000; 36: 97-108

Nucci MR, Granter SR, Fletcher CD Cellular angiofibroma: a benign neoplasm distinct from angiomyofibroblastoma and spindle cell lipoma. Am J Surg Pathol 1997; 21: 636-44

Nucci MR, Young RH, Fletcher CD Cellular pseudosarcomatous fibroepithelial stromal polyps of the lower female genital tract: an unrecognized lesion often misdiagnosed as a sarcoma. Am J Surg Pathol 2000; 24: 231-40

Obermair A, Koller S, Crandon AJ, Perrin L. Nicklin JL. Primary Bartholin gland carcinoma: a report of seven cases. Aust NZ J Obstet Gynaecol 2001; 41: 78-81

Oliva E, Quinn TR, Amin MN, Eble JN, Epstein JI, Srigley JR, Young RH. Primary malignant melanoma of the urethra: a clinicopathologic analysis of 15 cases. Am J Surg Pathol 2000; 24: 785-96

Oliva E, Young RH Clear cell adenocarcinoma of the urethra: a clinicopathologic analysis of 19 cases. Mod Pathol 1996; 9: 513-20

Ordonez NG, Manning JT, Luna MA. Mixed tumour of the vulva: a report of two cases probably arising in Bartholin's gland. Cancer 1981; 48: 181-6

Ortiz-Rey JA, Martin-Jimenez A, Alvarez C, De La Fuente A. Sebaceous gland hyperplasia of the vulva. Obstet Gynecol 2002; 5 (pt2) 919-21

Panizzon RG Vulvar melanoma Semin Dermatol 1996; 15: 67-70

Pelosi G, Martignoni G, Bonetti F. Intraductal carcinoma of mammary-type apocrine epithelium arising with a papillary hydradenoma of the vulva. Report of a case and review of the literature. Arch Path Lab Med 1991; 115: 1249-54

Piura B, Gemer O, Rabinovich A, Yanai-Innbar I Primary breast carcinoma of the vulva: case report and review of the literature. Eur J Gynaecol Oncol 2002; 23: 21-24

Preti M, Mezzetti M, Robertson C, Sideri M. Inter-observer variation in histopathological diagnosis and grading of vulvar intraepithelial neoplasia: results of an European collaborative study. BJOG; 107: 594-9.

Preti M, Micheletti L, Massobrio M, Shin-ichi Ansai Wilkinson EJ Vulvar Paget disease: one century after first reported. J Lower Gen Tract Dis 2003; 7: 122-135

Prevot S, Hugol D, Audouin J, Diebold J, Truc JB, Decroix Y, Poitout P. Primary non Hodgkin's malignant lymphoma of the vagina. Report of 3 cases with review of the literature. Pathol Res Pract. 1992 Feb;188(1-2):78-85

Rastogi BL, Bergman B, Angervall L. Primary leiomyosarcoma of the vagina: a study of five cases. Gynecol Oncol. 1984 May;18(1):77-86

Ridley CM, Frankman O, Jones ISC, Pincus S, Wilkinson E, New nomenclature for vulvar disease; international society for the study of vulvar disease. Hum Pathol 1989; 20: 495-496

Robertson DI, Maung R, Duggan MA Verrucous carcinoma of the genital tract: is it a distinct entity? Can J Surg 1993; 36: 147-51.

Saad AG, Kaouk JH, Kaspar HG, Khauli RB Leiomyoma of the urethra: report of 3 cases of a rare entity. Int J Surg Pathol 2003; 11: 123-6

Santillan A, Montero AJ, Kavanagh JJ, Liu J, Ramirez PT Vulvar Langerhans histiocytosis: a case report and review of the literature Gynecol Oncol 2003; 91: 241-6

Scurry J, Brand A, Planner R, Dowling J, Rode J. Vulvar Merkel cell tumor with glandular and squamous differentiation. Gynecol Oncol. 1996 Aug;62(2):292-7.

Seibel JL, Prasad S, Weiss RE, Bancila E, Epstein JI Villous adenoma of the urinary tract: a lesion frequently associated with malignancy. Hum Pathol 2002; 33: 236-41

Sert MB,Onsrud M, Perrone T, Abbas F, Currie JL. Malignant rhabdoid tumor of the vulva: Case report Eur J Gynaecol Oncol 1999; 20: 258-61

Sison-Torre EQ, Ackerman AB Melanosis of the vulva. A clinical simulator of malignant melanoma. Am J Dermatol Pathol 1985; 7 Suppl: 51-60

Solano T, Espana A, Sola J, Lopez G Langherhans' cell histiocytosis on the vulva. Gynecol Oncol 2000; 78: 251-4

Stefanato CM, Finn R, Bhawan J Extramammary Paget disease with underlying hidradenoma papilliferum: guilt by association Am J Dermatopathol 2000; 22: 439-42

Sutphen R, Galan-Gomez E, Koussef BG Clitoromegaly in neurofibromatosis. Am J Med Genet 1995; 30: 325-30

Turan C, Ugur M, Kutluay L, Kukner S, Dabakoglu T, Aydogdu T, Ergun Y, Cobanoglu O. Vulvar syringoma exacerbated during pregnancy. Eur J Obstet Gynecol Reprod Biol. 1996 Jan;64(1):141-2

Van Beurden M, de Caren AJ, de Vet HC, Blaauwgers JL, Drilleburg P, Gallee MP, de Kraker NW, Lammes FB, ten Kate FJ The contribution of MIB 1 in the accurate grading of vulvar intraepithelial neoplasia. J Ckin Pathol 1999; 52: 820-4

Van Beurden M, ten Kate FW, Tjong-A-Hung SP, de Craen AJ, van der Vange N, Lammes FB, ter Schegget J Human papillomavirus DNA in multicentric vulvar intraepithelial neoplasia. Int J Gynecol Pathol 1998; 17: 12-6

Van Beurden M, van der Vange N, ten Kate FW, de Craen AJ, Schiltuis MS, Lammes FB Restricted surgical management of vulvar intraepithelial neoplasia 3: Focus on exclusion of invasion and on relief of symptoms. Int J Gynecol Cancer 1998; 8: 73-77

Van der Putte Apoeccrine glands in nevus sebaceous Am J Dermatopathol 1994; 16: 23-30

Van der Putte SC, Toonstra J, Hennipman A Mammary Paget's disease confined to the areola and associated with multifocal Toker cell hyperplasia. Am J Dermatopathol 1995; 17: 487-93

Van der Putte SC, van Gorp LH Adenocarcinoma of the mammary-like glands of the vulva: a concept unifying sweat gland carcinoma of the vulva, carcinoma of supernumerary mammary glands and extramammary Paget's disease J Cutan Pathol 1994; 2: 157-63

Van der PutteSC Mammary-like glands of the vulva and their disorders. Int J Gynecol Pathol 1994; 13: 150-60

Van der Velden J, Hacker NF. Prognostic factors in squamous cell cancer of the vulva and the implications for treatment. Curr Opin Obstet Gynecol. 1996 Feb;8(1):3-7

Vang R, Medeiros LJ, Silva EG, Gershenson DM, Deavers M. Non-Hodgkin's lymphoma involving the vagina: a clinicopathologic analysis of 14 cases. Am J Surg Pathol 2000; 24: 719-25

Vang R. Medeiros LJ, Malpica A, Levenback C, Deavers M. Non-Hodgkin's lymphoma involving the vulva. Int J Gynecol Pathol. 2000; 19:236-42

Wechter ME, Gruber SB, Haefner HK et al. Vulvar melanoma: a report of 20 cases and review of the literature. J Am Acad Dermatol 2004; 50:4:554-62.

Weiss S, Amit A, Schwarz MR, Kaplan AL Primary choriocarcinoma of the vulva. Int J Gynecol Cancer 2001; 11: 251-4

Wick MR, Goellner JR, Wolfe JT 3rd, Su WP Vulvar sweat gland carcinomas Arch Pathol Lab Med 1985; 109: 43-7

Yin C, Chapman J, Tawfik O Invasive mucinous (colloid) adenocarcinoma of ectopic breast tissue in the vulva: a case report. Breast J 2003; 9: 113-5

Young S, Leon M, Talerman A, Teresi M, Emmadi R. Polymorphous low grade adenocarcinoma of the vulva and vagina: a tumor resembling adenoid cystic carcinoma. Int J Surg Pathol 2003; 11: 43-9.

Yu-Huei H. et al Vulvar syringoma: a clinicopathologic and immunohistologic study of 18 patients and results of treatment. J Am Acad Dermatol 2003; 48: 735-739

Chapter 14

8. NON-NEOPLASTIC CYSTS AND SWELLINGS

246. EPIDERMAL INCLUSION CYST (IMPLANTATION DERMOID)

Epidermal inclusion (implantation dermoid) cyst refers to a type of vulvar or vaginal cyst arising from traumatic implantation of squamous epithelium. They are not to be confused with those resulting from embryological inclusion during ectodermal fusion (see dermoid cyst **9**). The latter are rare. Cysts due to epidermal implantation from obstetric trauma are common.

Clinical features

Epidermal inclusion cysts resulting from obstetric trauma are found in or adjacent to the introitus and are of little clinical significance. They are not painful and are seldom larger than a centimetre or so. They are commonly encountered during a second or subsequent birth when they rupture or are incised to reveal creamy contents which at first resembles pus. The woman may find the cyst herself and request its removal, usually because of concern over the differential diagnosis.

Pathology

Implantation dermoids contain granular basophilic material and are lined by non-keratinising squamous epithelium. The lack of laminated keratin and a granular layer in their epithelial lining distinguishes implantation dermoids from epidermal cysts of infundibular origin, seen in the hair bearing area of the vulva.

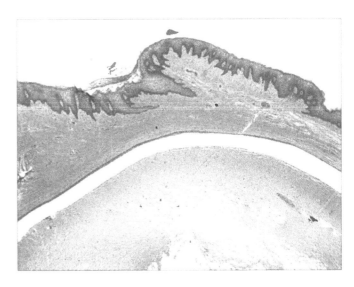

Figure 14.1. Implantation dermoid, vagina. The cyst lies in the lamina propria and contains basophilic debris.

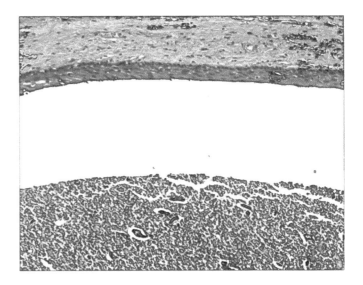

Figure 14.2. Implantation dermoid, vagina. Higher power view showing the basophilic debris in which there are scattered, small, darker bodies (squames) and its lining by non-keratinizing squamous epithelium.

Treatment

These cysts can be easily excised or shelled out under local anesthesia but treatment is seldom required.

247. SKIN TAG (ACROCHORDON)

The skin tag is a common, harmless, non-neoplastic vulvar excrescence. It could be looked upon as a malformation of hair bearing skin. It is easily confused with condyloma acuminatum, which it resembles.

Clinical features

Most often, the skin tag is noted on routine examination, the woman unaware of its presence. This skin disorder can be found in most adults, increasing in number with age. They are commonly found on the vulva and groin. Occasionally, acrochordons may become uncomfortable if large or on a long stalk. Fear of warts is a common reason for seeking advice.

The skin tag is seldom more than a centimetre in width, is flesh coloured, wrinkled and commonly on a stalk. Although arising from the hair bearing skin on and adjacent to the vulva, it does not have hair.

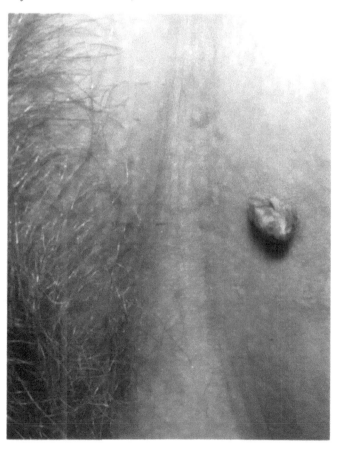

Figure 14.3. Acrochordon.

Diagnosis

Skin tags do not take up 5% acetic acid any differently to the surrounding skin. This may help distinguish them from condylomata acuminata, if there is doubt.

Histologically, skin tags are composed of an overgrowth of dermal collagen. There may be an admixture of fat (nevus lipomatosis) and, in a minority of cases, a dermal nevus. The epidermis varies from normal to changes resembling a seborrheic keratosis or lichen simplex chronicus.

Treatment

As the skin tag alters very little with time, treatment is not all that necessary. Ligation of the stalk with any suture material or destruction with liquid nitrogen are relatively simple, painless forms of treatment. Otherwise they may be snipped off under local anesthesia with an absorbable suture for hemostasis.

248. FIBROEPITHELIAL POLYP

Fibroepithelial polyps (FEP) are benign polyps found in the vagina and on the vulva. Such FEPs need to be distinguished from the common skin tags above (also known as fibroepithelial polyps) which occur all over the body, but especially in skin creases (including the vulva) in middle aged and older individuals. Lower female genital tract FEPs are common and most frequently seen in the vaginas of women in their reproductive years. They are believed to be reactive hyperplasias rather than true neoplasms. There is an increased incidence of FEPs in pregnancy and other hyperestrogenic states and rarely in association with chronic lymphedema. FEPs may be single or multiple, smooth or fronded, and show great size variation. While many are small (<1cm) and discovered incidentally, there are rare examples of vulvar tumors weighing more than 1kg.

"pseudosarcomatous", but despite their worrying appearance, behave benignly. In difficult cases, the presence of stellate and multinucleate cells as well as spindle cells, lack of a clear boundary with the overlying epithelial-stromal interface and increased cellularity in the centre of the lesion serve to distinguish FEPs from other benign mesenchymal lesions.

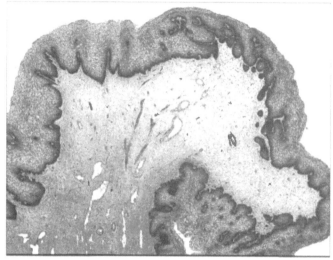

Figure 14.5. Vaginal fibroepithelial polyp composed of a proliferation of stroma covered by normal squamous epithelium.

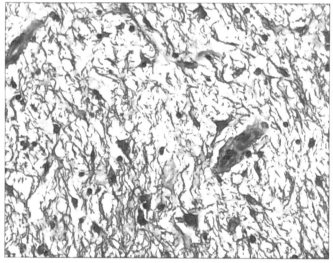

Figure 14.6. Vaginal fibroepithelial polyp under higher power showing its loose fibrous matrix containing a lowly cellular proliferation of stellate and spindle myofibroblasts.

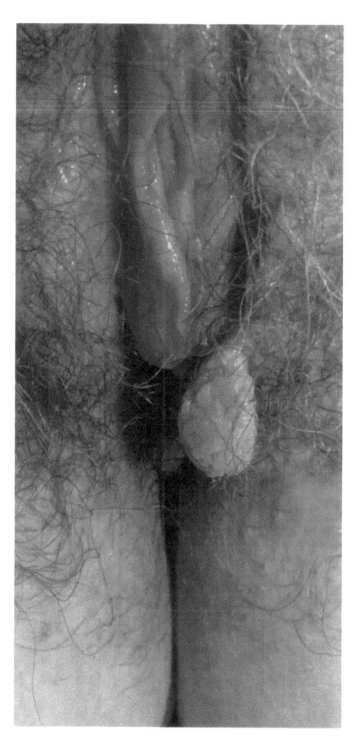

Figure 14.4. Fibroepithelial polyp of labium majus.

Pathology

The polyps are formed by proliferations of the hormone-receptor positive subepithelial stromal cells of the distal female genital tract and are covered by normal squamous epithelium. Rarely, in pregnancy, FEPs show increased cellularity, marked atypia and moderate mitotic activity. Such atypical FEPs have been termed

Treatment

FEPs are usually excised. While FEPs are perfectly benign, they may recur if incompletely excised.

249. JUVENILE HEMANGIOMAS

Hemangiomas are a common, benign vascular lesion of infants. They must be differentiated from vascular malformations (10). The majority are focal and involve areas of embryonal fusion, more commonly on head and neck than vulva. Occasionally, they are segmental, diffuse and may ulcerate and bleed with infection. Recently, two antigens (Glut 1 and Lewis Y) have been shown to be diagnostic of these lesions. Glut 1 is a placental antigen raising the possibility of a disorder of angiogenetic factors or that these hemangiomas represent placental emboli.

Clinical Features

These lesions, also known as strawberry or cavernous hemangiomas, depending on their appearance, are seen at birth or appear in the first few weeks of life. They are red or purple, raised soft lumps, varying from a couple of millimetres across to involving most of the vulva and rarely extending into the vagina. They rarely keep growing beyond early childhood, following which, most regress. In the absence of infection or bleeding, they cause little discomfort, but serious hemorrhage from them is possible.

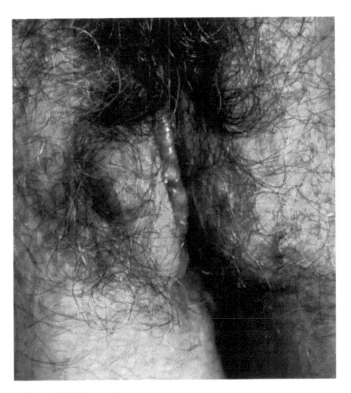

Figure 14.7. Hemangioma.

Pathology

The abnormal vessels are dermal or, dermal and subcutaneous. The lesions begin as lobulated highly cellular proliferations of plump endothelial cells with inapparent lumina. As the lesion maximizes, the vascular lumina become more obvious and the endothelial cells flatten. With regression, vessels disappear and are replaced by fibrous tissue and fat.

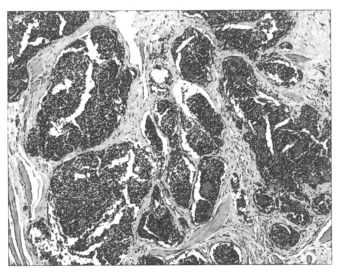

Figure 14.8. Hemangioma of vulva. composed of a circumscribed collection of large, thin-walled blood vessels in the dermis.

Treatment

Most will not require treatment due to spontaneous regression. When ulceration or functional complications occur, the following have all been used successfully: oral prednisolone (3 mg per kg), pulse dye laser, surgical excision, interferon and imiquimod.

250. ANGIOKERATOMA

Angiokeratomas are vascular lesions characterised by dilated, superficial dermal capillaries associated with epidermal hyperplasia. They are not true neoplasms but malformations or acquired telangiectases of pre-existing blood vessels. Angiokeratomas are divided into a widespread form (angiokeratoma corporis diffusum) and localised forms. The widespread form is an X linked lysosomal disorder usually occurring in males, but women who are carriers may develop the disease. Fordyce's angiokeratoma, one of the localised forms, is the type that generally occurs on the vulva (and scrotum). The pathogenesis of the Fordyce-type of angiokeratoma appears to be raised venous pressure. Part of the evidence for this assertion comes from the scrotum, where there is a strong association with surgical procedures such as inguino-crural hernioplasty, which may compromise the venous drainage.

Clinical features

Vulvar angiokeratomas are uncommon. They are usually unilateral and multiple and occur in the young as well as the older woman. They appear as red-blue, papular lesions and measure less than 1cm. In most cases, they are asymptomatic, but intermittent bleeding, pruritus, pain and occasional ulceration have been described. An analogous condition to "red scrotum" due to diffuse angiokeratomas has not, to our knowledge, been described on the vulva. Angiokeratomas tend to worsen in pregnancy.

Pathology

The epidermis shows hyperkeratosis and acanthosis and there is papillomatosis. The superficial dermis shows one of more greatly dilated capillaries lined by normal endothelial cells. The abnormal vessels may give the illusion of actually being within the epidermis.

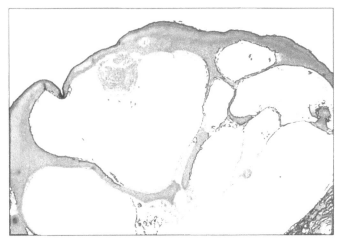

Figure 14.10. Angiokeratoma showing greatly dilated thin-walled vessels closely applied to the epidermis.

Treatment

In asymptomatic patients, management need only include reassurance and follow-up observation. Surgical excision, electrodessication, or argon laser for local removal of the lesions may be useful in symptomatic women.

251. PYOGENIC GRANULOMA

This uncommon lesion of unknown cause can occur at any age but may be associated with pregnancy. It is usually seen as a solitary, red papule, a centimetre or two in diameter, which bleeds profusely with minor trauma. It seems to be a capillary hemangioma arising from trauma. It may be confused clinically with amelanotic melanoma.

Excision needs to be adequate or recurrence may occur. Alternatively, the lesion may be curetted and the base diathermied.

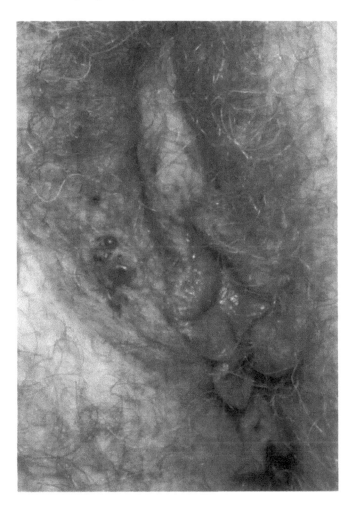

Figure 14.9. Angiokeratoma.

252. CAMPBELL DE MORGAN (CHERRY) ANGIOMA

The Campbell de Morgan spot or cherry angioma is the common red papule seen on the trunk of the older patient. Measuring 1 to 5 mm in diameter, they may extend on to the vulva. They do not require treatment.

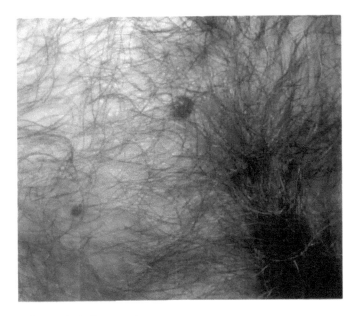

Figure 14.11. Cherry angioma.

EDEMA

The loose subcutaneous tissue of the vulva renders it prone to edema in the presence of systemic fluid retention or inflammation from infection or chemical irritation. Angioedema (usually allergic) is discussed in Chapter 10. Gross vulvar edema is most commonly seen in pregnancy, particularly when complicated by preeclampsia and in severe vulvovaginal candidiasis. Virtually any severe inflammatory disorder, trauma or disease state producing an increase in extravascular fluid volume can produce vulvar edema.

LYMPHEDEMA

Lymphedema is a variant of subcutaneous tissue swelling arising from disturbance of lymphatic outflow resulting in dilatation of lymphatics and extravasation of lymph. Filariasis (32) may be the commonest cause of vulvar lymphedema worldwide. Other causes include Milroy's disease (11) and lymphadenectomy as part of the treatment of gynecological cancer.

253. ACQUIRED LYMPHANGIOMA (LYMPHANGIOMA CIRCUMSCRIPTUM)

Lymphangioma circumscriptum is not a true tumor but a localised dilation of lymphatic channels that arises from lymphatic obstruction. It may be congenital or acquired. In a recent review, it was found that congenital vulvar lymphangioma circumscriptum has been reported in 11 patients and acquired lymphangioma 20 times. The congenital form includes patients with Milroy's disease and Turner's syndrome. The acquired type is most frequently seen after post-operative pelvic irradiation for carcinoma of the cervix but it is also seen in association with infection (filariasis, lymphangioma venereum, tuberculosis), Crohn's disease and hidradenitis suppurativa.

Clinical features

The condition is not painful but presents with a swelling of the vulva that may ooze clear fluid. The swelling is likely to be covered with vesicular lumps that may rupture easily, discharging lymph. The lesion may involve a small part of the vulva or all of it. Its appearance can be confused with herpes or condylomata.

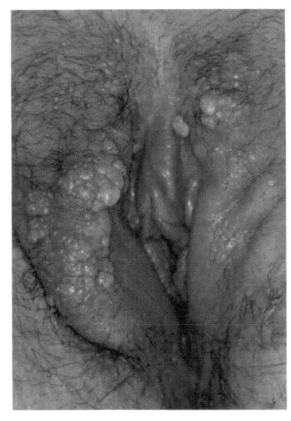

Figure 14.12. Lymphangioma circumscriptum 10 years after radical hysterectomy for carcinoma of the cervix.

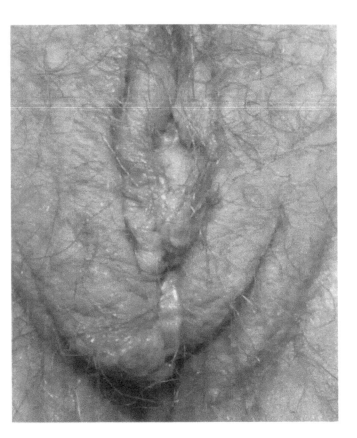

Figure 14.13. Lymphangioma circumscriptum in a patient with Turner's syndrome.

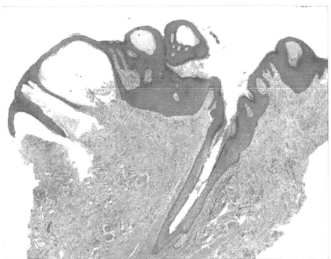

Figure 14.14. Lymphangioma circumscriptum of the vulva. Dilated vascular spaces are seen, closely associated with a hyperplastic epidermis.

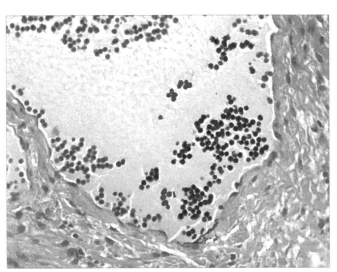

Figure 14.15. Lymphangioma circumscriptum of the vulva showing a markedly dilated capillary containing lymphocytes and lymph.

Pathology

The diagnosis is often first made histologically as the lesions may resemble condylomata due to associated hyperkeratosis and acanthosis of the dermis. The dermis shows a collection of dilated lymphatics and edema. Collections of chronic inflammatory cells may reflect previous episodes of cellulitis, but the pathologist should make a careful search for granulomas or even collections of intravascular macrophages, which suggest Crohn's disease or the Miescher-Melkerssohn- Rosenthal syndrome. The histological differential diagnosis is angiokeratoma because of traumatic translocation of red cells into lymphatics, although there is no problem clinically distinguishing angiokeratoma because of its red-blue color.

Treatment

Excision deep enough to include the deeper lymphatic channels and primary closure can be curative. However, the disease tends to recur as the underlying problem of lymphatic insufficiency usually cannot be corrected. Laser has been advocated.

254. VARICOSE VEINS

Varicose veins of the vulva resemble the common varices of the lower limb. They are of little clinical significance, however, other than in relation to pregnancy which heralds their appearance in almost all cases. The pathogenesis of vulvar varices is relatively complex compared to the leg because of the link to pregnancy and the venous drainage of the vulva (internal pudendal, obturator, superficial and deep external pudendal and round ligament veins). They generally develop independently of lower limb varices.

Clinical features

Women with vulvar varices become aware of them after the first trimester. They produce localised pruritus, pain and a sensation not unlike vaginal prolapse, relieved by recumbency.

The diagnosis is usually obvious because the outline of the grossly distended veins is visible through the skin. If the varices are present deeper in the dermis, the diagnosis may not be so obvious and such deep varices have been confused with hernia.

Rarely, vulvar varices have been complicated by thrombosis or hemorrhage in pregnancy.

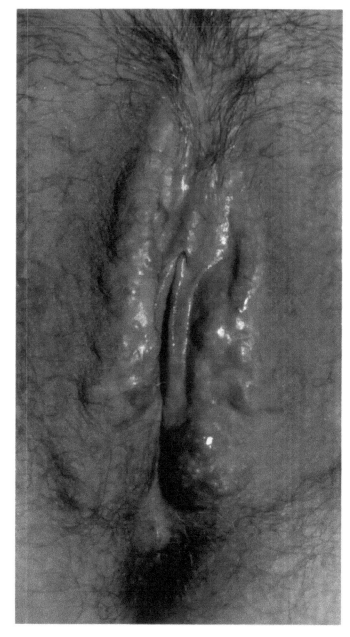

Figure 14.16. Varicose veins in pregnancy.

Treatment

There is very little that can be done for vulvar varices in pregnancy and little that needs to be done after delivery. Women often need reassurance that uncontrollable bleeding is not a significant risk. Discomfort from the varices may necessitate more time spent recumbent during the pregnancy. Ligation with or without excision of varices is rarely required in the more complicated case. Injection with 1% sodium tetradecyl sulfate with subsequent compression has been used successfully for treatment after pregnancy.

255. ANGIOLYMPHOID HYPERPLASIA WITH EOSINPHILIA

Angiolymphoid hyperplasia with eosinophilia (ALHE) is an uncommon tumor-like proliferation of blood vessels, lymphocytes and eosinophils of unknown cause. It is found more commonly on the heads of young adults but there are a handful of reports of this benign, papular disorder appearing only on the vulva.

Clinical features

Pruritus is the presenting symptom and then the lumps are found. They occur on the labia and may be single or multiple. They are reddish nodules less than 1 cm in diameter.

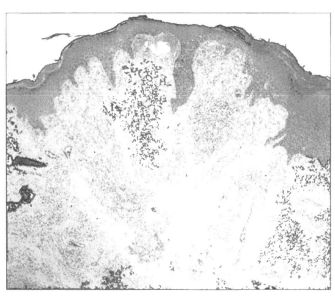

Figure 14.18. Angiolymphoid hyperplasia with eosinophilia, perineum. There are lobules of close-packed vessels and an inflammatory infiltrate in the dermis.

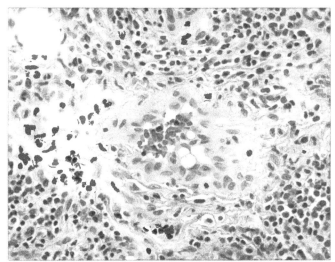

Figure 14.19. Angiolymphoid hyperplasia with eosinophilia showing a blood vessel lined by hobnail epithelioid endothelial cells, with a surrounding infiltrate of lymphocytes and eosinophils.

Treatment

Many treatments have been tried. Excision and suture may be the most successful with the lowest recurrence rate.

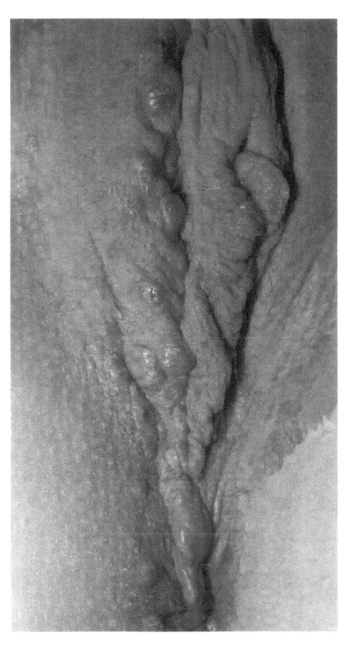

Figure 14.17. Angiolymphoid hyperplasia with eosinophilia.

256. EPIDERMOID CYST (EPIDERMAL INFUNDIBULAR CYST)

Epidermoid cysts (also known as infundibular or follicular cysts) are due to cystic dilatation of the infundibulum of a hair follicle, presumably as a result of obstruction. In the past, they were also known as "sebaceous cysts" on account of their slightly offensive, semisolid off-white contents. This material, however, is keratin, not sebaceous secretion. The offensive smell is due to bacterial overgrowth.

Clinical features

Epidermoid cysts are pain free and usually only noticed incidentally. They occur on the vulva most commonly in the labia majora, not vestibule or clitoris, because of their origin from follicles. They are usually small, 5 to 10 mm in diameter, occasionally up to 20 mm and often multiple. They are very superficial and, containing keratin, may appear slightly pale yellow. Their punctum may or may not be detectable. They rarely become infected.

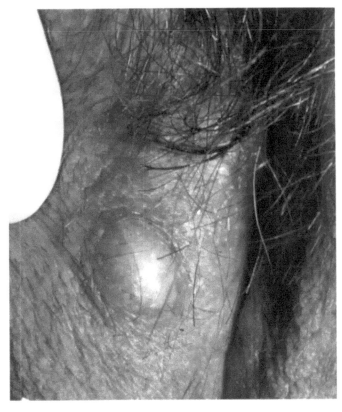

Figure 14.21. Solitary epidermal cyst.

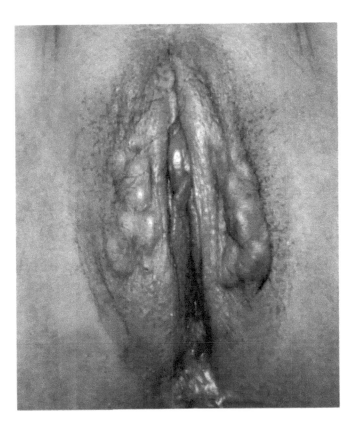

Figure 14.20. Epidermal cysts.

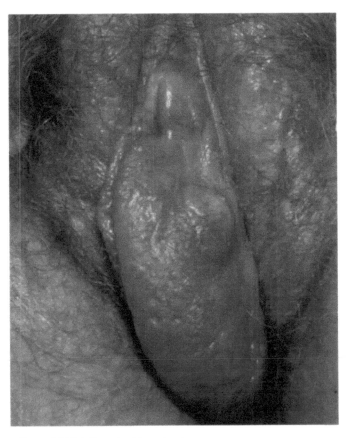

Figure 14.22. Inflamed epidermal cyst.

Pathology

The cyst may be intradermal or straddle the dermis and subcutis. The cyst is filled with laminated keratin and lined by keratinising squamous epithelium with a granular cell layer. The cyst may show evidence of rupture, where the epithelial lining is replaced by a foreign body granulomatous reaction to keratin. It may be secondarily infected and show acute or chronic inflammation. A thick cuff of fibrosis follows rupture or infection. Occasionally, multiple epidermal cysts are seen.

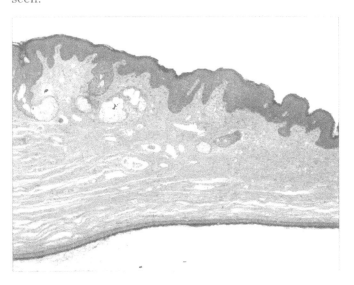

Figure 14.23. Epidermoid cyst. The dermis shows the top of a cyst lined by keratinizing squamous epithelium, which looks thinner than the epidermis.

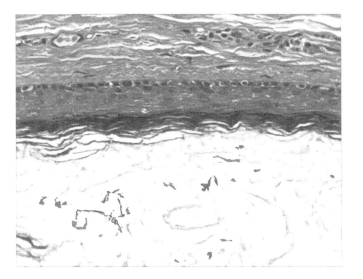

Figure 14.24. Epidermoid cyst. The cyst contains keratin and is lined by keratinizing squamous epithelium.

Treatment

It is not necessary to treat epidermal cysts and reassurance as to their harmless nature is all that is required. Women occasionally request their removal for cosmetic or other reasons, a simple procedure under local anesthesia.

257. ENDOMETRIOSIS

Ectopic endometrial glands and stroma (endometriosis) most commonly occur in the pelvis but the condition has been reported in numerous other sites including, rarely, cervix and vagina.

Vaginal endometriosis has been reported as a cause of bleeding after hysterectomy.

In these cases speculum examination reveals a red lesion of varying size, which bleeds on contact, at the vault. The condition has also been reported in episiotomy scars, presumably resulting from decidual implantation. It can cause a tender swelling in such a case. Because of the estrogen dependency of endometriosis, the patient is likely to be premenopausal or on estrogen replacement. Likewise, patients with an ovarian cycle may notice cyclical fluctuations of symptoms of the endometriotic lesion.

The main significance of superficial deposits of endometrium on the cervix is the diagnostic confusion that may occur with cervical cytology. Thus, endometriosis has been responsible for reports of glandular dysplasia, atypical glandular cells of unknown significance (AGUS), adenocarcinoma in situ or even invasive adenocarcinoma. Ectopic endometrium does occasionally become malignant.

Pathology

Endometriosis requires the identification of endometrioid glands and cellular stroma. Numerous small blood vessels, fresh hemorrhage and hemosiderin may be present. The endometriotic tissue usually appears inactive, but may be functional. Usually, the diagnosis is straightforward, but may be difficult when very small foci contain only cellular stroma or when the cellular stroma becomes fibrotic and unrecognisable as endometrioid stroma. The glands and stroma mark with estrogen and progesterone receptors and the stroma with CD10. Cutaneous deciduosis is a variant of endometriosis which normally occurs in cesarean surgical scars and presents in a subsequent pregnancy, but has also been described in the vulva.

Treatment

Symptomatic lesions visible to the naked eye are best excised for diagnostic as well as therapeutic reasons.

258. ECTOPIC BREAST

Ectopic breast and breast-like tumours are occasionally seen in the vulva. There is some dispute about the origin of vulvar breast tissue. In the time-honoured theory, vulvar breast tissue represents a failure of complete regression of the milk line. The milk line (mammary line or ridge) from which the breasts develop, is a line of vestigial breast tissue extending from the axillae, down the length of the front of the trunk, to the upper medial thigh and encroaching on the anterior vulva.

Vestigial breast tissue in the vulva is a rare cause of vulvar lump. It characteristically presents during pregnancy and enlarges during lactation. A common presentation is the "lactating adenoma" in the puerperium. This ectopic breast tissue will be situated in the labia anteriorly and can be bilateral. It is subject to the same disease processes as the normally situated breast, including fibrocystic disease, benign and malignant tumors.

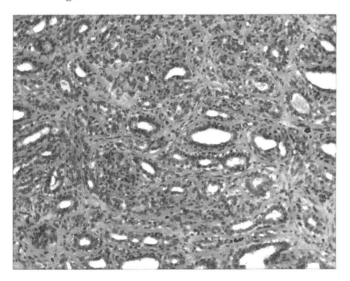

Figure 14.25 . Ectopic breast in labium majus. It is composed of a proliferation of close-packed breast lobules.

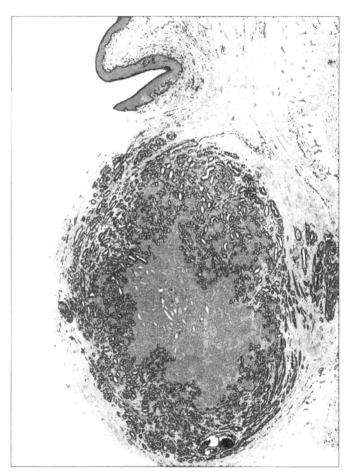

Figure 14.26. Ectopic breast in labium majus forming a nodular proliferation of glandular tissue.

259. BARTHOLIN'S DUCT CYST

The cyst arising from the duct of Bartholin's gland is the commonest large vulvar swelling and is the likely forerunner of Bartholin's abscess (**48**). It results from obstruction of the duct by infection, inspissated mucus or occasionally, surgical trauma. In most cases, however, the cause of the obstruction is unknown. The cyst usually arises from the duct of the gland and is unilocular. It may involve one or more acini and will then be found to be multilocular.

Clinical features

The patient, usually a young adult, will be aware of a lump which may enlarge with sexual arousal. In the early stages of its development it may collapse with expulsion of mucus. It is almost always unilateral. Providing the cyst is not infected, it is not particularly painful. It may be large enough to interfere with intercourse.

Examination reveals a spherical swelling beneath the posterior end of the labium minus usually 2 to 5 cm in diameter, occasionally larger. The anatomical site is an important sign - always the posterior end of the labium minus.

Pathology

Bartholin's duct cysts are lined by squamous, transitional, mucinous, ciliated, or flattened, non-specific epithelium. The presence of lobular mucinous glands next to the cyst should be sought to confirm the Bartholin's rather than vestibular gland origin of the cyst. There may be associated chronic inflammation and fibrosis.

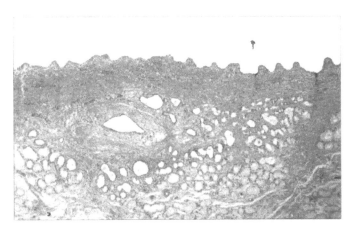

Figure 14.27. Bartholin's duct cyst. The collapsed cyst is lined by wrinkled and thinned transitional mucosa, with Bartholin's mucinous glands in the wall. There is no inflammation.

Treatment

A Bartholin's duct cyst that is not infected is relatively harmless. Surgery is advisable, however, because they frequently become infected, are unlikely to disappear spontaneously except in the short term, and are easiest to operate on at their largest.

Numerous procedures have been advocated but marsupialization (described in **48**) is permanent and should not result in any functional impairment or subsequent tenderness.

260. BARTHOLIN'S GLAND HYPERPLASIA

Swelling of Bartholin's gland for disorders other than duct obstruction and cyst formation is rare. Apart from neoplasia, such swellings do occur. Nodular hyperplasia, associated with chronic inflammation, is a cause of enlargement. It may or may not be painful. Nodular hyperplasia occurs at a mean age of 35 years (19-56) and presents as a mass, up to 4cm, in the region of Bartholin's gland. The diagnosis may become apparent when the surgeon incises the mass expecting the usual gush of mucus or mucopus and finds solid tissue. Excision of the entire gland should then be undertaken.

Pathology

Nodular hyperplasia appears as a mass of normal appearing lobular Bartholin's tissue. It lies adjacent to areas of cysts, chronic inflammation, fibrosis and atrophy, suggesting it may be a compensatory hyperplasia.

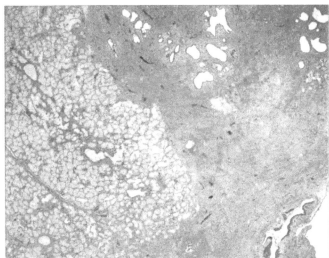

Figure 14.28. Bartholin's gland lobular hyperplasia. A post-inflammatory mass is composed of enlarged lobules of mucinous acini. These lie side by side with fibrosis, duct dilatation and complete loss of acini.

261. PERINEAL HERNIA

Rarely, as the result of a congenital or acquired defect in the pelvic diaphragm, bowel can herniate through the diaphragm producing a perineal hernia. It presents as a soft, reducible swelling of the perineum and/or a labium majus. Its treatment is likely to require an abdomino-perineal surgical approach.

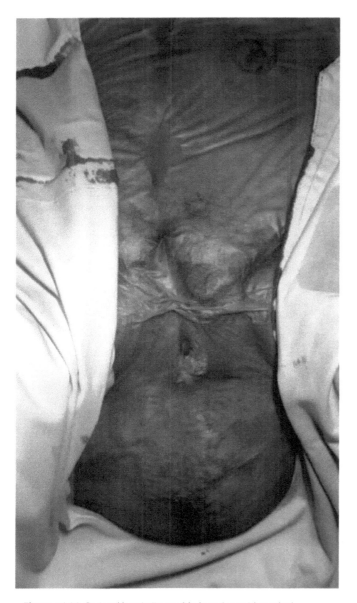

Figure 14.29. Perineal hernia (in an elderly patient with marked lichenification at the introitus).

263. NODULAR FASCIITIS

Nodular fasciitis is an unusual, reactive fibroblastic, tumor-like condition of soft tissue, whose chief importance is that it may mimic sarcoma clinically and histologically. It has a widespread occurrence in mesenchymal tissues. In the lower urogenital tract, it is seen most commonly in the bladder, where it was first described as "post-operative spindle cell nodule". It may also be rarely seen in the vulva and vagina. It may arise without antecedent trauma.

Histologically, it appears as a proliferation of plump myofibroblasts forming sweeping fascicles associated with edema, a little hemorrhage and a few lymphocytes.

It is a benign condition, curable by simple excision.

264. CYSTS OF VESTIBULAR GLANDS

The vestibule is surrounded by mucinous glands of which Bartholin's stand apart as the largest and most developed. The rest are tiny and are named "vestibular glands" or "minor vestibular glands". An autopsy study found 1 to more than 100 glands in 9 of 19 vulvas. It is uncommon for vestibular glands to give rise to clinical disorders. Nevertheless, they can become obstructed and form cysts and rarely, may be the seat of neoplasms.

Clinical features

Vestibular cysts are occasionally found in adolescents or women in the reproductive years who may be nulliparous. They present as one or more, small (2 to 30 mm), lumps which may or may not be painful. They are found anywhere in the vulvar vestibule including the medial aspect of the labia minora and may pedunculate. They contain thick mucus or pus.

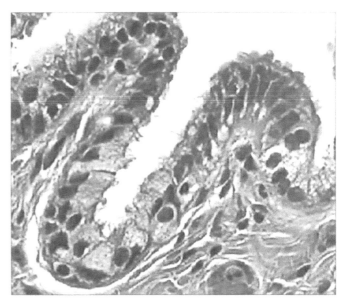

Figure 14.31. Vaginal mullerian cyst. A mixture of endocervical-like mucous cells and ciliated cells line the cyst.

Treatment
Excision is only necessary if they give rise to symptoms. There is no surgical plane of dissection around them.

265. CARUNCLE
The urethral caruncle (Latin: small piece of flesh) is a relatively common lesion of the urethral meatus usually found incidentally during a gynecological examination. Occasionally, it does give rise to symptoms necessitating treatment. It is almost always found in estrogen deficient women, suggesting shrinkage of the tissues surrounding the urethra has caused its mucosa to protrude through the meatus.

Clinical features
A minority of women with symptoms from their caruncle will complain of urethral pain, dysuria, dyspareunia and/or bleeding.

The caruncle appears as a red, fleshy lump, usually less than 1 cm in diameter and found on the posterior margin of the urethral meatus. They may pedunculate, rendering them more subject to trauma.

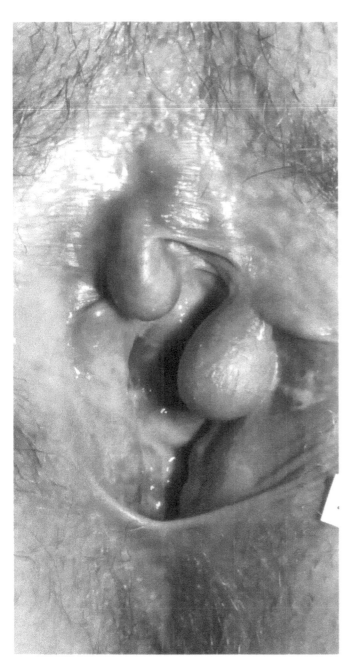

Figure 14.30. Vestibular cysts that have become pedunculated to a varying degree.

Pathology
The cysts are lined by benign mucinous, ciliated or mixed mucinous and ciliated epithelium.

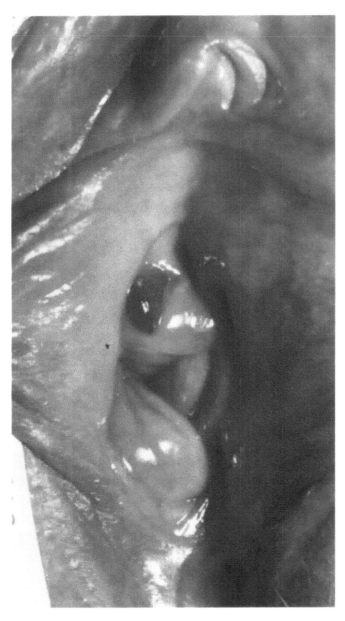

Figure 14.32. Urethral caruncle.

266. URETHRAL PROLAPSE

Urethral prolapse (which may be a pronounced form of the above mentioned caruncle) is associated with estrogen deficiency. It is most commonly found in children and postmenopausal women. The clinician unfamiliar with urethral prolapse is likely to find the condition's appearance alarming.

Clinical features

The patient will present with a lump, surprisingly not particularly tender, bleeding and/or difficulty voiding.

At the urethral meatus will be found a red, doughnut shaped lump of alarming size. It may be partially necrotic friable, bleed on contact and resemble a malignancy. Gentle probing, if in doubt, will demonstrate the urethral meatus at or near its centre.

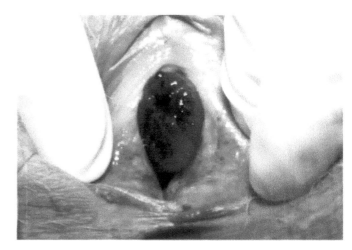

Figure 14.33. Urethral prolapse.

Pathology

The difference between a caruncle and urethral prolapse is that the caruncle also shows glandular structures or islands of epithelium

Treatment

Estrogen replacement, topical or systemic, may relieve the woman's awareness of the caruncle. Failing that, simple excision with a couple of 4/0 absorbable sutures for hemostasis should be curative. Diathermy of the caruncle has also been recommended.

Pathology

The diagnosis is clinical and the pathology is non-specific, with features of congestion, edema, hemorrhage and non-specific inflammation.

Treatment

Excision is relatively simple. Gentle traction is exerted on the prolapse and an absorbable suture is inserted from side to side traversing the urethral lump where it emerges from the urethra. The prolapsed tissue is then excised where the urethra meets the vestibule. The suture in the urethral lumen is then located, pulled out, cut and tied each side as the first of the sutures necessary to unite urethral mucosa to vestibular skin. Postoperative urinary retention may occur.

267. PARAURETHRAL CYSTS
After 6 weeks, the female embryo's urogenital sinus demonstrates numerous outgrowths representing the homologue of the prostate. The two largest, which are found adjacent to the urethral meatus, are called Skene's glands. Several others remain next to the urethra in a more or less vestigial form. These paraurethral glands are subject to infection, particularly with the gonococcus, obstruction and cyst formation. Rarely, they may be the seat of benign and malignant neoplasms.

Clinical features
There are two types of paraurethral cyst: congenital and acquired. The congenital type has a reported incidence of 1 in 2000 to 1 in 7000 live female births. These are usually diagnosed in the newborn. As they generally resolve spontaneously, a conservative approach is recommended, especially in paraurethral cysts of newborn without complications and symptoms. Needle aspiration and marsupialization are also effective. The least aggressive therapy is recommended. Surgery has been performed in cases that fail to resolve spontaneously after a 6 month observation period.

The acquired type of paraurethral cyst is very common. It may present as a lump but they are usually asymptomatic. It has an incidence of 1-6% in published post mortem data and surgical series. A prospective ultrasound study in a large cohort of asymptomatic women identified paraurethral cysts in 2.9% of 140 subjects. In this study, ultrasound allowed rapid definition of the site, size and vascularity of the lesion.

Pathology
Paraurethral cysts are lined by mucinous epithelium.

Treatment
Excision is the treatment of choice in the symptomatic woman. The urethra should be demarcated with a catheter and carefully avoided. Excision should not be attempted in the presence of acute inflammation which may require incision and drainage, culture and appropriate antibiotics.

268. SUBURETHRAL DIVERTICULA
Suburethral diverticula may be congenital, when muscle is found in their wall, or acquired. The latter have no wall muscle and probably arise from rupture of an inflamed paraurethral cyst into the urethral lumen. Diverticula have a demonstrable communication with the urethra, whereas paraurethral cysts (see above) do not.

Clinical features
Diverticula are prone to inflammation and may produce pain on intercourse or with voiding. Other symptoms include postmicturition dribbling, urethral discharge, recurrent cystitis and awareness of a lump.

Most diverticula are situated next to the lower two thirds of the urethra but may occasionally be situated beneath the trigone. They may be up to 8 cm. in diameter and thus seen on parting the labia but are usually smaller. Pressure on the diverticulum can bring about emptying into the urethra of contents, varying from clear urine to thick pus.

There is an association between urethral diverticulum and the rare urethral malignant tumor, clear cell carcinoma, with 2/3 of such carcinomas arising within a diverticulum in the largest series.

Diagnosis
The urethral opening of a diverticulum should be demonstrable by urethroscopy, micturating cystourethrography or urethrography, preferably with a double balloon catheter.

Inflammation and fibrosis may obscure the underlying histology. The diverticula are lined by transitional or squamous epithelium. A stain that distinguishes fibrous tissue from smooth muscle, such as the Masson Trichrome, may help separating congenital from acquired diverticula but frequently there is so much post-inflammatory change, such a distinction is difficult.

Treatment

Excision of these diverticula has the potential to be complicated by fistula formation, stress incontinence, urethral stricture, recurrence and persistence of symptoms.

The principles of treatment are to free the sac by dissection and remove it where it empties into the urethra. The urethral defect must be closed with 3/0 absorbable sutures with another layer of sutures plicating the urethral fascia over the closure. Redundant vaginal skin is excised prior to closure of the vagina. An indwelling urethral catheter or suprapubic catheter will be required for 4 to 6 days.

269. NEPHROGENIC ADENOMA

Nephrogenic adenomas are small, benign, pink, exophytic growths of glandular epithelium seen throughout the urinary tract, including the urethra, but most commonly in the trigone of the bladder. They occur over a wide age range. Previous renal tract surgery is a predisposing factor. Elegant recent studies in patients who have had a renal transplant from a person or cadaver of the opposite sex have shown that nephrogenic adenomas are formed by implants of tubular cells shed from the kidney.

Pathology

Nephrogenic adenoma is a benign glandular proliferation. Less than 10% of cases contain clear cells. It is distinguished from clear cell carcinoma by no more than mild atypia, none or rare mitoses, the absence of necrosis, absence of p53 staining and a low Ki-67 index.

REFERENCES

Agarwal-Antal N, Zimmermann J, Scholtz T, Noyes RD, Leachman SA. A giant verruciform xanthoma J Cutan pathol 2002; 29: 119-24

Argenta PA. Bell K. Reynolds C. Weinstein R. Bartholin's gland hyperplasia in a postmenopausal woman. [Review] [8 refs] Obstetrics & Gynecology. 90(4 Pt 2):695-7, 1997 Oct.

Azzena A, Ferrara A, Castellan L, Quintieri F, Salmaso R. Vaginal endometriosis. Two case reports and review of the literature on rare urogenital sites. Clin. Exp. Obst. Gyn. 1996; 23(2): 94-98.

Bruckner A, Frieden I. Hemangiomas of infancy. J Am Acad Dermatol 2003; 48:477-493.

Ceylan H, Ozokatan BH, Karakok M, Buyukbese S Paraurethral cyst: is conservative management always appropriate. Eur J Pediatr Surg 2002; 12: 212-4

Cohen PR, Young AW Jr, Tovell HM Angiokeratoma of the vulva: diagnosis and review of the literature. Obstet Gynecol Survey 1989; 44: 339-46

Connolly SB, Lewis EJ, Lindholm JS, Zelickson BD, Zachary CB, Tope WD Management of verruciform xanthoma. J Am Acad Dermatol 2000; 42: 343-7

Da Rosa G, Barra E, Gentile R, Boscaino A, Di Prisco B, Ayala F. Verruciform xanthoma of the vulva: case report. Genitourin Med 1989; 65: 252-4

Ekberg O. Nordblom I. Fork FT. Gullmo A. Herniography of femoral, obturator and perineal hernias. Fortschritte auf dem Gebiete der Rontgenstrahlen und der Nuklearmedizin. 143(2):193-9, 1985 Aug.

Fair KP, Patterson JW, Murphy RJ, Rudd RJ Cutaneous deciduosis J Am Acad Dermatol 2000; 43: 102-7

Foushee JH. Reeves WJ. McCool JA. Benign masses of Bartholin's gland. Solid adenomas, adenomas with cyst, and Bartholin's gland with varices and thrombosis or cavernous hemangioma. Obstetrics & Gynecology. 31(5):695-701, 1968 May.

Jappe U, Zimmermann T, Kahle B, Petzoldt D Lymphangioma circumscriptum of the vulva following surgical and radiological therapy of cervical cancer. Sex Transm Dis 2002; 29: 533-5

Jensern LM, Aabech J, Lundvall F, Iversen HG Female urethral diverticulum. Clinical aspects and a presentation of 15 cases. Acta Obstet Gynecol Scan 1996; 75: 748-52

Koenig C, Tavassoli FA Nodular hyperplasia, adenoma and adenomyoma of Bartholin's gland Int J Gynecol Pathol 1998; 17: 289-94

Linck D. Hayes MF. Clitoral cyst as a cause of ambiguous genitalia. Obstetrics & Gynecology. 99(5 Pt 2):963-6, 2002 May.

Markham S, Carpenter SE, Rock JA. Extrapelvic endometriosis. Obstet Gynecol Clin N Am 1989; 16:193-219.

Metry DW, Herbert AA. Benign cutaneous vascular tumors of infancy. When to worry. What to do. Arch Dermatol 2000; !36:905-14.

Mohta A. Bhargava SK. Congenital perineal hernia: report of a case. Surgery Today. 34(7):630-1, 2004.

Mohsin SK, Lee MW, Amin MB, Stoler MH, Eyzaguirre E, Ma CK, Zarbo RJ Cutaneous verruciform xanthoma: a report of five cases investigating the etiology and nature of xanthomatous cells. Am J Surg Pathol 1998; 22: 479-87

Mu XC, Tran TA, Dupree M, Carlson JA Acquired lymphangioma of the vulva mimicking genital warts. A case report and review of the literature. J Cutan Pathol 1999; 26: 150-4

Ninia JG, Goldberg TL. Treatment of vulvar varicosities by injection-compression sclerotherapy and a pelvic supporter. Obstet Gynecol 1996; 87:786-8.

North PE et al. Glut 1 - a newly discovered immunohistochemical marker for juvenile haemangiomas. Human Pathology 2000; 31:11-22.

Pradhan S, Tobron H Vaginal cysts: a clinicopathological study of 41 cases. Int J Gynecol Pathol 1986; 5: 35-46

Pfeifer JD, Barr RJ, Wick MR Ectopic breast tissue and breast-like sweat gland metaplasias: an overlapping spectrum of lesions J Cutan Pathol 1999; 26: 190-6

Poon FW. Lauder JC. Comment. Finlay IG.Perineal herniation. [see comment] Clin Radiol. 1993 Oct;48(4):290; PMID: 8243014 Clinical Radiology. 47(1):49-51, 1993 Jan.

Requena L, Sangueza OP Cutaneous vascular anomalies. Part I Hamartomas, malformations, and dilatation of pre-existing vessels J Am Acad Dermatol 1997; 37: 523-49

Sah SP, Yadav R, Rani S Lymphangioma circumscriptum of the vulva mimicking genital wart: a case report and review of the literature. J Obstet Gynecol Res 2001; 27: 293-6

Schwartz RA. Tarlow MM. Lambert WC. Keratoacanthoma-like squamous cell carcinoma within the fibroepithelial polyp. Dermatologic Surgery. 30(2 Pt 2):349-50, 2004 Feb.

Sinha A, Warwick AP. Vaginal vault endometriosis de novo, associated with hormone replacement therapy. Journal of Obstetrics and Gynecology 2004; 24(2): 190-2.

Schiller PI, Itin PH Angiokeratomas: an update. Dermatology 1996; 193: 275-82

Van der Putte Sc, van Gorp LH Cysts of mammary-like glands in the vulva. Int J Gynecol Pathol 1995; 14: 184-8

Vang R, Connelly JH, Hammill HA, Shannon RL Vulvar hypertrophy with lymphedema: a mimicker of aggressive angiomyxoma Arch Pathol Lab Med 2000; 124: 1697-9

Vlastos AT, Malpica A, Follen M. Lymphangioma circumscriptum of the vulva: a review of the literature. Obstet Gynecol 2003; 101: 946-54.

Chapter 15

9. FUNCTIONAL DISORDERS

A. Disorders of Sensation

270. DYSESTHESIA (VULVODYNIA)

Female genital dysesthesia (FGD) refers to unpleasant genital sensation, usually described as burning, pain, rawness or stinging, in the absence of clinical signs and with negative laboratory investigations. The term vulvodynia (derived from vulvo-, vulva -odynia, pain) has become fashionable but is confusing because it is often used in relation to painful vulvovaginal disease such as inflammatory disorders or sexual dysfunction. FGD is specific and is the preferable term. Related terms are hyperesthesia, meaning an unpleasant, heightened awareness of sensation and allodynia where there is an inappropriate perception of a stimulus, for example, light touch felt as pain.

Dysesthetic or focal pain syndromes occur elsewhere in the body but predominate in the head and neck and urogenital regions. This has given rise to terms such as glossodynia, carotidynia, orchidynia, prostatodynia, coccygodynia and proctodynia. In most of these disorders, the cause of the pain is conjectural. The totally subjective nature of the disorder renders scientific investigation particularly difficult to perform.

At its 2003 congress in Brazil, the International Society for the Study of Vulvovaginal Disease subdivided dysesthesia, which they referred to as vulvodynia, as shown in Table 1. The usefulness of such a subdivision remains to be demonstrated.

Table 1

Vulvodynia (ISSVD 2003)
1. Generalised
   - i. Provoked
   - ii. Unprovoked
2. Localised
   - a. Vestibulodynia
       - i. Provoked
       - ii. Unprovoked
   - b. Clitorodynia
       - i. Provoked
       - ii. Unprovoked

The question inevitably arises with a patient diagnosed with FGD as to whether or not the complaint is psychosomatic in origin. In most cases, the likely origin of the disorder will be multifactorial, usually some physical and/or psychological trauma in the past occurring in a psychologically vulnerable individual.

It is essential to diagnose FGD correctly or the patient may be worsened by inappropriate treatments, especially surgery.

Clinical features

The presenting symptom of FGD is discomfort of sufficient severity to constitute a major issue in the patient's life. The discomfort is most commonly described as a burning sensation. Other descriptions include simply pain, stinging or sensations of rawness or dryness. The sensation can be felt all around the vulva or within the vagina. Pruritus is not a feature of FGD and there is no desire to scratch or rub. Localisation tends to be imprecise. It commonly interferes with sitting so that secondary back complaints can result from sitting awkwardly.

Detailed history taking is essential and commonly will relate the onset of the complaint to some traumatic event. This event will be sexual abuse in only a minority of cases. Primary sexual dysfunction is a common initiating cause as is a prolonged episode of an inflammatory disorder such as recurrent candidiasis, in remission when the patient is seen. A past history of vulvar surgery, especially with laser and diathermy, vaginal repair and surgery to adjacent areas, such as inguinal herniorrhaphy may be obtained. Perhaps surprisingly, obstetric trauma alone does not seem to initiate FGD. Particularly in the older woman, there may be no apparent initiating event.

These patients are either not sexually active when seen or usually avoid sex because of the pain.

By definition, clinical examination reveals no abnormality. It is often informative to give the patient a swab stick and ask her to indicate the site of maximal discomfort. She is unlikely to be able to do so with precision or consistency.

Clinical depression will be present in many of these women and needs to be addressed.

Diagnosis
FGD is largely a clinical diagnosis but some investigations are necessary to exclude an organic cause for, or contributing factor to, the pain. A vaginal swab and possibly biopsy might be necessary.

Formal psychological assessment and/or a detailed sexual history will need to be considered.

Treatment
No topical application is of any benefit to FGD. A total lack of response to topical corticosteroids is almost a feature of the disorder. The patient needs to be specifically warned to avoid topical applications and physical treatments, such as ice packs, which only have the potential to produce an inflammatory response and exacerbate the pain.

Patients with FGD tend to be demanding on the clinician's time and patience. Skilful communication is essential in their management. Generally, they can be reassured that, with time, provided that there is no recurrence of the initiating trauma, the pain will gradually resolve. Resolution is not in a linear manner but with exacerbations of diminishing frequency and severity and she needs to be warned about this.

Drugs which have been found useful in the treatment of FGD include amitriptyline and gabapentin. The former

is the time honored treatment but the dosage may need to be increased to levels which produce side effects (drowsiness, dry mouth). Acupuncture has also been used for FGD with some success.

Other measures that will be necessary for the management of the more difficult case include psychotherapy, sexual counseling, hospital admission (for closer observation and ease of drug management) and regional nerve blockade.

271. PUDENDAL NEURALGIA
The pudendal nerve arises from the second, third and fourth sacral nerves. It passes behind the sacrospinous ligament just medial to the ischial spine where it is best localised and most accessible to injection. It then enters the pudendal canal on the medial side of the pudendal artery on the lateral wall of the ischiorectal fossa. Finally it branches to supply the clitoris, labia, perineum and anus. Pain arising in this distribution is called pudendal neuralgia. Its cause may be diabetic neuropathy, post-herpetic, post-surgical or compression by neoplasm. Most commonly, however, the pain arises for no known reason.

Clinical features
Pudendal neuralgia occurs in adult or elderly women. The pain tends to be gradual in onset and chronic. It may be unilateral or bilateral. Unlike the woman with genital dysesthesia, the patient with pudendal neuralgia can usually localise her pain to part or all of the area supplied by this nerve.

Unless she does have one of the causes listed above, examination findings will be negative. Depression is commonly found in these women.

Diagnosis
The diagnosis is usually made clinically. If there is doubt, injection of 5-10 ml. of 1% lignocaine around the nerve just medial to the ischial spine (usually palpable vaginally) should provide instant relief.

Electrophysiological testing has been used measuring the distal latency time of the nerve with a

St Mark's Hospital electrode. Electromyography of the anal sphincter has also been used to investigate these patients.

Treatment

Drug treatment as for dysesthesia is worth trying firstly. If unsuccessful, pudendal nerve blockade with long-acting agents such as bupivacaine with adrenaline, with or without a corticosteroid, is successful in many cases but might need to be repeated. Phenol may be used but is probably best done under CT guidance because of the added risks when it is used.

Limited success has been achieved with surgical decompression and transposition of the nerve through a gluteal approach.

272. SOMATOFORM DISORDER

Somatization is the tendency to experience, conceptualize and communicate mental states and distress as physical symptoms or altered bodily function and is a very common reason for seeking medical attention. The term somatoform disorder is used by the American Psychiatric Association in its Diagnostic and Statistical Manual of Mental Disorders (DSM-IV) to encompass various types and grades of somatization. These include somatization disorder, where there are several listed symptoms, pain disorder which may overlap with dysesthesia (270), hypochondriasis and body dysmorphic disorder. In all cases the symptoms are not intentionally produced or feigned and appropriate clinical and laboratory investigation will not provide an explanation for the symptoms.

The vulva and vagina are commonly targeted by the somatizer. Thus, an appreciation of this group of mental disorders is essential to assist in the woman's recovery and prevent unnecessary and inappropriate investigation and treatment. To complicate the issue, it must not be forgotten that somatization may coexist with or overlie organic disease. Furthermore, some of these patients will have other psychiatric disorders including anxiety disorder, affective disorder, personality disorder and psychosis.

Clinical features

All clinicians will have seen the less severe forms of somatization occurring, usually sporadically at times of stress, from childhood to old age. For example, the woman who feels guilty about a sexual relationship may perceive an alteration in the odor and/or volume of her vaginal secretions. In its more severe form, somatization disorder presents in the middle decades in women who are often well educated and have a history of unhappy personal and marital relationships. They will have a long history of numerous symptoms in the genital region including discharge, soreness and pain, bad odor, dysuria and concerns about appearance of the area. Sexual dysfunction or complete avoidance of sex is virtually universal.

The patient will often present the symptom in a bizarre manner such as providing carefully wrapped specimens of matter allegedly found in her underwear. One patient of this author even brought her own microscope with her to demonstrate such a specimen. They will also have several diagnoses of their own, now expanded by the internet. These include Candida sensitivity, multiple allergies, non-albicans yeast infections especially with *C. glabrata* and various other infections.

Often, one or more of the extragenital 'fashionable' diseases, including chronic fatigue syndrome, irritable bowel syndrome, fibromyalgia, vitamin or mineral deficiency, severe premenstrual syndrome or temporomandibular joint syndrome, is present. In all cases their symptoms will have become a primary focus in their lives often to the degree of rendering them unemployed and care dependant. They will have seen numerous doctors and/or alternative care practitioners, many of whom will have unintentionally or otherwise colluded with them and performed multiple investigations and treatments, often including, regrettably, surgery. Many become litigious and some resort to hazardous self-treatment. One patient of this author (and several of his colleagues) had attempted her own vulvectomy by ligating portions of her labia minora with a needle and thread.

Clinical examination findings will be negative or reveal relatively minor conditions, such as low grade prolapse or estrogen deficiency, incapable of producing symptoms of the type and severity of which the patient complains.

Likewise, investigations, especially microbiology and ultrasound, will be negative or have findings which do not properly explain the symptoms. The commonest of these misleading investigation reports include non-albicans yeasts and bacteria not pathogenic in this setting, such as Streptococci, Staphylococci and coliforms.

The diagnosis of a somatoform disorder is made on the history.

Treatment

It is important to remember that these patients suffer from various forms of anxiety and are emotionally fragile. Often anger is apparent but this may mask severe insecurity. The patient must not be belittled or dismissed.

The common, minor degrees of somatoform disorder will respond to correct diagnosis, explanation, reassurance and, ideally, linking the onset of the complaint to some particular stress.

The severer forms of somatoform disorder are likely to be beyond the skill of the average gynecologist, dermatologist or general practitioner. Unfortunately, these patients are likely to deny any psychological basis to their diagnosis making appropriate referral to a psychiatrist or psychologist difficult or impossible. They are notorious for asking themselves "What if the doctor is wrong?" Nevertheless, doctors working in this area must learn to make the diagnosis of somatoform disorder, avoid spurious diagnoses and *refrain from treating what the patient does not have*. One doctor should integrate the management of these difficult cases and all involved must avoid entering debate with the patient as to whether the condition is organic or functional.

B. Sexual disorders

Sexual dysfunction is highly relevant in the management of vulvovaginal disease for three reasons: Firstly, sexual dysfunction itself may present as an apparently organic genital disorder, most commonly with the complaint of dyspareunia. Secondly, every woman with an uncomfortable vulvar disorder will develop sexual dysfunction if the disorder lasts long enough. Finally, secondary sexual dysfunction can impair the recovery or exacerbate an organic genital disorder. The latter is a likely mechanism in the majority of cases of so-called 'vestibulitis syndrome' (see Modes of Presentation).

Sexual dysfunction is classified according to the phase (or phases) of the sexual cycle which has become disordered and, importantly in the context of genital complaints, whether the disorder is lifelong (primary) or acquired (secondary). The sexual cycle, comprehensively described by Masters and Johnson (and later by Kaplan) in the 1960's, consists of a phase of desire progressing to arousal then orgasm and satisfaction. Disturbances of arousal and pelvic floor muscle activity during sex are the aspects of greatest importance in the context of this manual.

20% to 50% of women are said to have disturbance of one or more phases of sexual response but a sexual disorder only needs to be considered present if the woman is unable to participate in a sexual relationship *as she would wish*. Women frequently complain to the gynecologist about perceived deficiency in sexual function, most commonly lack of desire for sexual intercourse. In many of these cases, their perceived inadequacy is based on the apparent needs of their partners or the usually inappropriate depiction of female sexuality by the media. This gives rise to unreal expectations.

An adequate sexual history is a prerequisite for the management of the patients. If the clinician is comfortable asking the questions and an adequate explanation for their need is given, the patient is unlikely to mind answering them. Often, the detailed sexual history is best left until after the examination which may indicate the need for such a history. The commonest sex related questions used by this author are: "Have you used artificial lubricants with intercourse?", "Are you still able to enjoy sex?", "Are you able to achieve a climax with intercourse?", "Are you able to achieve a climax with masturbation?", "Have you ever experienced a sexual climax?" and "Have you had any bad sexual experiences?"

273. AROUSAL DISORDER

Sexual arousal in the female produces changes in the vagina and vulva necessary in most women for penetration to be comfortable and pleasurable. The most important of these are natural lubrication arising mainly from filtered capillary fluid transuding between the intercellular spaces of the vaginal epithelium, clitoral erection and swelling of the labia minora, relaxation of the muscles of the pelvic floor and increase in vaginal volume. It is generally a much slower process in the female than the equivalent arousal and erection in the male. Furthermore, it is a mechanism that is much more easily switched off in the female than in the male. Arousal disorder is said to occur when this process fails to take place when the woman wishes or expects it to, with consequent physical or emotional distress.

Clinical features

Arousal disorder presents to the gynecologist as both cause and a result of genital discomfort. Dyspareunia is the commonest complaint. The discomfort is felt at the introitus when penetration is attempted, that is, superficial dyspareunia. It is usually associated with friction from the lack of lubrication. Less commonly (more likely in the parous woman), deep dyspareunia from lack of vaginal expansion is of greater concern.

Examination findings are usually negative. Occasionally, small lacerations may be seen, usually in the sulci medial and lateral to the labia minora and/or the fourchette. Repeated attempts at penetration in the absence of arousal will often produce chronic introital erythema.

Diagnosis

The diagnosis is made on the sexual history which needs to be appropriate to the particular presentation.

Special investigations have been devised but, in practice, are probably only applicable in a research setting. These include vaginal photoplethysmography, measures of clitoral and labial temperature and oxygenation, vaginal and clitoral Doppler and blood flow measures and vaginometry.

Treatment

Any organic cause of genital discomfort, such as infection or dermatosis, must be sought and treated before any improvement in sexual function can be expected. If the woman has had such a cause which has been long-standing, it can be useful to warn her that sexual function is likely to be the last facet of her recovery.

When sexual dysfunction is the primary diagnosis, its treatment should be in most cases, but not all, within the abilities of the average women's health practitioner. Linking the complaint to causes such as domestic or work stress can be beneficial as can be the management of depression when it is present. Couple counseling is the ideal management, with the emphasis on non-penetrative sexual pleasuring.

It is inadvisable to recommend artificial lubricants for these patients for two reasons: Firstly, water based gels are especially capable of producing or exacerbating contact dermatitis because of the preservatives they contain. Secondly, with appropriate counseling and modification of sexual behavior, natural lubrication should be possible and the woman should be advised to avoid penetration until this is achieved. Strategies likely to be helpful in this regard are couple counseling, encouraging the patient to communicate her sexual needs to her partner and to consider the inclusion of mutual masturbation and oral sex in the couple's sexual routine.

274. VAGINISMUS

Vaginismus refers to the involuntary spasm of the muscles surrounding the vaginal introitus occurring during attempts at sexual penetration or attempting insertion of objects such as tampons or specula, resulting in personal distress. Vaginismus can be primary (as in non-consummation of marriage) or secondary (frequently seen with chronic or recurrent vaginal infections).

Clinical features

Dyspareunia is by far the commonest symptom of vaginismus. Non-consummation and/or primary infertility are other presentations. It is rare for pregnancy to occur without penetration. The term for this rare situation is fecundatio ab extra.

The patient with primary vaginismus is unlikely to have successfully used tampons. Untreated, as with most sexual disorders, the condition will self-perpetuate because repeated attempts at penetration in the presence of the levator ani contraction is associated with increasing pain. As levator tone increases in this condition, the pain usually experienced with penetration may become chronic.

An attempt to ascertain the cause of the vaginismus should be made by sensitively, asking about any past experiences that might have been responsible. These include childhood abuse or unwanted sexual contact. However, many women with vaginismus will have no such history or evidence of any psychological problem.

Gynecological examination may be difficult or impossible because of the levator spasm. Unfortunately, a painful gynecological examination is one of the recognized causes of vaginismus.

In severe cases, an attempt at examination will produce more than levator spasm. The patient may bring her legs together and lift her buttocks off the couch rendering any further attempt impossible. Women who demonstrate vaginismus in the sexual situation do not always demonstrate the muscle spasm in the clinical situation and vice versa.

Nevertheless, some form of examination is essential, if not at the first consultation then at a subsequent one, in case there is a contributing organic cause. The examination must never be forced upon the patient. It should at least be possible to obtain a swab from the vagina, looking for inflammatory activity.

If a speculum cannot be inserted, the examiner should attempt to gently insert one finger, when the contracted ridge of levator will be felt just within the introitus posteriorly. Pressure on this ridge just above the fourchette will reproduce the pain that the patient experiences during attempts at sex. Fissuring of the fourchette in these cases is common because the fourchette is a site of trauma with attempts at entry against the contracted levator.

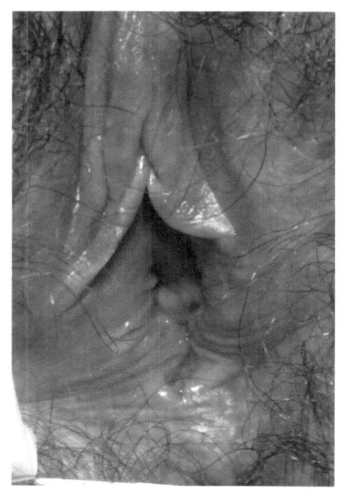

Figure 15.1. Fourchette fissure in a patient with vaginismus.

Diagnosis

The diagnosis of vaginismus is largely made on clinical grounds. This should be straightforward with primary vaginismus. It may be difficult with secondary vaginismus when the cause might be infection or an epithelial disorder. Appropriate microbiology, cytology of vaginal contents looking for an erosive disorder and/or biopsy may be necessary.

Treatment

Any underlying cause of vaginismus must be sought and treated. Any significant psychopathology must be appropriately managed as must any inflammatory disorder.

Where vaginismus is the primary diagnosis, self exploration is the modern method of management. The patient is given a lesson on the anatomy of the levator ani and then taught to insert her own fingers into the vagina, perhaps while showering, and practice squeezing and relaxing on her fingers to increase her conscious control over the muscle. This has the added benefit to her of restoring her confidence and dispelling the impression many of these women have that their vagina is abnormally narrow ("pencil vagina").

Only when she can comfortably insert two (preferably three) fingers should she attempt penile penetration. This should only be attempted in a high state of arousal or after having been brought to orgasm by masturbation and assuming a position on top of her partner so that she has full control over rate and depth of penetration. To quote this manual's psychologist: "There is no gain with pain!"

Electromyographic biofeedback has been successfully used in the management of vaginismus. There are no controlled trials to indicate that it has any advantage over the self-exploration technique described above. Graduated rubber or glass dilators have been used in the past but lack the educational advantage of the patient using her own fingers.

There is no place today for surgery for vaginismus. The Fenton procedure, where a longitudinal incision through the perineal body is sutured transversely to enlarge the introitus, was performed extensively in the past. It is bad treatment because it was strictly symptomatic, added surgical to emotional trauma and frequently failed. When it did permit penetration, sexual dysfunction almost always persisted.

Another advocated treatment we advise against is the use of topical anesthetic. This treatment is counterproductive and not relevant to female sexuality. The vulva is a sexual organ and its function as such is reliant on the sense of touch. Unlike male sexuality, which usually focuses on penetration as the end goal, female sexuality focuses on external sensations for arousal and resolution. Therefore, although an anesthetic cream may prevent pain, it also prevents any sense of pleasure. If penetration is at all painful for the woman, she should be advised not to attempt it but to focus upon other sources of sexual pleasure.

275. ORGASMIC DISORDER

Orgasmic disorder is defined as "...the persistent or recurrent delay in, or absence of, orgasm following a normal sexual excitement phase" (DSM IV), which causes the woman distress. However, orgasm itself is largely the result of a subjective sense of heightened arousal and requires sexual stimulation appropriate to the individual woman's preference. Therefore, in many instances where a woman complains of, or is diagnosed as having this 'disorder', she may not have had appropriate stimulation for her needs.

Women with this complaint alone are seen rarely compared with those with arousal disorder as defined above. Orgasmic disorder does not have the tendency to present as a suspected vulvovaginal disorder and the complaint usually emerges in discussion about other aspects of genital function.

REFERENCES

Baram DA. Sexuality, Sexual Dysfunction, and Sexual Assault. Chap. 11 in Novak's Gynecology. 13th ed., editor Berek JS. International. Lippincot Williams & Wilkins, 2002

Basson R et al. Report of the International Consensus Development Conference on Female Sexual Dysfunction: Definitions and Classifications. J Urol 2000; 163(3):888-99.

Graziottin A, Castoldi E, Montorsi F, Salonia A, Maga T. Vulvodynia: The Challenge of "Unexplained" Genital Pain. Journal of Sex and Marital Therapy 2001; 27:503-512.

Marin MG, King R, Dennerstein G, Sfameni S. Adverse behavioral and sexual factors in chronic vulvar disease. Am J Obstet Gynecol 2000; 183:34-38.

Marin MG, King R, Dennerstein G, Sfameni S. Dyspareunia and Vulvar disease. JReprod Med 1998:43L 952-958

Singh BS. Managing Somatoform Disorders. Medical Journal of Australia 1998; 168:572-7.

Slowinski J. Multimodal Sex Therapy for the Treatment of Vulvodynia: A Clinician's View. Journal of Sex and Marital Therapy 2001; 27:607-613.

Stewart DE. The Changing Face of Somatization. Psychosomatics 1990; 31(2)153-8.

Wesselmann U, Reich SG. The Dynias. Seminars in Neurology 1996; 16(1):63-74.

Index

1

19- s-igm fta abs, 133

5

5-fluorouracil, 210

A

abscess, 125
acantholysis, 23, 138, 174, 175, 179, 180
acanthosis nigricans, 197
accidental trauma, 208
aciclovir, 139
acne inversa, 188
acquired immunodeficiency syndrome, 144
acquired lymphangioma, 268
acrochordon, 264
acrodermatitis, 196
acrodermatitis enteropathica, 197
actinomyces israelii, 128
actinomycosis, 128
acute vulvar ulcer, 53
addison's disease, 195, 201
adenocarcinoma, 251
adenocarcinoma in situ (cervix-like), 251
adenocarcinoma of the female urethra, 256
adenoid cystic carcinoma, 235, 262
adenosquamous carcinoma, 251
adhesion molecules, 22, 174, 176, 179, 180
adrenal insufficiency, 195
aggressive angiomyxoma, 240, 253
agonadia, 105
AIDS, 110, 117, 143, 144, 145, 146, 147, 242, 253
allergens relevant to vulva, 184
allergic contact dermatitis, 149

allopurinol, 178
amebiasis, 25, 116
ameboma, 116
amphotericin b, 117
ampicillin, 128, 134
amyloidosis, 198
anaerobes, 75
androgen receptors, 73
angioedema, 184, 268
angiokeratoma, 98, 266
angiolymphoid hyperplasia with eosinphilia, 271
angiomyofibroblastoma, 240, 252
angiosarcoma, 242, 253
angry patient, 42
ano-genital granulomatosis (vulvitis granulmatosa), 181
anticandidal drugs, 122
anticonvulsants, 178
antihistamines, 185
antimalarial therapy, 173
antimony, 117
aphthous ulceration, 186
apoptotic keratinocytes, 168, 169
arousal disorder, 287
asthma, 15, 151
asymptomatic, 79
atopic dermatitis, 151
atrophic vaginitis, 14, 15, 16, 93, 94, 95, 168, 171
atrophy, 18, 24, 25, 93
atypical leiomyoma, 243
atypical melanocytic nevus of genital tract, 237
autoantibodies, 161, 171, 174
azathioprine, 179, 188
azithromycin, 131

B

bacitracin, 127
bacterial vaginosis, 134
Bacteroides species, 75, 134
Bartholin's gland, 63, 70, 127
Bartholinitis, 127, 133
Bartholin's duct cyst, 274
Bartholin's gland carcinoma, 234

Bartholin's gland hyperplasia, 275
basal cell carcinoma, 228
basal layers, 65, 69, 73, 217, 218, 220
basaloid papilloma, 215
basement membrane zone (bmz), 23
BCC, 228
B-cell lymphoma, 247
Behcet's disease, 25
Behcet's syndrome, 188
benign familial chronic pemphigus, 180
benign mixed tumor, 234, 251
bexarotene, 248
Bifidobacterium, 129
bilharziasis, 113
biopsy, 13, 16, 23, 30, 48, 49, 50, 69, 92, 113, 116, 120, 129, 139, 141, 152, 155, 160, 161, 163, 164, 174, 176, 181, 184, 185, 196, 200, 201, 208, 219, 221, 224, 228, 236, 247, 249, 250, 284, 289
Birbeck granules, 72
blastoconidia, 117, 122
bleeding, 79
blistering disorders, 174, 176, 180
blisters, 23, 24, 25, 50, 79, 118, 137, 139, 149, 174, 175, 176, 177
boil, 125
bowenoid papulosis, 201, 216
Bowen's disease, 216
brachytherapy, 250
breast-like carcinoma, 231, 234
breast-like tumors, 231
breslow system, 238
bronze diabetes, 201
bubo, 130, 134
bulbospongiosus, 63, 64
bullous erythema multiforme, 178
bullous pemphigoid, 175
burning, 79
burning vulva syndrome, 14

C

C. guilliermondii, 122
C. krusei, 122
C. parapsilosis, 122
calcinosis, 199
Calymmatobacterium
    granulomatis, 130, 131
Campbell de Morgan spot, 268
candida, 18, 19, 26, 75, 117, 120,
    122, 123, 146, 149, 156, 157,
    195, 285
Candida albicans, 18, 19, 26, 75,
    122, 156, 157, 195
Candida albicans vulvovaginitis,
    117
Candida glabrata, 18, 122
candidiasis, 14, 15, 16, 24, 25, 95,
    117, 118, 120, 121, 124, 141,
    144, 145, 149, 150, 153, 155,
    180, 195, 268, 283
capillaritis, 54
carbuncle, 125
carcinoma in situ, 216, 249, 256
carcinosarcoma, 252
Carney's complex, 235
Carney's syndrome, 239
caruncle, 277
ccr5, 144
ceftriaxone, 130
cellular angiofibroma, 239
cellulitis, 125
cephalosporins, 128, 130
cercaria, 113
cervical ectropion, 15
cervical mucus, 18, 75
cervicitis, 133
cestodes, 114
chancre, 25, 130, 132, 133
chancroid, 25, 130, 134
cherry angioma, 268
chicken pox, 139
Chlamydia trachomatis, 128, 134,
    146, 160
Chlamydia trachomatis
    oculogenital infection, 133
chloramphenicol, 134

chondroid syringoma, 234
chromogranin, 73, 229, 252
Chung's levels, 238
cicatricial pemphigoid, 176
circinate vulvitis, 160
cisplatin, 229
Civatte bodies, 168
CK20, 73
Clark's levels, 238
Clark's nevus, 237
classification, 55
clear cell carcinoma, 102, 234, 235,
    251, 256, 279, 280
clindamycin vaginal cream, 136,
    171
clinicopathological diagnosis, 53
clitoral amputation, 211
clitoral cysts, 211
clitoris, 30, 31, 59, 60, 61, 62, 63,
    64, 65, 67, 70, 94, 97, 103,
    104, 105, 134, 150, 154, 157,
    190, 195, 205, 210, 211, 272,
    284
clitorodynia, 283
clotrimazole, 121, 125, 129
clue cell, 19, 135
cmv, 139, 146
CO2 laser, 30, 180, 219, 249, 258
coeliac disease, 179
coliforms, 75, 95, 125, 286
collagen xvii, 175, 176
colposcope, 17, 67
colposcopy, 30, 219, 221, 249
communication, 53
complex aphthosis, 26, 186, 188,
    191
condylomata acuminata, 92, 140,
    203, 227, 258, 260, 264
congenital adrenal hyperplasia,
    104, 105, 195
congenital lymphedema (Milroy's
    disease), 98
contact dermatitis, 149
contact urticaria, 184
coproporphyrin, 129
corpora cavernosa, 63, 70

Corynebacteria, 75, 129
Corynebacterium diphtheriae, 129
Corynebacterium minutissimum,
    129
crabs, 109
Crohn's disease, 25, 55, 182
crust, 23, 52, 116, 152, 209
cutaneous T-cell lymphoma, 24,
    247
cyclosporin, 170, 186, 188
cyst of the canal of Nuck
    (hydrocele of the vulva), 97
cystosarcoma phyllodes, 231
cysts of vestibular glands, 276
cytokines, 72, 151, 157, 182, 197
cytology, 17, 29, 49, 94, 115, 161,
    168, 171, 219, 249, 273, 289
cytomegalovirus, 139

D

damaging self care, 36
damaging sexual behavior, 37
danazol, 196
dapsone, 179, 188
Darier's disease, 25, 55, 179
deep compartment, 63
deep external pudendal arteries,
    64
delayed hypersensitivity reaction,
    149
denileukin diftitox, 248
depot medroxyprogesterone
    acetate, 15, 121, 136
dermatitis, 15, 23, 24, 25, 26, 34,
    36, 37, 51, 52, 53, 56, 93, 94,
    95, 113, 117, 119, 122, 143,
    149, 150, 151, 152, 153, 155,
    156, 157, 160, 177, 179, 180,
    191, 192, 196, 197, 208, 287
dermatitis artefacta, 208
dermatitis enteropathica (de), 197
dermatitis herpetiformis, 179
dermatofibrosarcoma
    protruberans, 241
dermatophyte, 26, 123
dermis, 22

dermoid cyst, 97
DES, 102, 251
desmoglein 3, 174
desmosomes, 22, 152
desquamative inflammatory vaginitis, 54, 170
DFSP, 241
dhobie itch, 123
diabetes mellitus, 117
diaper dermatitis, 149, 151
diathermy, 30, 93, 142, 188, 210, 215, 249, 283
diazoxide, 196
didelphic uterus, 100
diethylcarbamazine, 114
diethylstilbestrol, 102
differentiated VIN, 219
diffuse large cell B cell lymphoma, 255
dimorphic yeast, 117
diphtheria, 129
diphtheria antitoxin, 130
diplococci, 128
diptheria, 25
discharge, 15, 79, 170
discomfort, 14, 16, 34, 44, 48, 79, 98, 125, 137, 140, 149, 156, 166, 171, 196, 211, 266, 283, 284, 287
Donovan bodies, 131
Donovania granulomatis, 130
donovanosis, 25, 130, 131
double vagina, 101
double vulva, 97
doxycycline, 134
ducts, 59, 60, 62, 63, 64, 76, 97, 100, 102, 188
DVIN, 219, 220, 221, 222, 227
dysesthesia, 283
dysgerminoma, 105
dyspareunia, 45, 79, 118, 127, 161, 287, 288
dysplastic naevus syndrome, 236
dystrophy, 54, 160, 197, 216
dysuria, 79

E

E coli, 131
EVB, 140
ecchymoses, 23, 161, 162, 163
echinococcosis, 114
Echinococcus granulosus, 114
Echinococcus multilocularis, 114
ecology, 75
econazole, 121
ectopic breast, 274
ectopic ureter, 103
eczema, 25, 120, 149, 151
edema, 268
EIA, 144
ejaculate, 75, 76
elephantiasis, 113
ELISA, 113, 114, 116
EMPD, 231, 232
endogenous dermatitis, 149
endometrial stromal sarcoma, 255
endometrioid carcinoma, 234, 251
endometrioid stromal sarcoma, 234
endometriosis, 234, 273
Entamoeba histolytica, 116
enterobiasis, 112
Enterobius vermicularis, 112, 145
Enterococcus, 75
enzyme linked immunoabsorbent assay, 113
epidermal inclusion cyst, 263
epidermal infundibular cyst, 272
epidermis, 22
epidermoid, 272
epidermoid cyst, 272
epidermolysis bullosa, 180
Epidermophyton floccosum, 123
epispadias, 103
epithelial desquamation, 75
epithelioid sarcoma, 246
Epstein Barr virus, 140
erosion, 15, 19, 20, 25, 49, 79, 161, 165, 166, 167, 170, 176, 212, 213

erosions, 23, 24, 25, 56, 114, 150, 160, 170, 173, 174, 176, 177, 178, 180
erosive/ulcerative rashes, 49
erysipelas, 125
erythema, 16, 23, 24, 25, 26, 118, 122, 125, 126, 137, 149, 150, 151, 160, 175, 182, 184, 196, 197, 203, 246, 287
erythema multiforme, 178
erythemato-squamous (red and scaly) lesions, 24
erythrasma, 24, 129
erythromycin, 127, 129, 130, 134
erythroplasia of Queyrat, 216
esthiomene, 134
estradiol, 95, 171, 195
estriol pessaries, 95
estrogen deficiency, 93, 195
estrogen excess - iatrogenic, 195
estrogen receptors, 73
exogenous, 149
external genitalia development, 60
extracellular matrix protein 1, 161, 192
extramammary Paget's disease, 231

F

factitial dermatitis, 208
famciclovir, 139
female circumcision and related procedures, 210
fibroadenoma, 231
fibrocystic disease, 231
fibroepithelial polyp, 264
fibrolipoma, 244
FIGO staging, 224
filariasis, 113
fissuring, 15, 79, 118, 150, 154, 157, 161
fistula, 104
fluconazole, 122
fluke, 113
follicle stimulating hormone, 195

folliculitis, 125
Fordyce spots, 91
foreign body, 184, 212
foreign body granuloma, 184
fossa navicularis, 62
fourchette, 15, 62, 65, 67, 134, 161, 205, 207, 224, 287, 288
Fox-Fordyce disease, 188
frenulum of the clitoris, 62, 65, 67
FSH, 95, 195
furuncle, 125

G

Gardnerella vaginalis, 19, 75, 134
Gartner's duct cyst, 102
genital herpes, 136, 139
genital hygiene, 44
genital melanocytic macule, 252
genital melanotic macules, 235
genital tract development, 59
genital tubercle, 59, 60
giant cell scc, 221
giant condyloma, 142, 258
giant condyloma of Buschke-Loewenstein, 142, 227
Giemsa, 17, 116, 130, 131, 138
glucagonoma, 25, 196, 203
glucagonoma syndrome, 196
Glut 1, 266, 281
glycogen, 73, 75
gonadal agenesis, 105
gonadal development, 59
gonadal dysgenesis, 104, 105
gonadoblastoma, 105
gonadotrophin, 195
gonorrhea, 128
Gorlin's syndrome, 228
graft versus host disease, 160, 173
Graham's adhesive tape test, 112
granular cell tumor, 244, 255
granuloma, 130, 133, 146, 181, 183, 246
granuloma inguinale, 130
granuloma venereum, 130
granulomas, 181, 183

granulomatous diseases, 181
granulomatous vulvitis, 55, 181, 192
griseofulvin, 124
group b streptococci, 75
Grover's disease, 179
gumma, 132
guttate morphea, 160
guttate scleroderma, 160

H

HAART, 145
Haemophilus ducreyi, 130
Hailey and Hailey disease, 25, 179, 180
Hand-Schuller-Christian syndrome, 246
Hansemann cells, 131
Hart's line, 62, 73
hay fever, 15, 151
hearing impaired patient, 42
hemagglutination assay, 133
hematometra, 99
hemochromatosis, 201
Henoch-Schonlein purpura, 185
hereditary hemorrhagic telangiectasia, 98
hermaphroditism, 105
herpes gestationis, 177
Herpes hominis 8 virus, 242
herpes simplex, 25, 136, 138, 139, 144, 178
herpes simplex virus, 136
herpes zoster, 25, 139
herpesvirus infection, 136
hibernoma, 244
hidradenitis suppurativa, 188
hidradenoma papilliferum, 230
highly active antiretroviral therapy(haart), 145
histology of the vulva, 65
HIV, 116, 133, 138, 140, 144, 145, 146, 157, 169, 186, 192, 199, 201
HIV western blot, 144
hives, 184

HLA DR, 72
homosexual patient, 42
hormone receptors, 72, 73
hormone replacement therapy, 16, 121, 195
HPV, 69, 102, 140, 141, 142, 144, 180, 215, 216, 219, 220, 221, 227, 234, 235, 249, 250, 256
HSV, 136, 139
human herpesvirus, 139
human immunodeficiency virus, 144
human immunodeficiency virus disease, 136
human itch mite, 110
human leukocyte antigen, 72
hydatid disease, 114
hymen, 62
hypermelanosis, 201
hyper-pigmentation, 201
hypertrophic lp, 169
hypomelanosis, 199
hypo-pigmentation, 24, 199
hypospadias, 103

I

ichthyosis, 23
IgA nephritis, 185
IgE, 151
IgG fluorescent treponemal antibody absorption test, 133
IgG FTA Abs, 133
imidazole, 121, 122, 151
imidazoles, 122, 123, 124, 149
imiquimod, 142, 145, 210, 233, 258, 266
immunobullous diseases, 174, 175, 179
immunochromographic strip testing, 116
immunofluorescence, 50, 138, 160, 175, 176, 177, 185
immunoglobulin, 179, 198
immunosuppressives, 152, 186
imperforate anus, 104

imperforate hymen, 99
impetigo, 25, 125
implantation dermoid, 263
incidental finding, 79
including beta blockers, 157
infantile eczema, 151
infibulation, 210, 211
inflammatory bowel disease, 182, 185
inguinal groin, 65
inguino-femoral lymphadenectomy, 224, 239, 250
instructions for self care, 44
internal pudendal artery, 64
interpreter, 41, 42
intersex, 104, 105
intertrigo, 156
intraepithelial neoplasia of urethra, 256
invasive carcinoma arising from intraepithelial Paget's disease, 233
ipsilateral inguino-femoral lymphadenectomy, 224
irradiation, 210
ischiocavernosus, 63, 64
ischiocavernosus muscles, 63, 64
isosexual precocity, 195
itch, 15, 24, 26, 34, 38, 110, 112, 123, 140, 149, 153, 155, 156, 161, 192
itch-scratch cycle, 26, 38, 153, 156
itraconazole, 122, 124
ivermectin, 112

J

juvenile hemangiomas, 266

K

kala azar, 116
Kaposi's sarcoma, 32, 144, 242, 253
keratin barrier, 23
keratinising, 221, 222
keratinising scc, 221

keratinocytes, 22
keratoacanthoma, 228
keratosis follicularis, 179
ketoconazole, 117, 122, 125
Klebsiella granulomatis, 130
Klinefelter's syndrome, 105
Kobner phenomenon, 210
KOH, 124, 125
kraurosis vulvae, 160

L

labia majora, 61
labia minora, 62
labial adhesions, 92, 94
labial adhesions in infancy, 92
lactating adenoma, 231, 274
Lactobacillus spp, 75
Langerhan's cell histiocytosis, 25, 246
Langerhans' cells, 22, 67, 72
Langhans' giant cells, 132
large labia minora, 91
laryngeal papillomatosis, 140
laser, 16, 30, 93, 98, 140, 142, 165, 188, 199, 210, 213, 219, 266, 267, 283
laser surgery, 165
latex agglutination, 116
LCR, 128, 133
leiomyoma, 242, 253, 256
leiomyosarcoma, 31, 242, 243, 253, 258, 261
Lleishmania, 116
lentigo, 236
Letterer-Siwe syndrome, 246
leucocytoclastic vasculitis, 185
leukoplakia, 153, 160
Lewis, 191, 266, 280
Lewis Y, 266
LGV, 134
LGV complement fixation, 134
lichen aureus, 54
lichen planus, 19, 24, 25, 49, 52, 53, 54, 94, 160, 161, 164, 167, 168, 169, 170, 171, 172, 173, 174, 199, 210, 218

lichen sclerosus, 22, 23, 24, 26, 52, 53, 54, 56, 160, 162, 163, 164, 191, 192, 196, 198, 199, 209, 216, 219, 221, 222, 227, 243
lichen sclerosus et atrophicus, 160, 164
lichen simplex chronicus, 153
lichenification, 24, 109, 150, 151, 159, 163, 168, 276
lichenoid dermatitis, 160
ligand chain reaction, 128
limitations of pathological diagnosis, 51
linear IgA bullous dermatosis (LABD), 177
lipoma, 244
liposarcoma, 245
Lipschutz ulcer, 53, 186
lithium, 157
longitudinal septum, 100
lump, 79
lupus erythematosus, 25, 173
lymph nodes, 65, 72, 129, 131, 181, 221, 224, 226, 228, 246, 247, 260
lymphangioma circumscriptum, 268
lymphatic drainage, 64
lymphedema, 98, 268
lymphogranuloma, 25, 113, 133, 134
lymphogranuloma inguinale, 134
lymphogranuloma venereum, 25, 134
lymphoma, 247, 257

M

macules, 79, 201
maculopapular rashes, 49
malakoplakia, 131
Malassezia furfur, 124, 157
malformations, 97, 104
malignant granular cell tumor, 244

malignant melanoma, 238, 252, 256
malignant tumors of urethra, 256
Malt, 72, 76
maturation index, 75
Mayer-Rokitansky-Kuster-Hauser syndrome, 101
mebendazole, 113
melanocytes, 22, 67, 72, 200, 201, 215, 236, 237, 238, 239, 252, 256
melanocytic nevus, 236, 237
melanoma in situ, 238, 252
melanosis, 235
Melkersson-Rosenthal syndrome, 55
menopausal woman, 42
menstrual flow, 75, 99, 211
Merkel cell tumor, 228
Merkel cells, 66, 72, 76, 229, 260
mesonephric duct, 59
mesonephros, 60
metastatic and direct spread to the urethra, 257
metrifonate, 113
metronidazole, 114, 115, 116, 136
miconazole, 121, 129
microfilariae, 114
Mierscher-Melkersson-Rosenthal syndrome, 181
minocycline, 134, 201
minoxidil, 196
mobiluncus species, 75, 134
modes of presentation, 79
mole, 236
molluscum contagiosum, 143
mononucleosis, 140
mons pubis, 61
mucinous adenocarcinoma, 235
mucinous carcinoma, 251
mucous glands, 70
mucous membrane pemphigoid, 176
mucous membrane pemphigoid(cicatricial pemphigoid, 176

mucous patches, 132
mullerian adenosarcoma, 255
mullerian duct, 59, 100
mullerian papilloma, 251
mupirocin, 127
Mycobacterium tuberculosis, 131
mycophenolate mofitil, 179
mycoplasmas, 75
mycosis fungoides, 247, 259
myeloproliferative disease, 185
myofibroblastic cells, 68, 69, 73

N

nappy rash, 149
necrolytic migratory erythema, 196
necrotising fasciitis, 126
Neisseria gonorrhoeae, 128
neomycin, 127, 149, 157
nephrogenic adenoma, 280
nerve supply, 65
neurofibroma, 243, 255
neurofibrosarcoma, 244
nevus flammeus, 98
niridazole, 113
nitrogen mustard, 248
nits, 109, 110, 125
NME, 196, 197
nodular fasciitis, 276
non-albicans yeast infection, 122
non-Hodgkin's lymphoma, 255
nucleic acid test, 141
nystatin, 121, 157

O

oblique septa result, 100
obstetric trauma, 205
odor, 15, 79
office pathology, 17
orgasmic disorder, 289
Osler's disease, 98
other immunobullous diseases, 179
ovarian dysgenesis, 105
oxamniquinine, 113
oxyuriasis, 112

P

P. humanus humanus capitus, 109
Paget's cells, 232
Paget's disease, 31, 50, 73, 216, 231, 232, 233, 234, 257, 258, 259, 261
pain, 15, 16, 17, 25, 35, 37, 44, 54, 79, 94, 99, 125, 128, 130, 137, 139, 140, 149, 183, 207, 208, 210, 211, 220, 256, 267, 270, 272, 277, 279, 283, 284, 285, 288, 289
papillary squamotransitional cell carcinoma, 250
papular acantholytic genitocrural acantholysis, 179
papular acantholytic genitocrural dermatosis, 55
papular urticaria, 184
papules, 26, 79, 130, 140, 160, 166, 177, 179, 181, 184, 188, 229, 236, 243
parabasal cells, 18, 75
paramesonephric duct, 59
paraneoplastic pemphigus, 175
parasitophobia, 110
paraurethral cysts, 279
pathologist's report, 50
pautrier microabscess, 248
PCR, 114, 115, 116, 128, 130, 131, 133, 134, 138, 139, 140, 141
pediatric, 79, 106, 107, 213, 214, 260
pediculocides, 110
Pediculosis pubis, 109
Pediculus humanus capitus, 109
pemphigus and variants, 174
pemphigus foliaceus, 175
pemphigus vegetans, 175
pemphigus vulgaris, 174, 175, 191
penicillin, 127, 128, 129, 130, 133, 184, 185
pentamidine isethionate, 117
pentavalent antimonial drugs, 117
peptostreptococci, 134
perineal body, 64

perineal hernia, 276
perineal membrane, 63, 64
perineum, 63
peri-orificial dermatitis, 26
permethrin, 110, 112
phenolphthalein, 174
phenytoin, 196
phimosis of the clitoral hood, 161
physiological discharge, 93
piedra, 125
pigmented purpuric dermatosis, 54
pilonidal sinus complex, 190
pimicrolimus, 152, 170, 201
pinworm, 112
piperazine, 113
pityriasis versicolor, 124
Pityrosporum, 157
plaques, 23, 24, 116, 131, 173, 174,
    175, 177, 181, 184, 215, 247
plasma cell vulvitis of Zoon, 171
plasmacytoma, 257
pleomorphic adenoma, 229, 234,
    251
pneumatocyst, 97
podophyllin, 142, 210
podophyllotoxin, 142
poikiloderma, 210
polyarthritis, 185
polycystic ovarian syndrome, 196
polymerase chain reaction, 51, 131,
    132, 133, 140
polymorphous eruption of
    pregnancy, 177
posterior root ganglia, 139
post-operative spindle cell nodule,
    276
potent antiseptic, 127
povidone iodine, 127, 144
praziquantel, 113
precocious puberty, 195
premalignant Paget's disease, 231
prevention of sexual problems, 44
prickle cell, 65, 67, 141, 152, 209,
    237, 252
primarily extragenital, 79
primary irritant dermatitis, 149

primitive cloaca, 59
processus vaginalis peritonei, 97
progesterone receptors, 73, 274
Propionibacterium, 128
prostatic carcinoma, 256
prostatic type adenocarcinomas,
    256
prostatic type and clear cell
    carcinoma, 235
protease inhibitors, 145
pruritic urticarial papules and
    plaques of pregnancy, 177
pruritus, 14, 18, 24, 38, 52, 79,
    109, 110, 112, 118, 122, 125,
    149, 151, 155, 157, 184, 188,
    195, 209, 216, 220, 229, 238,
    267, 270, 271, 283
pseudohyphae, 117, 118, 120, 121
psoriasiform dermatitis, 153
psoriasiform diaper rash, 157
psoriasis, 15, 24, 26, 51, 52, 120,
    121, 124, 144, 149, 152, 153,
    156, 157, 159, 160, 191, 192,
    200, 209
Pthirus pubis, 109, 110
pubic lice, 109
pudendal neuralgia, 284
PUPPP, 177
purpura, 23, 24, 185, 246
pyoderma gangrenosum, 185
pyogenic granuloma, 267
pyogenic vulvar infections, 125
pyrantel, 113
pyrvinium, 113

R

radical vulvectomy, 224
radioallergosorbent test, 184
radiotherapy, 29, 31, 210, 213, 225,
    226, 242, 245, 248, 250, 251,
    252, 255
rapid plasma reagin, 133
RAST, 184
recurrent scc of the vulva, 226
regional enteritis, 182
Reiter's syndrome, 160

religious order, 42
retained tampon, 212
rete ridges, 52, 53, 65, 67, 68, 74,
    153, 155, 159
retinitis, 140
retroviral agents, 145
retrovirus, 144
rhabdoid tumor, 245
rhabdomyoma, 253
rhabdomyosarcoma, 243, 254, 257
rifampicin, 117, 132, 134
ringworm, 123
RPR, 133

S

S. intercalatum, 113
S. japonicum, 113
S. mekongi, 113
S.haematobium, 113
SALT, 72, 76
sandfly, 116
sarcoidosis, 181
sarcoma botryoides, 243
Sarcoptes scabiei, 110, 111
scabies, 110
SCC, 219, 220, 221, 222, 223, 224,
    226, 227, 228, 233, 235, 249,
    250, 251
Schistosoma mansoni, 113
schistosomiasis, 113
schwannoma, 244, 255
sclerosis, 23
seatworm infection, 112
sebaceous carcinoma, 234
sebaceous glands, 65, 67, 91, 234
seborrheic, 54, 141, 142, 157, 197,
    215, 257, 264
seborrheic dermatitis, 157
seborrheic keratosis, 215
secondary tumors of the vagina,
    256
self-induced trauma, 208
senile wart, 215
sentinel lymph node biopsy, 224
sentinel nodes, 65, 225
sexual disorders, 286

sexual trauma, 207
Sezary cells, 247
Sezary syndrome, 247
shingles, 139
Skene's glands, 64
skin appendages, 30, 63, 65, 66, 231
skin tag, 264
small cell carcinoma, 235, 252
smooth muscle tumor of intermediate differentiation - vulva, 243
smooth muscle tumor, intermediate differentiation - vagina, 253
sodium fusidate, 127
soft chancre, 130
somatoform disorder, 285
spectinomycin, 128
spider angiomas, 98
spindle cell lipoma, 240, 244, 261
spindle cell scc, 221
spirochete, 132
splitting, 15, 79
spongiotic dermatitis, 149, 152
squamous cell carcinoma, 220, 250
squamous cell hyperplasia, 54
squamous dysplasia, 216, 249
SRY gene, 59, 105
Staphylococcus, 25, 75, 125, 126, 156
Staphylococcus aureus, 75, 125, 126, 156
Staphylococcus epidermidis, 75
Staphylococcus pyogenes, 125
steroid therapy, 165, 170
Stevens-Johnson syndrome, 178
stinging, 14, 24, 79, 283
stool microscopy, 112
stratum corneum, 22, 23, 24, 50, 65, 67, 110, 117, 120, 121, 124, 129, 175, 209
strawberry cervix, 114
streptococcal infection, 125, 127, 185
Streptococci, 95, 125, 286

Streptococcus pyogenes, 125
Streptococcus viridans, 75
suburethral diverticula, 279
sucking louse, 109
sulphur granules, 129
superficial angiomyxoma, 239
superficial cells, 18, 75
superficial compartment, 63
surface scale, 23
synaptophysin, 229, 252
synovial sarcoma, 245
synpatophysin, 73
syphilis, 25, 130, 132, 133, 134, 136, 144, 146, 147, 186
syringoma, 229

T

T cell lymphoma, 247, 255
T helper cells, 151
T. mentagrophytes, 123
tacrolimus, 152, 170, 201
tapeworms, 114
T-cell lymphoma, 247
telangiectasia, 24, 25, 98, 161, 210
terbinafine, 124
testicular dysgenesis, 105
testicular regression syndrome, 105
testosterone ointment, 196
tetracycline, 26, 128, 134
tetracyclines, 179, 189
TH1 cytokines, 157
threadworm, 112
tinea, 24, 123, 124
tinea cruris, 123
tinea incognito, 24, 123
tinea versicolor, 124
tinidazole, 115
Toker cells, 72, 73, 76, 260
topical testosterone, 165
torulopsis glabrata, 122
toxic epidermal necrolysis, 178
toxic shock syndrome, 126
TPHA, 133
transitional cell carcinoma, 235
transverse vaginal septa, 100

Treponema pallidum, 132, 133
Treponema pallidum hemagglutination assay, 133
tretinoin cream, 188
triamcinolone, 26, 157, 170, 173
trichloracetic, 142, 210
trichloracetic acid, 142, 210
trichofolliculoma, 234
trichomonads, 18, 19, 114, 115
Trichomonas, 114, 115
trichomoniasis, 114
trichomycosis, 129
Trichophyton rubrum, 123
Trichosporon beigelli, 125
tropical bubo, 134
tuberculosis, 131
Turner's syndrome, 105, 106, 268, 269
Tzanck test, 138

U

ulceration, 79, 113
ulcerative colitis, 182
ulcers, 16, 23, 25, 26, 49, 53, 116, 130, 131, 132, 134, 137, 145, 174, 182, 183, 185, 186, 187, 188, 192, 208, 228
ulcus vulvae acutum, 186
ureaplasmas, 75
urethra, 63, 74, 256
urethral meatus, 62
urethral plate, 59
urethral prolapse, 278
urinary tract development, 60
urogenital sinus, 59, 60, 99, 100, 101, 105, 279
urosacral septum, 59
urticaria, 23, 112, 184, 185, 191
urticarial vasculitis, 184
usually immuno-fluorescence, 174
UV therapy, 248

V

vaginal agenesis, 101
vaginal atresia, 101
vaginal hypoplasia, 101

vaginal intraepithelial neoplasia, 249

vaginal plate, 60, 99, 101

vaginal septa, 100

vaginal transudate, 75, 76

vaginectomy, 249, 250

vaginismus, 288

VAIN, 30, 54, 140, 216, 249, 250, 251, 256

valaciclovir, 139

varicella, 136, 139

varicella zoster virus, 136, 139

varicose veins, 270

vascular malformations, 98

vasculopathic disorders, 184

vasoactive intestinal peptide VIP, 73

VDRL, 133

venereal disease research laboratory, 133

venereum, 25, 113, 130, 133, 146, 268

venous drainage to the vulva, 64

verruciform xanthoma, 199

verrucous carcinoma, 227, 251

vesicobullous disorders, 174

vesico-urethral canal, 60

vestibular bulbs, 63

vestibular papillomatosis, 92

vestibule, 62, 68, 69, 205

vestibulitis syndrome, 14, 16, 34, 54, 55, 76, 118, 286

vestibulodynia, 283

villous adenoma, 256

VIN, 30, 50, 52, 54, 55, 140, 144, 163, 180, 216, 217, 218, 219, 220, 221, 222, 227, 231, 234, 249, 256

VIP, 73

vitiligo, 24, 200, 203

vulvar dystrophy with atypia, 216

vulvar dysuria, 14

vulvar intraepithelial neoplasia, 30, 54, 145, 216, 259

vulvar vestibulitis syndrome, 54, 79

vulvectomy, 67, 165, 224, 246, 250, 285

vulvitis circumscripta plasmacellularis, 171

vulvodynia, 14, 24, 34, 54, 79, 283, 290

vulvovaginogingival syndrome, 166

VZV, 139

W

warty basaloid VIN, 216

warty-basaloid SCC, 221

western blot, 144

wheal, 23

white piedra, 125

white spot disease, 160

Wickham's striae, 166

wolffian duct, 59

Wood's light, 129

Wright's stain, 17

Wuchereria bancrofti, 113

Y

yeasts, 75, 117, 122, 123, 124, 155, 157, 286

yolk sac tumor, 105, 255

Z

Ziehl-Neelsen staining, 132

zinc deficiency, 197

zinc neonate, 197

zoonosis, 116

Zoon's vulvitis, 171

CLASSIFICATION OF VULVOVAGINAL DISEASE

1. NORMAL VARIATIONS

VULVA
1. Fordyce spots
2. Large labia minora
3. Vestibular papillomatosis
4. Labial adhesions in infancy
VAGINA
5. Physiological discharge
6. Estrogen deficiency - atrophy

2. DEVELOPMENTAL ABNORMALITIES

NO SEXUAL AMBIGUITY
VULVA
7. Double vulva
8. Cyst of canal of Nuck
9. Dermoid cyst
10. Vascular malformations
11. Congenital lymphedema (Milroy's disease)
VAGINA
12. Imperforate hymen
13. Vaginal septa
14. Double vagina
15. Vaginal hypoplasia
16. Vaginal atresia
17. Vaginal agenesis
18. DES associated abnormalities
19. Cyst of Gartner's duct (cyst of mesonephric duct)
VULVOVAGINAL ABNORMALITIES ASSOCIATED WITH URINARY/ INTESTINAL TRACT ABNORMALITIES
20. Ectopic ureter draining into vagina
21. Epispadias
22. Hypospadias
23. Imperforate anus with vulvar or vaginal fistula
SEXUAL AMBIGUITY
24. Turner's syndrome
25. Klinefelter's syndrome
26. True hermaphroditism
27. Gonadal agenesis

3. INFECTIONS

PARASITES
ECTOPARASITES
28. Pediculosis pubis
29. Scabies
WORMS
30. Oxyuriasis
31. Schistosomiasis
32. Filariasis
33. Hydatid disease
PROTOZOA
34. Trichomoniasis
35. Amebiasis
36. Leishmaniasis
FUNGI
CANDIDIASIS
37. Candida albicans infection
38. Non-albicans yeast infection
DERMATOPHYTES
39. Tinea cruris
40. Pityriasis versicolor
41. White piedra
BACTERIA
PYOGENIC (STAPHYLOCCUS, STREPTOCOCCUS, COLIFORMS AND MIXED)
42. Impetigo
43. Folliculitis
44. Abscess
45. Cellulitis
46. Necrotizing fasciitis
47. Toxic shock syndrome
48. Infected Bartholin's duct cyst
GRAM NEGATIVE COCCI
49. Gonorrhea
GRAM POSITIVE BACILLI
50. Actinomycosis
51. Erythrasma
52. Trichomycosis
53. Diphtheria
GRAM NEGATIVE BACILLI
54. Chancroid
55. Donovanosis (granuloma inguinale)
56. Malakoplakia
MYCOBACTERIA
57. Tuberculosis
SPIROCHETES
58. Syphilis
MYCOPLASMAS - CHLAMYDIAL INFECTIONS
59. Chlamydial oculogenital infection
60. Lymphogranuloma venereum
BACTERIAL OVERGROWTH
61. Bacterial vaginosis
VIRUSES
DNA VIRUSES
62. Herpes simplex
63. Herpes zoster
64. Cytomegalovirus infection
65. Infectious mononucleosis
66. Human papillomavirus infection
67. Molluscum contagiosum
RNA VIRUSES
68. HIV infection

4. NON-INFECTIOUS DERMATOSES

SPONGIOTIC DERMATITIS
69. Irritant contact dermatitis
70. Allergic contact dermatitis
71. Atopic dermatitis
PSORIASIFORM DERMATITIS
72. Lichen simplex chronicus
73. Intertrigo
74. Psoriasis
75. Seborrheic dermatitis
76. Reiter's syndrome (circinate vulvitis)
LICHENOID DERMATITIS
77. Lichen sclerosus
78. Lichen planus
79. Desquamative inflammatory vaginitis
80. Vulvitis circumscripta plasmacellularis (Zoon's vulvitis)
81. Lupus erythematosus
82. Graft versus host disease
83. Fixed drug eruption
VESICOBULLOUS DISORDERS
Immunobullous:
84. Pemphigus and variants
85. Bullous pemphigoid
86. Cicatricial pemphigoid
87. Linear IgA disease of childhood
88. Stevens-Johnson disease (Erythema multiforme)
89. Toxic epidermal necrolysis (Erythema multiforme)
Non-immunological:
90. Darier's disease
91. Papular acantholytic genitocrural acantholysis
92. Benign familial chronic pemphigus (Hailey-Hailey disease)
93. Epidermolysis bullosa
GRANULOMATOUS DISEASES
94. Sarcoidosis
95. Anogenital granulomatosis (vulvitis granulomatosa, Mierscher-Melkerssohn-Rosenthal syndrome)
96. Crohn's disease
97. Foreign body
VASCULOPATHIC DISORDERS
98. Urticaria
99. Leukocytoclastic vasculitis: Henoch-Schonlein purpura
100. Neutrophilic dermatosis: Pyoderma gangrenosum
101. Aphthous ulcers
102. Behcet's disease

FOLLICULAR OCCLUSION
SYNDROMES
103. Fox Fordyce disease
104. Hidradenitis suppurativa (acne inversa)
105. Pilonidal sinus complex

5. ENDOCRINE AND METABOLIC DISORDERS AND DISORDERS OF PIGMENTATION

ESTROGEN
106. Estrogen therapy
107. Precocious puberty
108. Deficiency - sequelae
ANDROGEN
109. Adrenocortical syndromes
110. Topical testosterone induced virilization
GLUCAGON AND INSULIN
111. Glucagonoma syndrome (Necrolytic migratory erythema)
112. Acanthosis nigricans
METABOLIC DISORDERS
113. Zinc deficiency (Acrodermatitis enteropathica)
114. Amyloidosis
115. Ligneous vaginitis
116. Calcinosis
117. Verruciform xanthoma
DISORDERS OF PIGMENTATION
118. Vitiligo
119. Hyperpigmentation

6. TRAUMA

120. Obstetric
121. Sexual
122. Accidental
123. Self-induced
124. Surgical
125. Chemical
126. Radiation
127. Female circumcision and related procedures
128. Foreign body

7. NEOPLASMS

VULVA - EPITHELIAL
EPIDERMAL - SQUAMOUS
Benign
129. Seborrheic keratosis
Premalignant
130. Vulvar intraepithelial neoplasia (VIN, squamous dysplasia/carcinoma in situ) - common type (warty-basaloid)

131. Differentiated VIN
Malignant
132. Squamous cell carcinoma (SCC) - common type
133. Verrucous carcinoma
134. Keratoacanthoma
135. Basal cell carcinoma
EPIDERMAL - NEUROENDOCRINE
136. Merkel cell tumor
SKIN APPENDAGES AND ECTOPIC TISSUES
Eccrine glands:
137. Syringoma
138. Pleomorphic adenoma
139. Microcystic adnexal carcinoma
Apocrine and breast-like tumors:
140. Hidradenoma papilliferum
141. Fibroadenoma (Benign)
142. Cystosarcoma phyllodes (Benign)
143. Extramammary Paget's (EMPD - Premalignant)
144. Adenocarcinoma ex EMPD (Malignant)
145. Primary breast-like carcinoma (Malignant)
Hair follicles:
146. Trichofolliculoma
Sebaceous glands:
147. Sebaceous carcinoma
Endometriosis-derived epithelial neoplasms:
148. Endometrioid carcinoma
149. Clear cell carcinoma
MAJOR (BARTHOLIN'S) AND MINOR (VESTIBULAR) MUCINOUS GLANDS
150. Pleomorphic adenoma (Benign mixed tumor)
Malignant
151. Squamous cell carcinoma
152. Adenosquamous carcinoma
153. Mucinous adenocarcinoma
154. Salivary gland types adenocarcinoma - adenoid cystic carcinoma
155. Prostatic type carcinoma
156. Transitional cell carcinoma
VULVA - MELANOCYTIC
Benign
157. Genital melanocytic macule (melanosis)
158. Lentigo
159. Nevus (Mole) - common type
160. Atypical melanocytic nevus of genital tract
Premalignant
161. Melanoma in situ
Malignant

162. Melanoma
VULVA - MESENCHYMAL
FIBROBLASTS
Benign
163. Superficial angiomyxoma
164. Cellular angiofibroma
165. Angiomyofibroblastoma
Intermediate
166. Aggressive angiomyxoma
167. Dermatofibrosarcoma protruberans
Malignant
168. Fibrosarcoma
BLOOD VESSELS
Malignant
169. Kaposi's sarcoma
170. Angiosarcoma
SMOOTH MUSCLE
Benign
171. Leiomyoma (myxoid and epithelioid)
Intermediate
172. Smooth muscle tumor of intermediate differentiation (atypical leiomyoma)
Malignant
173. Leiomyosarcoma
SKELETAL MUSCLE
Malignant
174. Rhabdomyosarcoma (sarcoma botryoides)
NERVE
Benign
175. Neurofibroma - Neurofibromatosis
176. Schwannoma
177. Granular cell tumor
Malignant
178. Malignant peripheral nerve sheath tumor
179. Malignant granular cell tumor
FAT
Benign lipoma and variants
180. Spindle cell lipoma
181. Fibrolipoma
Malignant
182. Liposarcoma
SYNOVIUM
Malignant
183. Synovial sarcoma
UNKNOWN
Malignant
184. Rhabdoid tumor
185. Epithelioid sarcoma
186. Alveolar soft parts sarcoma
VULVA - HEMOPOIETIC AND LYMPHOID

HEMOPOIETIC
187. Langerhans' histiocytosis
188. Myeloid/monocytic leukemia
LYMPHOID
189. Non-Hodgkin's lymphoma
B cell:
190. Diffuse large cell B cell
lymphoma
191. Diffuse small cell B cell
lymphoma
T cell:
192. Peripheral T cell lymphoma
193. Cutaneous T cell lymphoma
VULVA - SECONDARY TUMORS
194. Gynecological
195. Non-gynecological
VAGINA - EPITHELIAL
SQUAMOUS
Premalignant
196. Vaginal intraepithelial
neoplasia (VAIN, squamous
dysplasia/carcinoma in situ)
Malignant
197. Papillary squamotransitional
squamous cell carcinoma
198. Verrucous squamous cell
carcinoma
GLANDULAR
Benign
199. Mullerian papilloma
200. Pleomorphic adenoma (benign
mixed tumor)
Premalignant
201. Adenocarcinoma in situ (cervix-
like) occurring in vaginal adenosis
Malignant
202. Clear cell adenocarcinoma
203. Endometrioid adenocarcinoma
204. Mucinous carcinoma
205. Adenosquamous carcinoma
206. Carcinosarcoma (MMMT)
UNDIFFERENTIATED/
NEUROENDOCRINE
207. Small cell undifferentiated/
neuroendocrine carcinoma
MELANOCYTIC
Benign
208. Genital melanocytic macule
(melanosis)
Premalignant
209. Melanoma in situ
210. Malignant melanoma
VAGINA - MESENCHYMAL
SPECIALISED GENITAL STROMA/
MYOFIBROBLASTIC
211. Cellular angiofibroma
212. Angiomyofibroblastoma
213. Aggressive angiomyxoma

BLOOD VESSELS
214. Kaposi's sarcoma
215. Angiosarcoma
SMOOTH MUSCLE
216. Leiomyoma
217. Smooth muscle tumor,
intermediate differentiation
218. Leiomyosarcoma
SKELETAL MUSCLE
219. Rhabdomyoma
220. Rhabdomyosarcoma
NEURAL
221. Neurofibroma
222. Schwannoma
223. Granular cell tumor
ENDOMETRIAL STROMAL
224. Endometrial stromal sarcoma
225. Mullerian adenosarcoma
**VAGINA - HEMOPOIETIC AND
LYMPHOID**
226. Non-Hodgkin's lymphoma
VAGINA - GERM CELL
227. Yolk sac tumor
VAGINA - SECONDARY
228. Secondary tumor
URETHRA - EPITHELIAL
SQUAMOUS
229. Squamous dysplasia/carcinoma
in situ
230. Squamous cell carcinoma
GLANDULAR
231. Villous adenoma
Adenocarcinoma:
232. Colonic type (associated with
villous adenoma)
233. Clear cell
TRANSITIONAL (UROTHELIAL)
234. Carcinoma in situ
235. Transitional cell carcinoma
236. Prostatic
NEUROENDOCRINE
237. Carcinoid
238. Small cell undifferentiated/
neuroendocrine carcinoma
URETHRA - MELANOCYTIC
239. Melanoma in situ
240. Malignant melanoma
URETHRA - MESENCHYMAL
241. Leiomyoma
242. Rhabdomyosarcoma (sarcoma
botryoides)
URETHRA - HEMOPOIETIC
243. Lymphoma
244. Plasmacytoma
**URETHRA - SECONDARY
TUMORS**
245. Metastatic and direct spread

8. NON-NEOPLASTIC CYSTS AND SWELLINGS

VULVA
EPIDERMAL
246. Epidermal inclusion cyst
(implantation dermoid)
DERMAL
247. Skin tag
248. Fibroepithelial (superficial
mesodermal) polyp
VASCULAR
249. Hemangioma
250. Angiokeratoma
251. Pyogenic granuloma
252. Campbell de Morgan (cherry)
angioma
253. Acquired lymphangioma
(lymphangioma circumscriptum)
254. Varicose veins
255. Angiolymphoid hyperplasia
with eosinphilia
SKIN APPENDAGES
256. Epidermoid cyst (epidermal or
infundibular cyst)
ECTOPIC TISSUES
257. Endometriosis
258. Ectopic breast
BARTHOLIN'S GLAND
259. Duct cyst
260. Lobular hyperplasia
PERINEUM
261. Perineal hernia
VAGINA
262. Fibroepithelial (superficial
mesodermal) polyp
263. Nodular fasciitis (postoperative
spindle cell nodule)
264. Mullerian cysts
URETHRA
265. Caruncle
266. Prolapse
267. Paraurethral cyst
268. Suburethral diverticulum
269. Nephrogenic adenoma

9. FUNCTIONAL DISORDERS

DISORDERS OF SENSATION
270. Dysesthesia (vulvodynia)
271. Neuralgia
272. Somatoform disorder
SEXUAL DISORDERS
273. Arousal disorder
274. Vaginismus
275. Orgasmic disorder

Chapter 7. Normal variations 91

Chapter 8. Developmental abnormalities 97

Chapter 9. Infections 109

Chapter 10. Non-infectious dermatoses 149

Chapter 11. Endocrine and metabolic disorders and disorders
              of pigmentation 195

Chapter 12. Trauma 205

Chapter 13. Neoplasms 215

Chapter 14. Non-neoplastic cysts and swellings 263

Chapter 15. Functional disorders 283

T - #0568 - 071024 - C308 - 276/216/14 - PB - 9780367391980 - Gloss Lamination